Photographic Atlas of Fetal Anatomy

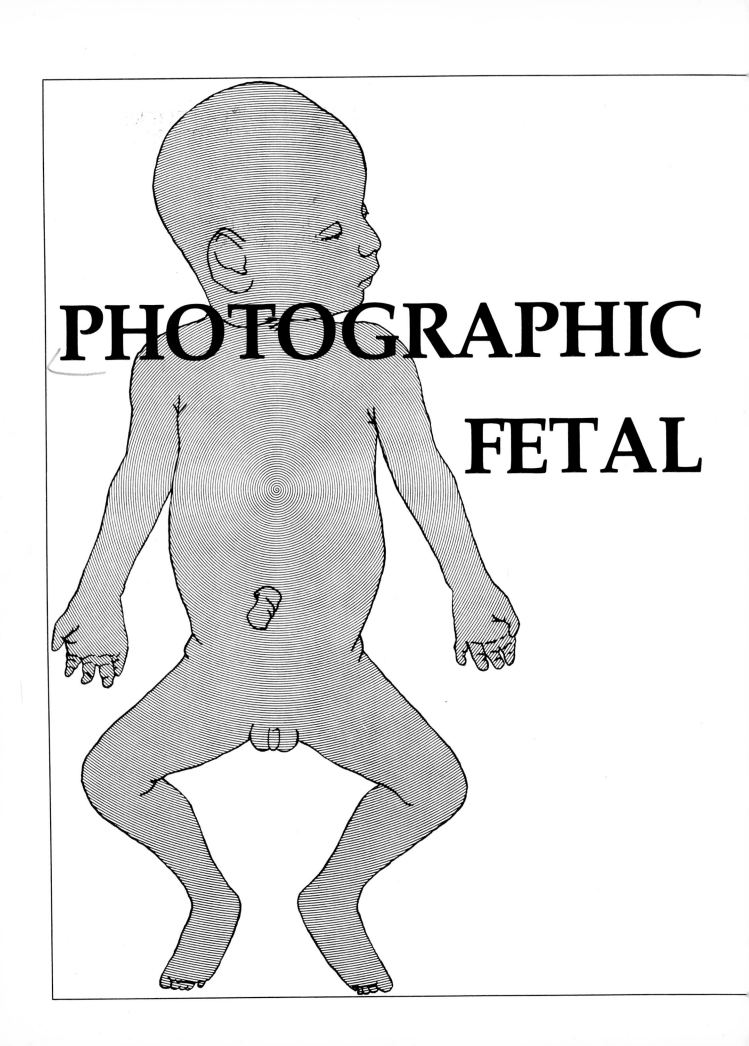

ATLAS OF ANATOMY

Wesley W. Parke, Ph.D.

Professor of Anatomy
Southern Illinois University
School of Medicine

University Park Press Baltimore • London • Tokyo

Library of Congress Cataloging in Publication Data
Parke, Wesley W.
Photographic atlas of fetal anatomy.

Includes index.
1. Fetus — Atlases. I. Title.
RG600.P35   611'.013'0222   75-1078
ISBN 0-8391-0600-9

CONTENTS

ACKNOWLEDGMENTS

Considerable credit and gratitude are due to the staff of University Park Press for their superb handling of the many technical difficulties inherent in the publication of a book of this type. The author is particularly indebted to Braxton D. Mitchell, general manager; Janet S. Hankin, production editor; and Paul H. Brookes, production manager, for their continual guidance, constructive criticism, and infinite patience in the preparation of the manuscript and plates. In addition, the kind consideration of Dr. Florence M. Foote, who helped to proofread the text pages, is much appreciated.

This book was prepared with the technical assistance of Angelina A. Sylvestro.

To Marie
who made it all possible
and who makes it all worthwhile

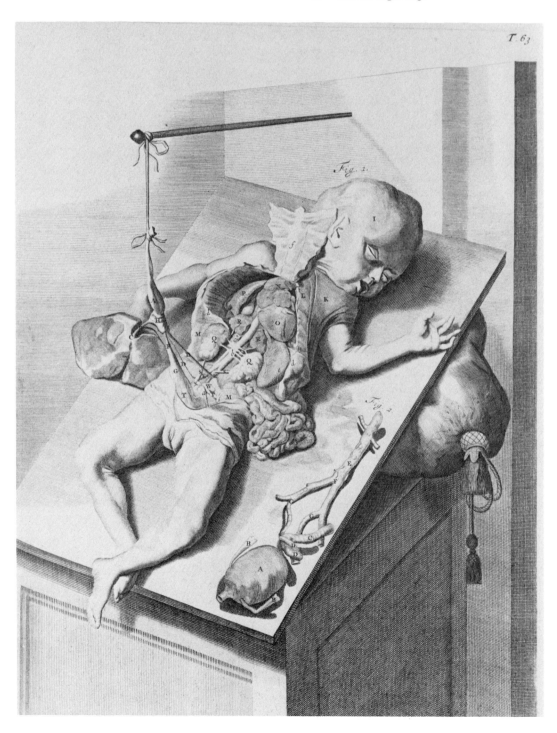

Figure 1. A photocopy of a plate in William Cowper's *Anatomia Corporum Humanorum* showing almost photographic realism in illustrating a dissection of a "foetus foeminae." Note the artistic embellishments to the background of this 16 × 12 inch engraving.

INTRODUCTION

Anatomy is a visual discipline that ultimately depends upon illustration to communicate its facts and concepts. Ever since morphologists first adorned the walls of prehistoric caves, they have continually attempted to convey graphically their impressions of anatomic details with variable accuracy.

With regard to both realism and esthetic rendering, the manual graphic depiction of anatomy seemed to have reached a peak in the 17th and 18th centuries. To this day, one cannot study the huge volumes from the Caldani studios or the Cowper engravings without wondering why more modern texts do not contain such excellent illustration. Considering the means by which these types of plates were usually produced, one comes to realize that the source of their authenticity lay in the objectivity of the illustrator, who, most often, was not the anatomist. This is particularly evident in much of the work of William Cowper (*Anatomia Corporum Humanorum*. Lugduni Batavorum. Published in 1739, 30 years after the death of the author) in which the two lower corners of a number of illustrations bear the names of both the artist and the engraver. Thus, it is apparent that although the dissections were prepared under Cowper's direction, an artist simply recorded the preparations exactly as they appeared to him, including soiled linen wrappings, dripping fluids and, in one plate, even a bothersome fly settled on the unembalmed flesh at the edge of a dissection. The academically detached attitude of the artist gave him an objectivity rivaled only by that of a camera.

In handling these early works it becomes obvious that it was the quest for exquisite detail that paradoxically restricted their usefulness. The limited number of engraving lines per inch required that they be executed in a large format (the Caldani plates measure 16 x 22 inches) and therefore bound into massive, unwieldy tomes that were very costly to produce. This latter factor severely limited the editions, and the high individual value kept the atlases out of both the dissection laboratories and the hands of students.

With the development of photoengraving in the latter half of the 19th century, one might have expected that this technologic advance would have greatly stimulated the direct use of photography in the production of accurate inexpensive anatomic illustration, but this has not been the case. Although there have been a number of attempts to produce photographic atlases, the results have generally proved disappointing, for dissections of the adult cadaver do not readily provide good photographic material. There is a decided lack of the necessary contrast in most preparations, and it is exhaustingly time consuming to clean the fields sufficiently. Furthermore, the specimens usually have to be kept moist, and wet, uneven surfaces produce a disconcerting number of highlights under intense illumination. It is not surprising that many specimens prepared for photography have been so painted and waxed that they look more like anatomic models, and many photographs have needed such extensive retouching that they virtually became drawings.

As a photographic subject, the fetus not only lacks a number of the drawbacks inherent in the adult material, but it provides several additional advantages. Vascular injection of the perinatal specimen is more rewarding since even the larger vessels have sufficiently thin walls to permit visualization of the injected medium. The serous membranes and fasciae are also quite transparent and allow the identification of underlying structures without further exposure. Size, however, is the greatest single advantage in the use of the fetus, for the ease with which this miniature cadaver may be manipulated under water and subjected to variable lighting conditions has furnished illustrations of anatomic fields with a clarity and contrast that could never be duplicated with adult specimens.

Figure 2. A photograph of the Leitz Reprovit II system with an attached Leica IIIf camera back. To the right is the cantilevered operating dissecting microscope with the Zeiss Ikon Contaflex camera attached. The instrumentation shown here provided the thousands of negatives and prints from which the illustrations in this work were selected.

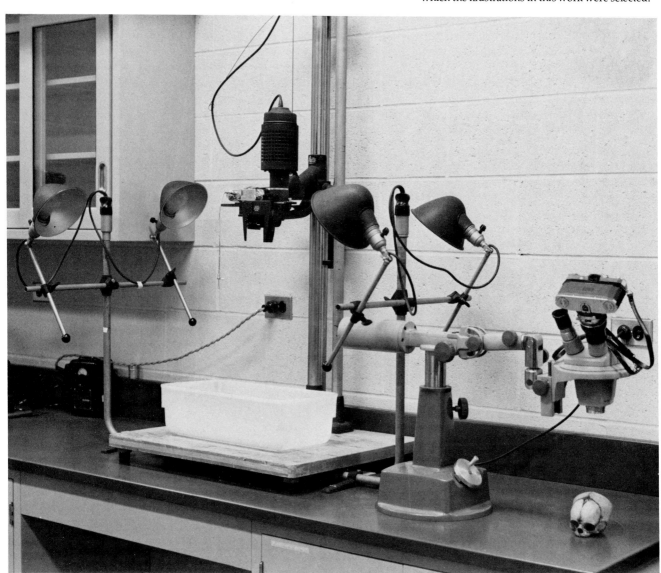

Therefore, the primary intention in the compilation of this volume of unretouched photographs was to enable both the experienced professional and the student to better comprehend the structure of the human body in general and to visualize that of the fetus in particular with an authenticity that is surpassed only by actual dissection. The descriptive text that accompanies each plate was not intended to be an exhaustive treatment but should serve as a guide to the better visual appreciation of the subject. Italics have been used in the text to suggest the core information presented and to enable the reader to scan the print and more easily identify the essential anatomic features under discussion.

The recent increase in the knowledge of genetic and developmental defects with the possibility of their early detection and a therapeutic intervention has made the fetus "Medicine's newest patient." As these interests have stimulated research in visualizing intrauterine fetal morphology and angiography, it is also hoped that this work will be a contribution to the emerging science of Fetology.

Technical Comments

Although the fetal stage of human development extends from the 7th week of gestation to parturition (usually about the 36th week), the illustrations and discussions in this volume, with very few exceptions, were derived from specimens delivered within the last 10 weeks of intrauterine life. Most of these selected cadavera were from the 26- to 30-week period, in which the fetus is generally considered independently viable and to a large measure developmentally complete, but has not yet acquired the late fetal deposits of fat that may obscure anatomic detail.

For the most part, the fetal cadavera used for dissection were injected with either natural white and colored latex or white synthetic Neoprene (E. I. DuPont Co., Wilmington, Del.) latex via an umbilical artery. Shortly after this vascular injection, the specimens were preserved by a dilute mixture of phenol, ethanol and glycerin injected into the body cavities and between the fascial planes of the trunk and limb musculature. Conventional dissection techniques provided the appropriate exposures.

Before the specimens were photographed, the prepared anatomic fields were washed repeatedly in tap water to remove as much loose and buoyant debris as possible, and the whole preparation was then placed in a plastic tank containing just enough water to provide complete coverage. Because most tap water is delivered at a pressure of approximately 60 pounds per square inch, it contains much dissolved gas that rapidly forms a layer of fine bubbles on the submerged material. This problem required that the immersion water be drawn at least 12 hours in advance and allowed to stand in open containers to gradually release the pressurized gasses in solution. Since anything more than minimal manipulations generated new debris, the required frequent changes of the immersion water proved to be the most tedious part of the procedure.

The versatile 35mm format was used exclusively throughout this work. Photomacrography was accomplished with a Leitz Reprovit II using a IIIf Leica camera back. Although the more recent Reprovit IIa with the M4 camera was available, the individually adjustable lamps found only in the older system offered a very necessary advantage. All of the frames taken with this system were exposed at an f/11 diaphragm setting. The immersion water gave but a single plane of light incidence that eliminated highlights, and the slight reflection from this surface was minimized by a polarized neutral-density filter rotated to the appropriate angle.

Where magnification was required, a cantilevered operating dissecting scope with an attached Zeiss Ikon Contaflex camera was employed. This single-lens reflex has an eyepiece adapter that threads directly to its standard 50mm lens and permits the use of its through-the-lens metering and electrically driven diaphragm. By selectively under- or overriding the specified ASA settings, this system provided negatives of remarkable quality with a minimal number of trial exposures.

As the length of exposure time was not a critical factor, Kodak Panatomic-X film (ASA 25) was utilized in all specimen photography. When developed in 1:1 dilutions of Kodak Microdol or D-76, at relatively cool temperatures (65 to 67 degrees Fahrenheit), this superb film gave the very fine-grained negatives required for enlarging. Most of the enlargements were printed on Kodak Polycontrast paper and developed in an Ektamatic processor. This entire system permitted the operator to take a rapid series of 35mm exposures with varying time and light conditions and furnished a series of variable contrast wet prints for quality assessment all within nearly 30 minutes. This time factor was no small consideration when it is realized that approximately only 1 out of 10 negatives was selected for printing, and only 1 of about 12 trial prints might prove suitable if the original dissection were finally judged satisfactory. In most cases, however, the whole procedure, from redissection to photoprocessing, was repeated several times.

For angiography the fetuses received vascular injections of a suspension of Micropaque (Damancy & Co. Ltd., Birmingham), a very finely divided barium sulfate powder.

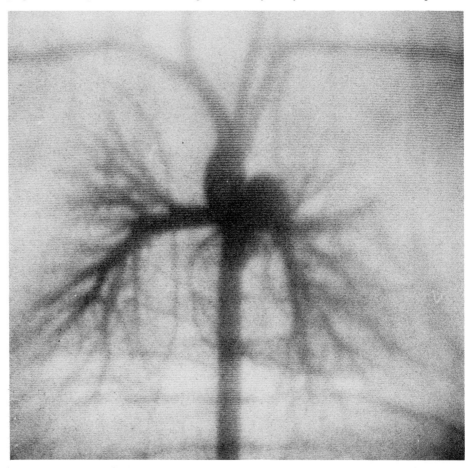

Figure 3. A photograph of a television readout from the electronic image intensifier monitoring the injection of Micropaque into a fetus. This fluoroscopic view enabled the immediate assessment of the progress and results of the injection. Note the transverse scanning lines of the television screen. This photograph was taken with Kodak Tri-X Pan film (ASA 400) with a f/2.4 diaphragm setting and a 1-second exposure.

This contrast medium was mixed with an approximately equal volume of water containing 1 percent gelatin. This last ingredient solidified under contact with a 0.5 percent addition of formalin to the previously mentioned embalming fluid. In a number of cases, the use of a Fairchild image intensifier facilitated the injection of the radiopaque medium. By connecting several feet of fine polyethylene tubing to the cannula in the umbilical artery, the operator could delicately control the pressure on the injection syringe from the safety of a shielded location while observing the intravascular progress of the medium on a television monitor. Thus, failures because of incomplete penetration or massive extravasation were immediately apparent.

The larger radiographic exposures involving the entire fetus were made by placing the injected specimen in a plastic tank that had a bottom of uniform thickness. Water was then added to the tank until the fetus was about three fourths submerged. The water provided a resistance to x-ray penetration that approximated that of the flesh. Thus, the much thinner areas at the ends of the extremities were not overexposed by the quantity of radiation required to adequately penetrate the head and trunk. The plastic tank and its immersed specimen were placed on top of a 14 × 16.5 inch fluorescent cassette loaded with Kodak Blue brand film, and irradiated with 50 milliamperes at 42 to 48 kilovolts for $1/10$ to $1/4$ second, depending on the size of the fetus. The beam distance for all radiograms was maintained at 40 inches from the cassette, and the head of the specimen was oriented toward the anode side of the cone of radiation to take advantage of the "heel effect," which produces a greater intensity of emanation in that half of the field.

Specific regional angiograms were taken by removing individual organs or trunk and body sections and placing them on mammography film cassettes. As the silver halide in this industrial-type film is potentiated by the direct effect of the x-rays, longer exposures were required. With a constant setting of 50 milliamperes at 50 kilovolts, the time varied from 10 to 40 seconds, depending on the thickness of the specimen. The angiograms obtained by this direct exposure had much sharper and finer detail than those produced within the fluorescent cassette.

For detailed enlargements of regional angiograms, the x-ray films were placed on an illuminated viewbox and photographed with the Leitz Reprovit II system.

"Fetus" or "Foetus"

The widespread use of variant spellings of the term *fetus* offers the writer a constant source of uncertainty as to the validity of his choice of the alternate forms.

Fetus was a word frequently used in classical Latin to indicate the recognizable prenatal form of a viviparous animal, a definition which generally still holds. Because it was a noun of the fourth declension, its plural spelling was identical to that of its nominative singular, but a diacritical mark was placed over the final vowel to indicate a change in its pronunciation to a long *u* (i.e., *fetūs;* however, to eliminate the need of the diacritic, the anglicized *fetuses* is acceptable). The Latin derivation of the word was based on an Indo-European root *fe,* which meant to bear or bring forth. This stem is recognizable in other cognate forms such as *feminine, female* and *femur.*

Since the term was taken directly from early classical Latin in both meaning and spelling, the source of the permutations *foetus* and more rarely *faetus* is somewhat of a mystery. That these are erroneous forms is readily admitted in the Oxford English Dictionary where it is stated that the "etymologically preferable spelling with the *e* in this word and its cognates is adopted in some dictionaries, but its actual use is almost unknown." It is obvious that this quote is primarily indicative of British writings, for the *e* form is now widely used in the United States. Nevertheless, the origin of the *oe* spelling is most intriguing, for it has enjoyed considerable antiquity. LaPrimaud (French Academy. 11.397. 1594) used it in the 16th century, and William Cowper (1666 to 1709) in the 17th and 18th centuries. The latter showed extended consistency in this when labeling a female stillborn as a *foetus foeminae*.

Although the literature fails to reveal the exact origin of the double vowel spelling, *Harper's Latin Dictionary* (1884) lists an early variation of the Latin root as *feo* (possibly a verb form?) which by simple vowel transposition could lead to the erroneous *foe-*. However, since the use of the *oe* form seems to have gained acceptance after the 15th century, a more probable source of the error may lie in the advent of printing. The early common usage of a single character of type for the Æ and Œ ligatures in Latin and Greek texts may have tempted the typesetters with an inclination toward elaborating manuscripts to substitute these for the single vowel.

Despite the present extensive use of the more complex *oe* spelling, it must be recognized as historically incorrect, and the shorter, true Latin version should be used exclusively.

Photographic Atlas of Fetal Anatomy

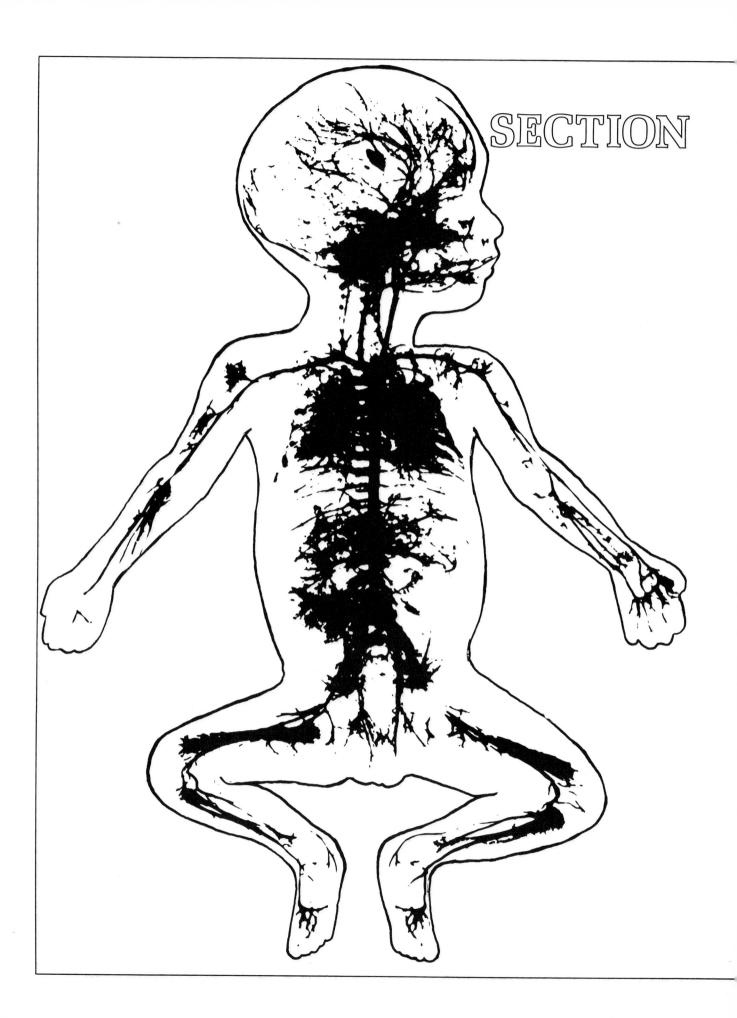

SECTION

ONE

COMPREHENSIVE OVERVIEWS WITH VENOUS AND ARTERIAL CIRCULATION

ANTERIOR SUPERFICIAL TOPOGRAPHY OF THE FETUS

The natural posture of the perinatal human approximates the "true anatomic position" more closely than that of the adult. In this position both the upper and lower limbs are supinated so that their embryologic and comparative preaxial borders face laterally and their postaxial borders face medially. Because this is the position in which the limbs grew from the sides of the body during the embryonic stages, the skin and muscles of the preaxial (lateral) parts of the limbs receive sensory and motor innervation from more rostral spinal nerves than do their corresponding postaxial (medial) regions. In the presented photograph of the anterior surface of the fetal body and the right lateral surface of the head, the body regions have been labeled to illustrate the topographic areas referred to in the deeper dissections of the body. All labels have adjectival endings indicating that they modify the noun "region."

This plate also illustrates the relative proportions of the fetal body in which the lower extremities are roughly the same length as the trunk, and the size of the head (from the adult frame of reference) is disproportionately large.

This particular plate shows a 34-week-old female fetus with the proximal section of the umbilical cord still attached. It should be noted that the labial swellings of the late fetal female are rather pronounced and may, at first glance, resemble scrotal sacs.

Plate 1   Anterior Superficial Topography   3

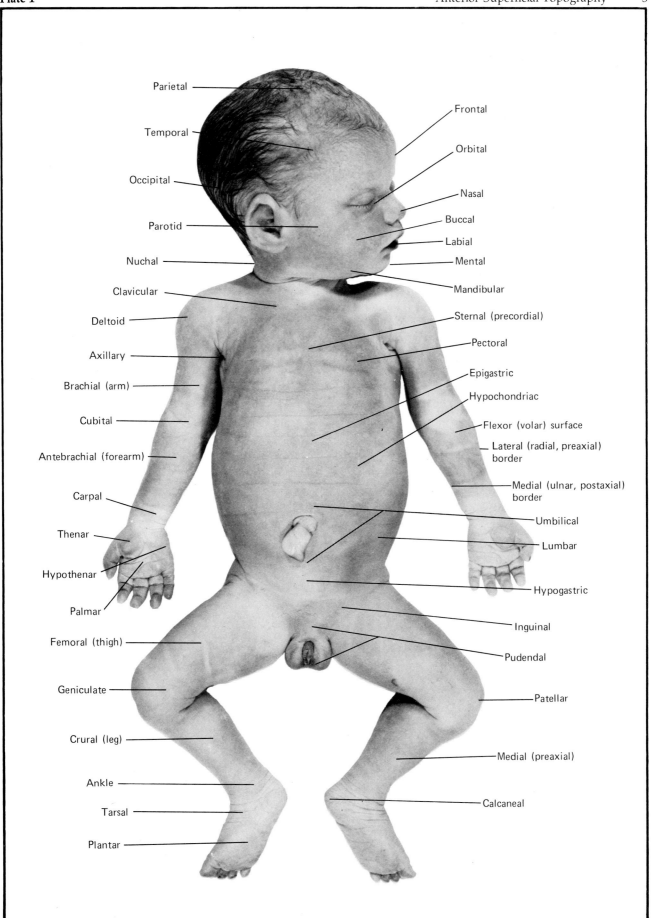

Parietal

Frontal

Temporal

Orbital

Occipital

Nasal

Parotid

Buccal

Labial

Nuchal

Mental

Clavicular

Mandibular

Deltoid

Sternal (precordial)

Axillary

Pectoral

Brachial (arm)

Epigastric

Hypochondriac

Cubital

Flexor (volar) surface

Antebrachial (forearm)

Lateral (radial, preaxial) border

Medial (ulnar, postaxial) border

Carpal

Thenar

Umbilical

Hypothenar

Lumbar

Palmar

Hypogastric

Femoral (thigh)

Inguinal

Pudendal

Geniculate

Patellar

Crural (leg)

Medial (preaxial)

Ankle

Tarsal

Calcaneal

Plantar

POSTERIOR SUPERFICIAL TOPOGRAPHY OF THE FETUS

This is a posterior view of the same specimen shown in the preceding illustration. Again the true anatomic position is revealed in the posture of the limbs.

The posterior aspect of the late fetus still accentuates the axial gradients of development that are so prominent in the earlier embryonic stages. In this respect, the head and upper limbs are developmentally more advanced than the caudal regions of the body, and the pectoral girdle that bears the upper members shows a greater resemblance to its definitive proportions. The pelvic girdle, gluteal region and lower limbs both structurally and functionally are less well developed. The abducted and flexed position of the lower extremities becomes modified postnatally when the bipedal stance is assumed.

Plate 2   Posterior Superficial Topography   5

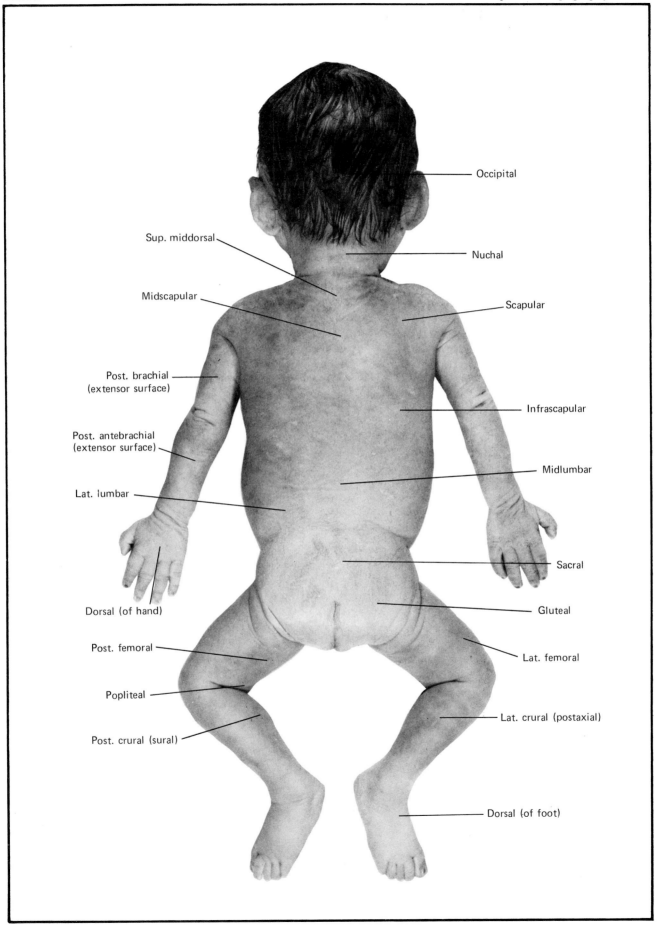

Occipital

Sup. middorsal

Nuchal

Midscapular

Scapular

Post. brachial
(extensor surface)

Infrascapular

Post. antebrachial
(extensor surface)

Midlumbar

Lat. lumbar

Dorsal (of hand)

Sacral

Gluteal

Post. femoral

Lat. femoral

Popliteal

Lat. crural (postaxial)

Post. crural (sural)

Dorsal (of foot)

THE SKELETON OF THE TERM FETUS

This commercial preparation of a fetal skeleton is mounted in a nonfetal posture with the legs extended and adducted, presumably for proportional comparison to the erect adult skeleton. However, it provides a good reference for the relative sizes of the various body regions.

With regard to the axial skeleton (skull, spine and rib cage), it should be noted that the head is as large as the width of the pectoral girdle. Although the fetal spine is presented as straight here, in reality it shows a large single curve of flexion from the skull to the lumbosacral junction. When the erect posture and bipedal locomotion are eventually perfected, the cervical and lumbar regions will assume compensatory curves of extension.

The fetal ribs are not directed obliquely downward as in the adult, and are therefore unable to provide the same degree of assistance to respiratory movements in the newborn as they do in later life.

Here the ossified parts of the skeleton are joined by dried and shrunken remains of cartilaginous articulations which no longer reveal the mechanics of the joints by the shapes and relations of the articular surfaces.

Plate 3   Skeleton of Term Fetus   7

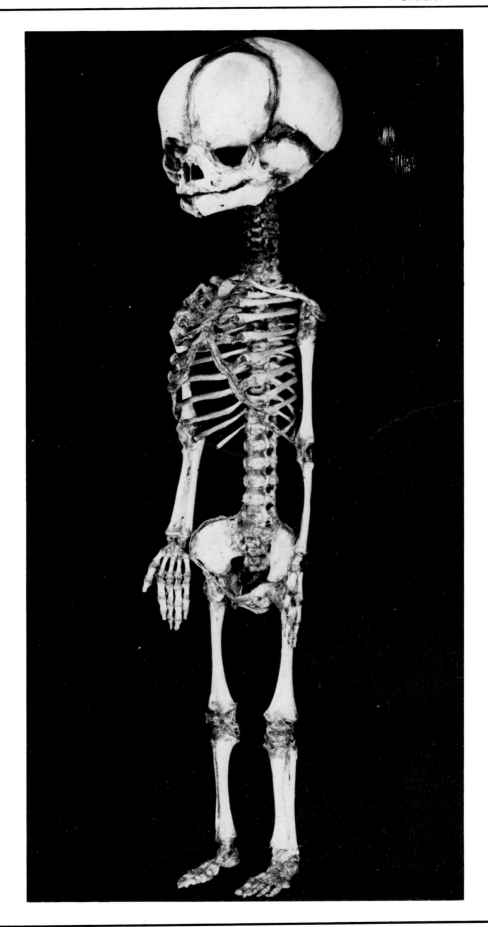

Plate 3

Radiogram
of the
Fetal Skeleton

This specimen shows the fetal skeleton in its normal posture but with a greater flexion of the legs; the flexion was required in order to place the whole subject on the x-ray cassette.

The primary centers of ossification for the diaphyses of all the long bones and the three centers for each vertebral element can be identified. Aside from the gradual expansion of the observable ossified areas, there has been little addition in the way of new ossification centers since the 16th week of gestation. Prior to birth, only the centers for the calcaneus and talus, which appear in the 6th and 7th months, respectively, represent the smaller bones. The one secondary center of ossification to appear during fetal life is seen here in the distal epiphyses of the femora. This center becomes visible at the onset of the 7th month and has thus been used as a medicolegal indication of fetal viability.

Inasmuch as the individual bones are labeled and discussed with their regional anatomy, this plate remains unlabeled and should be used to place the components of the different areas in their proper perspective.

One must realize that the unossified articular areas are radiolucent, and the bones therefore appear disconnected. However, each joint is functionally and anatomically expressed in a small cartilaginous model that closely approximates their definitive form. These are best seen in some of the following sectional views through various articular areas.

Plate 4   Radiogram of Fetal Skeleton   9

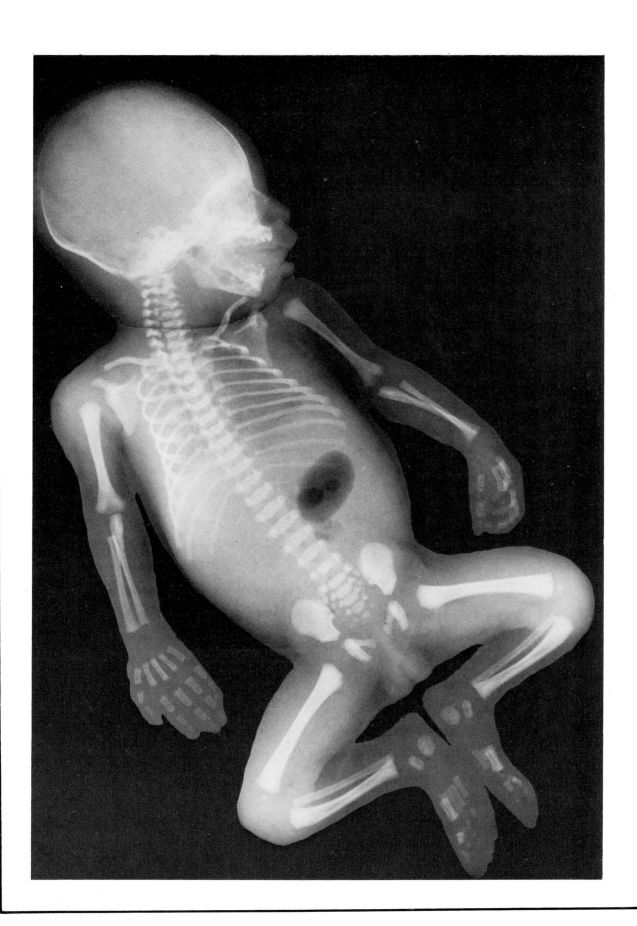

ANGIOGRAM OF THE ARTERIAL SYSTEM OF THE FETUS

In this plate, the entire arterial system of a 30-week-old female fetus is illustrated. The specimen represents the 14th attempt to inject the major parts of the whole arterial tree via one of the umbilical arteries. The primary technical difficulty resulted from the pressure required to force the finely divided suspension of barium sulfate throughout the entire system. Most frequently the cusps of the aortic and/or the pulmonary valves everted under the pressure and permitted filling of the ventricles and a retrograde injection of the venous system as far as the first competent valves. With the other unsuccessful cases, either rupture of a vessel would produce mass extravasation or the medium would not penetrate all regions uniformly. In the fortunate case shown here, the valves of the great vessels remained intact and the ventricles are outlined only by their coronary circulation. The medium penetrated all regions evenly to the extent of showing the fine arterial tufts at the ends of the digits (see enlarged angiogram of the hand). The peak pressure, however, did produce a slight choroidal extravasation that can be seen in the left ventricle of the brain.

Unlike the adult situation, the pulmonary arteries of the fetus are connected to the aorta by the ductus arteriosus, so that the medium delineated both the greater (systemic) and lesser (pulmonary) arterial systems.

Inspection of individual areas will show that this specimen reveals in detail all of the arteries that would be described in a comprehensive text of anatomy, including even the nutrient arteries within the bones.

Because the individual regions of this specimen have been enlarged and discussed in their various particulars throughout this atlas, the total picture here has not been labeled. Instead it remains as a reference illustration of the total complexity of the vascular system and a challenging review to one's knowledge of anatomy. If the student or practitioner of applied human biology can identify accurately the major vessels and the organs they supply that are so well depicted here, he may regard himself as an accomplished anatomist.

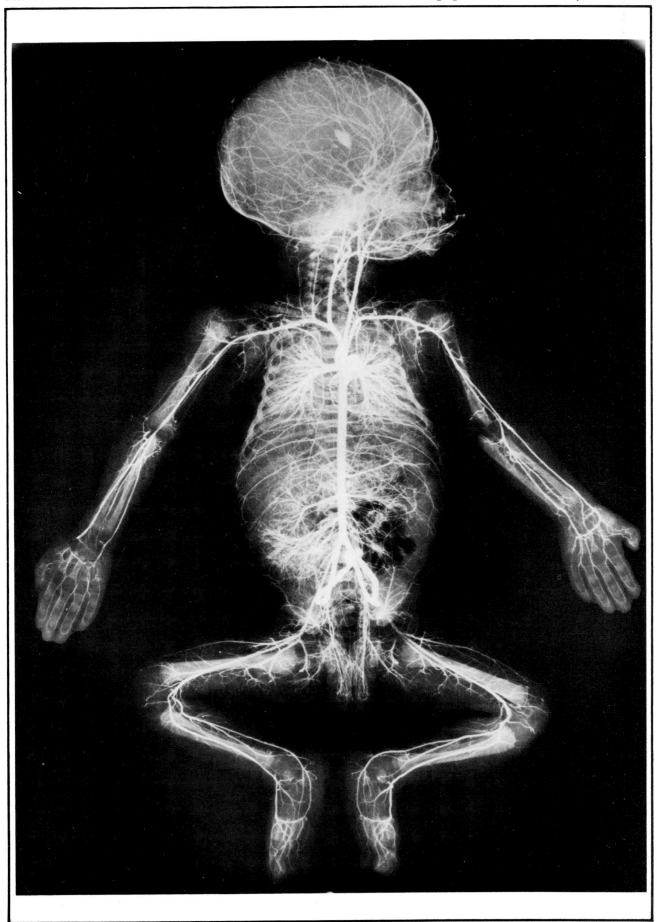

LATERAL ANGIOGRAM OF THE FETAL CIRCULATION

In this view of a doubly injected fetus, the contrast medium was introduced through the umbilical artery. It ascended the aorta and ruptured the aortic and pulmonary valves and descended into the major venous channels to outline the caval, portal and umbilical veins.

The double injection well illustrates the relations of the umbilical vessels to the rest of the fetal circulation and indicates the route of the blood to and from the placenta.

Both ventricles of the fetal heart discharge blood into the aorta. Some of the blood from the *left ventricle* supplies the head and upper extremities via the *aortic arch*, but the greater quantity enters the *descending aorta*. The blood from the *right ventricle* that eventually will be destined for the pulmonary circulation in the adult is shunted to the descending aorta by the *ductus arteriosus*. The descending aorta supplies the trunk, viscera and lower extremities, but a large percentage of its blood is passed through the *common iliac arteries* that lead to the *umbilical arteries* and placenta. The major functions that eventually will be accomplished by the digestive, respiratory and urinary systems are provided through the vascular exchange mechanisms of the placenta. The oxygenated nutritive blood returns to the fetus through the single *umbilical vein* and is shunted through the liver by the *ductus venosus*. The placental and caval venous blood is mixed where the ductus empties into the *inferior vena cava*, and the latter vessel returns it to the heart to recommence the cycle.

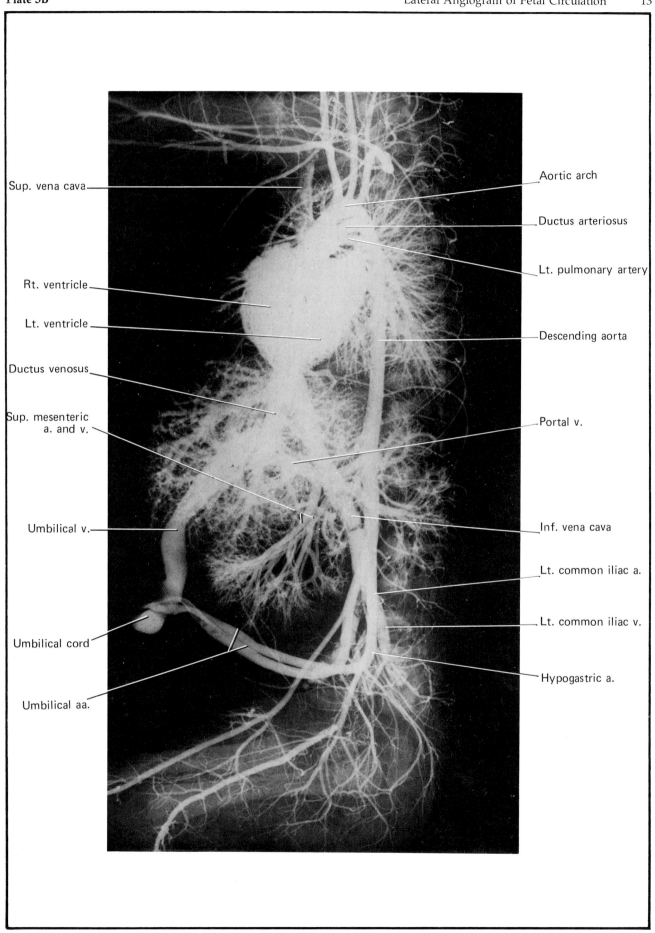

Sup. vena cava

Aortic arch

Ductus arteriosus

Lt. pulmonary artery

Rt. ventricle

Lt. ventricle

Descending aorta

Ductus venosus

Sup. mesenteric
a. and v.

Portal v.

Umbilical v.

Inf. vena cava

Lt. common iliac a.

Lt. common iliac v.

Umbilical cord

Umbilical aa.

Hypogastric a.

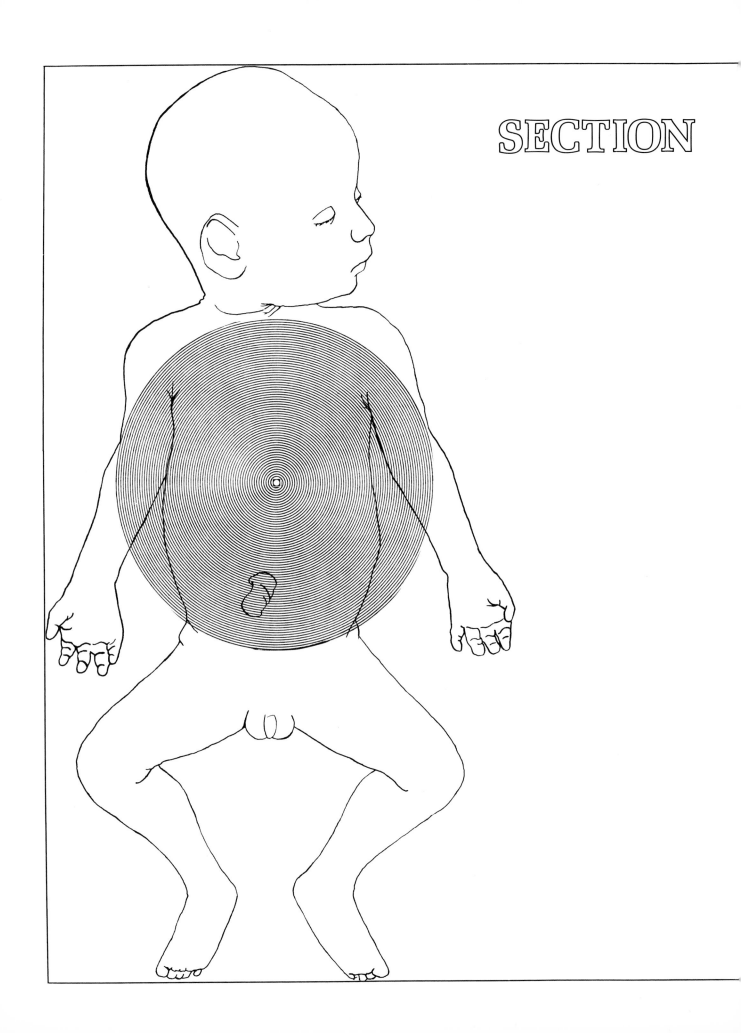

SECTION

TWO

UPPER EXTREMITY

DORSOLATERAL ASPECT OF THE SUPERFICIAL MUSCULATURE OF THE BODY

In this illustration the skin and most of the subcutaneous fat and fascia have been removed from the neck and trunk to provide an overview of the superficial musculature.

The thin *platysma muscle* sheaths the anterior surface of the neck from the clavicle to the inferior edge of the mandible and overlies the sternal and clavicular origins of the *sternocleidomastoid muscle*. The latter can be seen extending toward its insertion on the mastoid process behind the ear. The *great auricular nerve* that is sensory to most of the external ear and the skin behind it originates in the cervical plexus and courses upward across the sternocleidomastoid.

The intrinsic muscles of the back are a complex series of overlapping bundles that move the axial skeleton, and unlike most of the body musculature, they are innervated by the dorsal primary divisions of the spinal nerves. Because the greater part of the back is covered by the dorsal muscles of the shoulder girdle, the *splenius* in the posterior neck and the lower lumbar part of the *erector spinae* are the only intrinsic back muscles visible in this superficial exposure.

The extensive origin of the *trapezius muscle* can be traced from the occiput to the lower thoracic spines from where its fibers converge upon three regions of the shoulder. The part of the muscle that is of nuchal origin inserts on the lateral section of the clavicle and that of the upper and lower thoracic origins inserts on the acromion and spine of the scapula, respectively.

The broad *latissimus dorsi* contributes to the posterior wall of the axilla where its fibers coalesce to insert in the bicipital groove of the upper anterior part of the humerus. This muscle originates from the lumbodorsal fascia, an extensive aponeurotic sheet that is attached to the vertebral spines and covers the erector spinae.

In the triangular interval between the trapezius and latissimus, the *infraspinatus, teres minor* and *teres major muscles* may be seen, and the posterior part of the *deltoid* that originates from the scapular spine is well depicted.

The inferior fibers of the *rhomboid* are exposed at their insertion on the vertebral border and inferior angle of the scapula. The lower border of this muscle is almost imperceptible as it thins out to reveal a small triangular portion of the costal wall.

The toothlike projections of the *serratus anterior* may be seen extending from beneath the latissimus dorsi to interdigitate with the fibers of the *external abdominal oblique muscle*. The serratus inserts along the vertebral border of the scapula, but the greatest part of the muscle is attached to the inferior angle.

The external muscles of the pelvic girdle and lower extremity are also well illustrated. The origin and insertion of the *gluteus maximus* show how the contraction of this muscle serves to extend the hip. In the interval between the *iliac crest* and the upper edge of the maximus, the *gluteus medius* may be seen originating on the external surface of the ilium. The direction of its fibers leading to the greater trochanter proves this muscle to be an abductor of the hip.

The fascia lata, a tough investing membrane that ensheaths the anterior thigh muscles, has been left intact in this superficial dissection, and its role in the insertion of the *tensor fasciae latae* and part of the gluteus maximus is obvious.

Plate 6 Dorsolateral Aspect of Superficial Musculature 17

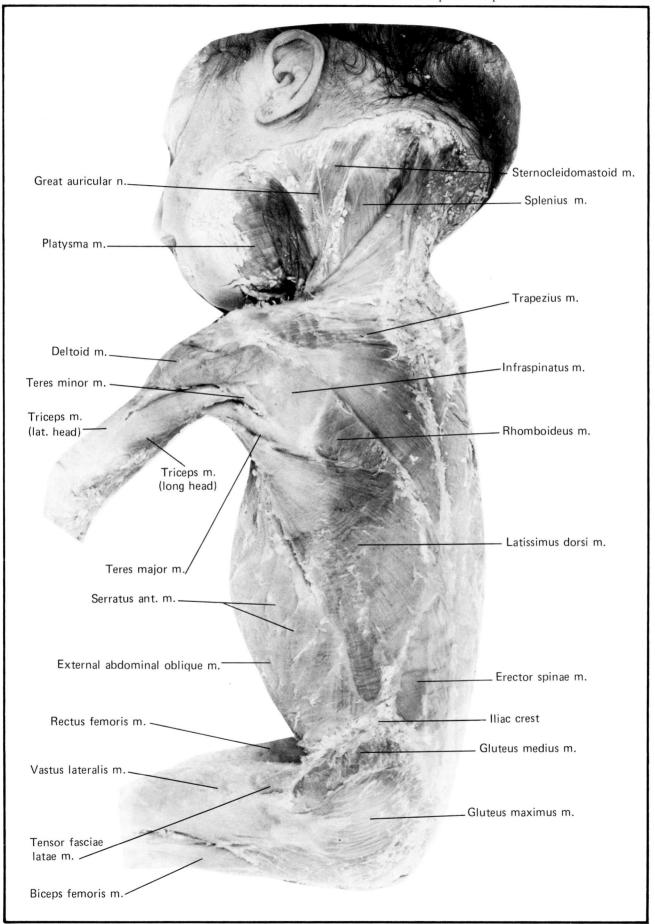

Great auricular n.

Platysma m.

Deltoid m.

Teres minor m.

Triceps m.
(lat. head)

Triceps m.
(long head)

Teres major m.

Serratus ant. m.

External abdominal oblique m.

Rectus femoris m.

Vastus lateralis m.

Tensor fasciae
latae m.

Biceps femoris m.

Sternocleidomastoid m.

Splenius m.

Trapezius m.

Infraspinatus m.

Rhomboideus m.

Latissimus dorsi m.

Erector spinae m.

Iliac crest

Gluteus medius m.

Gluteus maximus m.

X-RAY: OSTEOLOGY OF THE UPPER EXTREMITY

Although no secondary centers of ossification appear in the upper extremity before the end of gestation, the essential elements of the pectoral girdle and the shafts of all the long bones may be radiologically defined.

The *clavicle,* which is the first bone of the body to ossify during development, is shown as a recurved shaft connecting the sternum to the acromioclavicular point of the scapula. The major functional attachment of the shoulder to the trunk is by a suspension of musculature. Nevertheless, a skeletal connection to the vertebral column is indirectly provided through the clavicular articulation to the sternum and first rib.

The form of the *scapula* is revealed as a broad, thin blade reinforced by the thickened *axillary border* and spine. These structures afford better attachments for muscle origins and buttress the scapula against stresses transmitted through the glenohumeral joint.

The *coracoid* and *acromion processes,* yet to be enhanced by additional centers of ossification, can be seen at the lateral angle of the scapula.

The actual articular surfaces of the glenohumeral joint lie in the radiolucent area between the visibly calcified ends of the bones where a chondroid, spherical humeral head fits a matching shallow chondroid socket.

The distal end of the *humeral shaft* shows medial and lateral differences that indicate the positions of the grooved trochlea and ball-like capitulum that, respectively, support a hinge joint with the *ulna* and a pivot joint with the *radius.* The pivoting action of the radius permits its distal end to rotate over the fixed ulna to produce supination of the forearm.

The totally cartilaginous carpals are not visible here, but their support of the *metacarpals* and more distally dependent *phalanges* is obvious.

Plate 7   X-Ray: Osteology of Upper Extremity   19

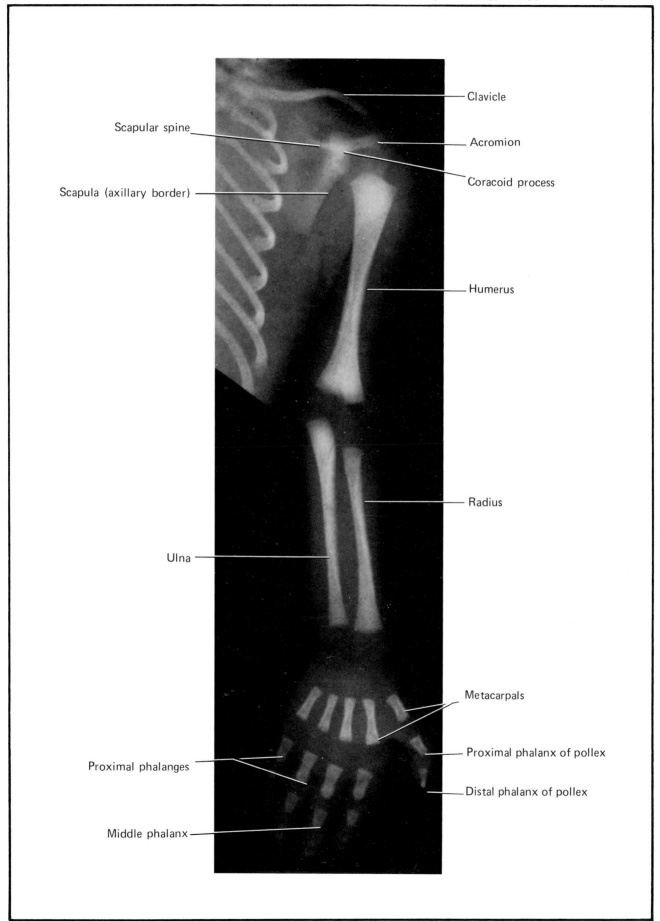

Clavicle

Scapular spine

Acromion

Coracoid process

Scapula (axillary border)

Humerus

Radius

Ulna

Metacarpals

Proximal phalanx of pollex

Proximal phalanges

Distal phalanx of pollex

Middle phalanx

ARTERIOGRAM OF THE UPPER EXTREMITY

A single arterial stem originates from the brachiocephalic trunk (right) or aortic arch (left) and extends from the mediastinum to the elbow with no abrupt change in caliber or course. However, in the atypical (5 percent) variation illustrated here, the distal end of the vessel splits to embrace the median nerve.

Solely for the convenience of description, this main artery of the upper limb is divided into three major sections named according to the region traversed. The subclavian artery is mostly mediastinal in its course and becomes the *axillary artery* at the outer margin of the first rib. It supplies branches to the neck and upper intercostals and serves the dorsal scapular region through the *transverse cervical* and *scapular arteries*.

The axillary artery is the main stem artery of the shoulder. It distributes branches to the pectoral and deltoid regions by way of the *thoracoacromial artery*, and to the medial wall of the axilla and the scapular muscles through the *lateral thoracic* and *subscapular arteries*.

The last of the major branches of the axillary artery are the *humeral circumflex arteries* that supply the shoulder joint. Distal to these, the origin of the *deep brachial artery* approximates the point where the stem vessel becomes the *brachial artery* that follows the medial intermuscular septum to the elbow. The triceps muscle receives most of its vascularity from the deep brachial artery as it follows the radial nerve around the humerus and terminates in collateral branches that join the *radial recurrent artery*.

It should be realized that mechanical principles usually require that the larger arteries pass over the flexor surfaces of joints, and the major vessels are therefore usually found coursing between the flexor muscles. This necessitates that extensors must be supplied by deep perforating branches such as the deep brachial and posterior interosseous arteries.

As the brachial artery crosses the elbow joint, it divides into the medial *ulnar artery* and the lateral *radial artery*. The larger ulnar division supplies the flexor mass of the medial epicondyle through a number of muscular branches, one of which is reflected proximally to anastomose with the ulnar collaterals as the *ulnar recurrent artery*. Also an ulnar derivative, the *common interosseous artery* immediately divides into anterior and posterior branches that course along their respective surfaces of the interosseous membrane as far distal as the carpal region.

Muscular rami from the radial artery and its recurrent branch, in conjunction with the *posterior interosseous artery*, form the major arterial supply to the antebrachial extensors.

Both the radial and ulnar arteries terminate by sending deep and superficial branches to the palmar arterial arches. These in turn provide vascularity to the hand and fingers through a series of *common* and *proper digital arteries*.

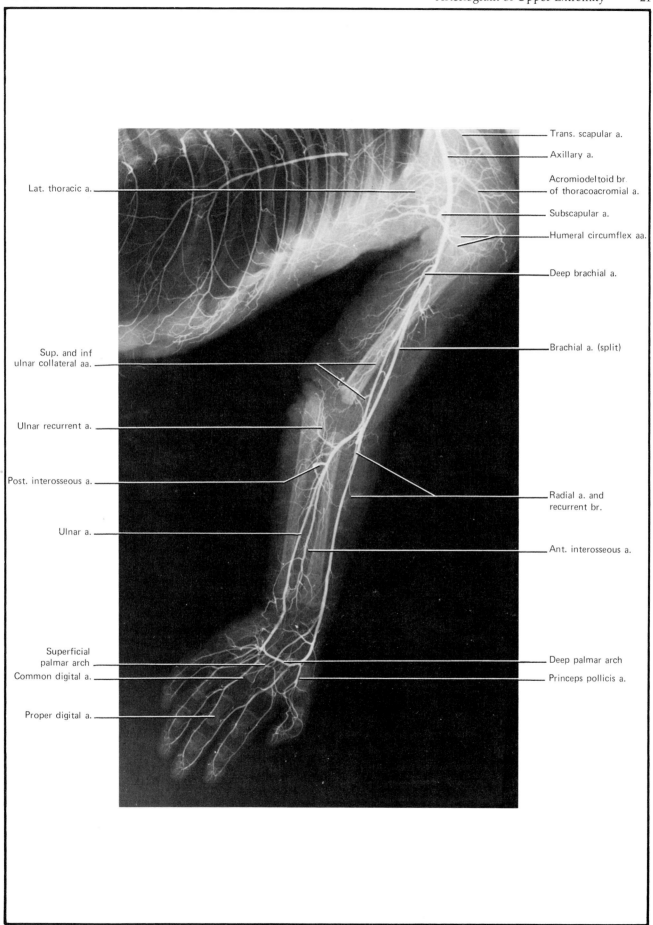

Trans. scapular a.

Axillary a.

Acromiodeltoid br. of thoracoacromial a.

Lat. thoracic a.

Subscapular a.

Humeral circumflex aa.

Deep brachial a.

Brachial a. (split)

Sup. and inf ulnar collateral aa.

Ulnar recurrent a.

Post. interosseous a.

Radial a. and recurrent br.

Ulnar a.

Ant. interosseous a.

Superficial palmar arch

Deep palmar arch

Common digital a.

Princeps pollicis a.

Proper digital a.

DORSAL ASPECT OF THE SHOULDER

The *trapezius* has been reflected from its insertion on the *acromion* and *scapular spine* to expose the descending branch of the *transverse cervical artery* and the *spinal accessory nerve*. The deeper *rhomboid* and *serratus anterior muscles* that serve to adduct, rotate and stabilize the scapula are also revealed. Both of these muscles insert along the entire extent of the vertebral border of the scapula, but the greatest part of the serratus muscle inserts into the inferior angle. The lateral reflection of the *deltoid muscle* has further exposed the *supraspinatus, infraspinatus* and *teres minor muscles* that insert on the greater tuberosity of the humerus beneath the *joint capsule.* Collectively they form the greater part of the rotator cuff which helps to stabilize the glenohumeral joint and to abduct and laterally rotate the humerus. The *teres major* originates on the inferior angle of the scapula to insert on the anterior surface of the humerus. As the long head of the *triceps* crosses this muscle posteriorly, it divides the interval between the axillary border of the scapula and the teres major into the *medial triangular space* and the *lateral quadrangular space.* The former gives access to the *circumflex scapular artery,* a branch of the subscapular artery that serves the muscles of the infraspinous fossa, while the latter space reveals branches of the *posterior humeral circumflex artery* accompanied by the *circumflex branches* of the *axillary nerve.*

The *deltoid muscle,* which has been dissected from its origins on the scapular spine and acromion, is separated from the joint capsule by the *subdeltoid bursa,* a space lined by synovial membrane that is continuous with the synovial cavity of the shoulder joint. The deltoid inserts on the deltoid tuberosity of the humerus and provides a powerful adduction of the brachium in addition to medial and lateral rotation.

The *latissimus dorsi muscle* that arises from the lumbodorsal fascia of the lower back has been divided, and its origin has been reflected to expose the ribs. Its distal one fourth has been trimmed but still remains attached to its insertion on the upper anterior surface of the humerus, whereby it produces extension and medial rotation of the brachium.

Well depicted here is the *triceps muscle,* a powerful extensor of the forearm that also provides adduction of the humerus by its long head. The medial or deep head of the triceps arises from the posterior surface of the humerus and is concealed by the long and lateral heads.

The diverse sources of the vascularity of the scapular muscles are well illustrated; shown are branches of the *transverse cervical, circumflex scapular, posterior humeral circumflex* and *intercostal arteries* that, with the deeper suprascapular vessels, form an anastomotic plexus to provide vascularity to the upper extremity that is collateral to the axillary artery.

Beneath the inferior angle of the scapula, intercostal muscles are evident. Normally only a small triangular section of the costal space shown here is evident before the trapezius and latissimus dorsi are reflected. Because it is the only area where musculature of the shoulder does not intervene between the skin and the costal wall, it affords a point where the chest sounds are easily heard and is therefore called the triangle of auscultation.

Plate 9   Dorsal Aspect of Shoulder   23

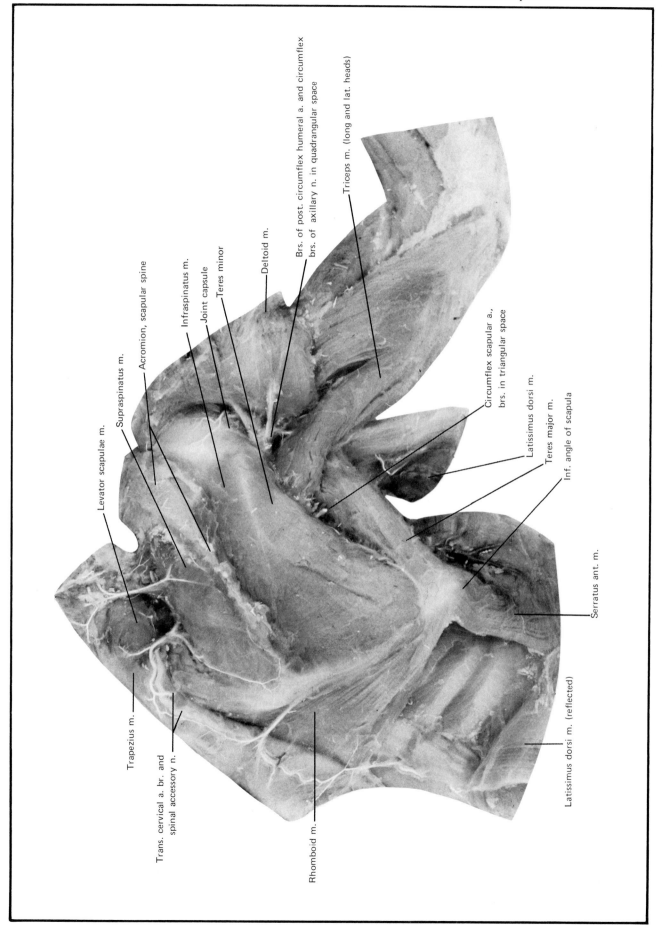

Brs. of post. circumflex humeral a. and circumflex
brs. of axillary n. in quadrangular space

Triceps m. (long and lat. heads)

Deltoid m.

Teres minor

Joint capsule

Infraspinatus m.

Acromion, scapular spine

Supraspinatus m.

Levator scapulae m.

Circumflex scapular a.,
brs. in triangular space

Latissimus dorsi m.

Teres major m.

Inf. angle of scapula

Serratus ant. m.

Trapezius m.

Trans. cervical a. br. and
spinal accessory n.

Rhomboid m.

Latissimus dorsi m. (reflected)

SUPERFICIAL POSTEROLATERAL ASPECT OF THE UPPER EXTREMITY

The convergence of the fibers of the *deltoid muscle* toward their insertion on the deltoid tuberosity of the humerus marks the upper extent of the *lateral intermuscular septum,* the fascial division between the brachial flexors and extensors. The lateral aspect of the long head of the *biceps brachii* is seen emerging beneath the deltoid, which covers its tendinous origin on the superior lip of the glenoid fossa.

The fascial attachment between the biceps and the *brachioradialis* has been divided to expose the *radial nerve,* which is a derivative of the posterior cord of the brachial plexus. This nerve leaves the axilla by penetrating the *triceps brachii* anterior and deep to its long head. After giving branches to the three heads of the triceps, the nerve perforates the lateral intermuscular septum and spirals around the lateral surface of the humerus. The nerve then courses between the tendon of the biceps and the brachioradialis, and after giving a motor branch to the latter, it enters the substance of the supinator muscle. Within this muscle the radial nerve divides into a deep motor branch and a superficial sensory branch.

The deep antebrachial branch of the radial nerve distributes motor branches to the extensors in the upper half of the forearm, but its terminal branch extends along the posterior surface of the interosseous membrane, accompanied by the dorsal interosseous artery, to terminate finally in an expansion over the dorsum of the wrist. Here it is a sensory nerve to the intercarpal joints.

In this figure it is apparent that the extensor muscles of the hand and wrist originate as a group from the *lateral epicondyle* of the humerus. The brachioradialis and the *supinator* may seem to be exceptions to this generalization because they are flexors and supinators of the forearm, but their innervation by the radial nerve indicates that they originally developed from the same embryonic primordium that produced the extensors.

Examination of the extensor surface shows that the small trianglar *anconeus muscle* originates from the dorsum of the lateral humeral epicondyle to insert on the proximal ulna. This extensor of the forearm is developmentally derived from the triceps muscle mass and is innervated by a branch of the motor nerve that supplies its medial head. It has been accurately described as a fourth head of the triceps.

Separation of the *extensor digitorum communis* from the brachioradialis shows the division between the superficial and deep groups of the antebrachial extensors. The extensor digitorum communis is the most conspicuous muscle of the superficial group. It may be traced down the midline of the dorsum of the forearm to its division into four tendons as it passes deep to the *extensor retinaculum.* The tendons expand over the back of the hand to reach the extensor assemblies of their respective digits. Through the intervals of these tendons the dorsal interosseous muscles and dorsal digital arteries may be observed.

Medially, on the ulnar side of the forearm, the *extensor digiti minimi* and the *extensor carpi ulnaris* may be discerned. The former assists the action of the fourth tendon of the extensor digitorum communis, and the latter inserts into the dorsal carpal region to extend and medially deviate the wrist.

On the lateral side of the forearm, the *extensors carpi radialis longus* and *brevis* are exposed. These pass deep to the antebrachial muscles of the thumb to insert on the bases of the second and third metacarpals, respectively.

The *abductor pollicis longus* and the *extensor pollicis brevis* spiral over the radius to reach the metacarpus of the thumb. The deeper *extensor pollicis longus* originates on the ulnar side of the forearm and passes under the *extensor retinaculum* to eventually insert on the base of the proximal phalanx of the thumb.

The superficial branch of the radial nerve courses over the structures mentioned above to distribute sensory endings to the skin over the dorsum of the thumb and the second and third digits.

Plate 10   Superficial Posterolateral Aspect   25

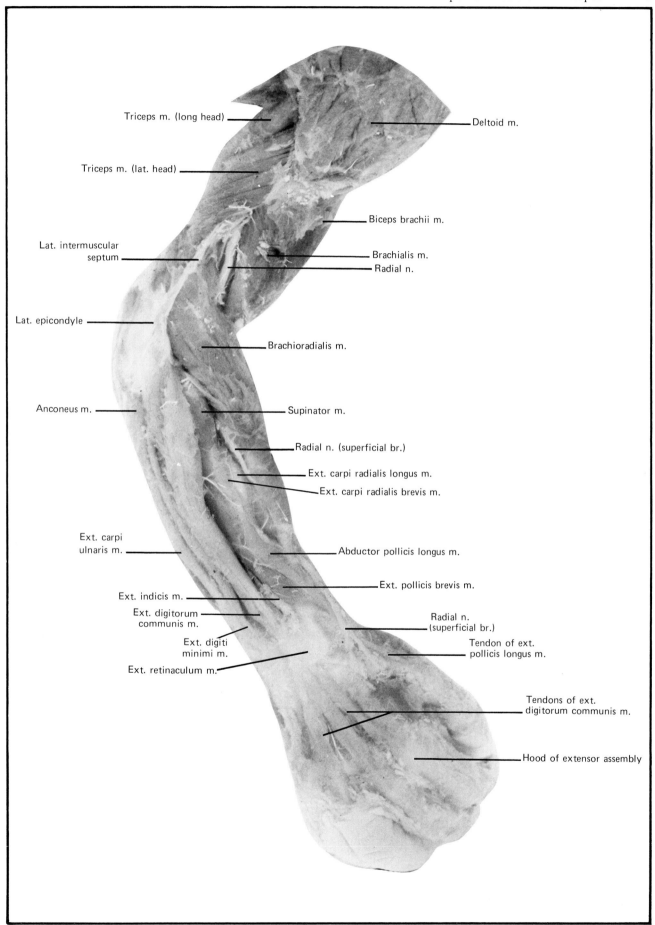

Triceps m. (long head)

Triceps m. (lat. head)

Lat. intermuscular septum

Lat. epicondyle

Anconeus m.

Ext. carpi ulnaris m.

Ext. indicis m.

Ext. digitorum communis m.

Ext. digiti minimi m.

Ext. retinaculum m.

Deltoid m.

Biceps brachii m.

Brachialis m.

Radial n.

Brachioradialis m.

Supinator m.

Radial n. (superficial br.)

Ext. carpi radialis longus m.

Ext. carpi radialis brevis m.

Abductor pollicis longus m.

Ext. pollicis brevis m.

Radial n. (superficial br.)

Tendon of ext. pollicis longus m.

Tendons of ext. digitorum communis m.

Hood of extensor assembly

SUPERFICIAL ANTERIOR ASPECT OF THE UPPER EXTREMITY

The upper extremity, including the anterior surface of the shoulder, has been stripped of its skin and superficial fascia to reveal the superficial flexor muscles and other readily accessible structures.

Proximally, the clavicular origin of the *deltoid* shows how the contraction of this segment of the muscle can produce medial rotation of the brachium in addition to abduction. The clavicular and sternal parts of the *pectoralis major* separated by a deep incisura are seen traversing the axilla to insert into the upper anterior surface of the humerus. Their medial rotation of the humerus and strong abduction of the brachium are evident by the direction of their fibers. The *pectoralis major* forms the anterior boundary of the axilla, and the *latissimus dorsi* and *coracobrachialis muscles*, respectively, form its posterior and medial boundaries.

Through the axilla passes the *axillary sheath* containing the axillary artery and the entwined derivatives of the brachial plexus. These structures enter the medial intermuscular septum, an irregular fascial attachment of the humerus that separates the extensor muscles of the triceps from the anterior flexors, the *biceps brachii* and the deeper *brachialis muscle.*

In the distal region of the medial intermuscular septum, its contents separate into the *median nerve* that overlies the *brachial artery*, the *medial antebrachial cutaneous nerve* and the more dorsally positioned *ulnar nerve*. The *musculocutaneous nerve* seen on the deep surface of the biceps is derived from the lateral cord of the brachial plexus in the axilla.

The anterior surface of the forearm shows that all of the flexors, with the exception of the *brachioradialis muscle*, originate from the medial condyle of the humerus. Of these, the most lateral, the *pronator teres*, can be seen passing from its origin, which embraces the median nerve, to its insertion deep on the upper one third of the radius. Overlying the insertion of the pronator teres are the *flexor carpi ulnaris* and the *palmaris longus*. The latter extends beyond the wrist joint to a broad fascial expansion, the *palmar aponeurosis*. Beneath the palmaris longus, the *flexor digitorum superficialis muscle* passes under the *palmar carpal ligament* to reach the medial four digits.

The *ulnar artery*, which is the primary source of the superficial arch, runs between the flexor digitorum superficialis and the flexor carpi ulnaris and is accompanied by the *ulnar nerve*. Both of these structures pass superficially to the base of the *hypothenar compartment* and are thus liable to injury in this region.

The *radial artery*, which may be observed lateral to the tendon of the *flexor carpi radialis*, passes dorsal to the carpals and the proximal phalanx of the thumb to supply primarily the deep palmar arch.

Plate 11   Superficial Anterior Aspect   27

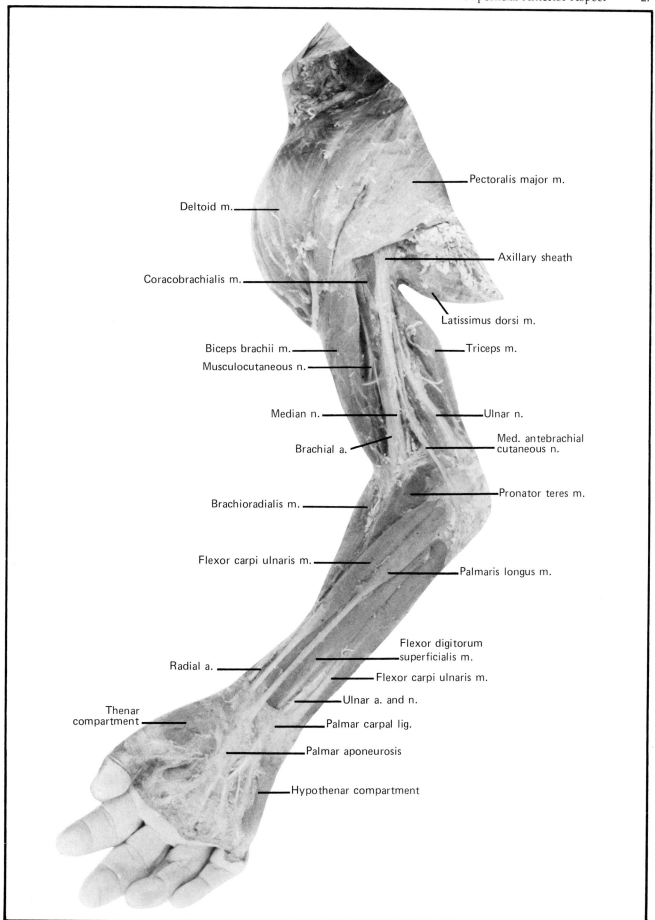

Pectoralis major m.

Deltoid m.

Axillary sheath

Coracobrachialis m.

Latissimus dorsi m.

Biceps brachii m.

Triceps m.

Musculocutaneous n.

Median n.

Ulnar n.

Med. antebrachial cutaneous n.

Brachial a.

Pronator teres m.

Brachioradialis m.

Flexor carpi ulnaris m.

Palmaris longus m.

Flexor digitorum superficialis m.

Radial a.

Flexor carpi ulnaris m.

Ulnar a. and n.

Thenar compartment

Palmar carpal lig.

Palmar aponeurosis

Hypothenar compartment

DEEP DISSECTION OF THE AXILLA

Removal of the clavicle and the upward reflection of the deltoid and pectoralis minor muscles have exposed the shoulder joint capsule, the acromial origins of the short head of the biceps, coracobrachialis and the contents of the axilla.

The subclavian artery becomes the *axillary artery* after passing over the first rib posterior to the *anterior scalene muscle*. The axillary artery in turn becomes the *brachial artery* as it enters the brachium.

At the base of the neck, the *transverse cervical, dorsal scapular* and *suprascapular arteries,* all branches of the subclavian artery, independently enter the axillary region. The major derivatives of the axillary artery are the *superior* and *lateral thoracic arteries,* the *thoracoacromial artery,* the *subscapular artery* and the *anterior* and *posterior humeral circumflex arteries.* The thoracoacromial artery here has a double origin, but the typical distribution to pectoral subclavian and acromiodeltoid regions may be discerned.

The subscapular artery descends along the posterior wall of the axilla to supply the scapular and *latissimus dorsi* muscles. A number of small, variable branches to the joint capsule and the upper brachial musculature arise from the distal section of the axillary artery, but the most important vessels in this region are the *anterior* and *posterior humeral circumflex arteries,* of which the anterior branch is visible traveling adjacent to the *radial nerve.*

Shortly after the brachial artery commences, it gives off the *deep brachial artery* that supplies the extensor muscles of the arm. This vessel spirals posteriorly and laterally around the shaft of the humerus in a course that approximates that of the radial nerve, and it terminates as superior collateral vessels above the elbow.

The interweaving of the anterior primary divisions of the fifth to eighth cervical and first thoracic spinal nerves forms the brachial plexus. In its course through the axilla the fibers of the individual spinal nerves undergo a series of unions and separations that form a number of more or less discrete nerve bundles that eventually give rise to the large nerves that enter the brachium. These bundles are successively called the roots, trunks, divisions and cords of the brachial plexus. Of the roots, the most superior from the fifth cervical nerve is visible here as it emerges posterior to

the anterior scalene muscle. Just proximal to this point it has given off contributions to the phrenic nerve and the dorsal scapular nerve. The fifth and sixth cervical roots unite as the *superior trunk* and can be seen giving rise to a split *suprascapular nerve* for the dorsal scapular muscles. The *middle trunk,* formed by only the seventh cervical root, and the *inferior trunk* that unites the eighth cervical and first thoracic roots are apparent just above the origin of the axillary artery.

The trunks separate into anterior and posterior divisions that reunite as cords that are named for their relation to the axillary artery. Thus the posterior divisions of the trunks pass deep to the artery to coalesce as the *posterior cord,* and the anterior divisions travel superolaterally and inferomedially to the artery to form, respectively, the *lateral* and *medial cords.*

The lateral cord, after giving a branch to the *median nerve,* becomes the *musculocutaneous nerve,* which penetrates the *coracobrachialis muscle* and provides motor branches to it and to the *biceps* and *brachialis muscles.*

Contributions from the lateral and medial cords fuse anterior to the artery as the large median nerve, which becomes the main motor supply to the muscles on the flexor side of the forearm and thenar eminence.

The axillary branches of the medial cord include the sources of the *medial brachial* and *medial antebrachial cutaneous nerves* that are sensory to areas on the medial surfaces of the arm and forearm.

Close to the medial wall of the axilla the *long thoracic nerve* descends to supply the serratus anterior muscle. This nerve originates from the combination of three slender posterior branches of the fifth, sixth and seventh cervical roots.

The only nerve supply to the brachium that is not derived from the brachial plexus consists of some sensory fibers to a small area of the skin on the upper medial aspect of the arm. These fibers are derived from the *intercostobrachial nerve,* a lateral branch of the second intercostal nerve that may be noted extending across the axilla toward the medial intermuscular septum of the brachium.

The veins of the axillary region have been removed in this dissection. The large, thin walled axillary vein had lain anterior to the axillary artery, where it received branches from both the deep and superficial veins of the arm. It became the subclavian vein upon passing over the first rib anterior to the anterior scalene muscle.

Plate 12

Deep Dissection of Axilla   29

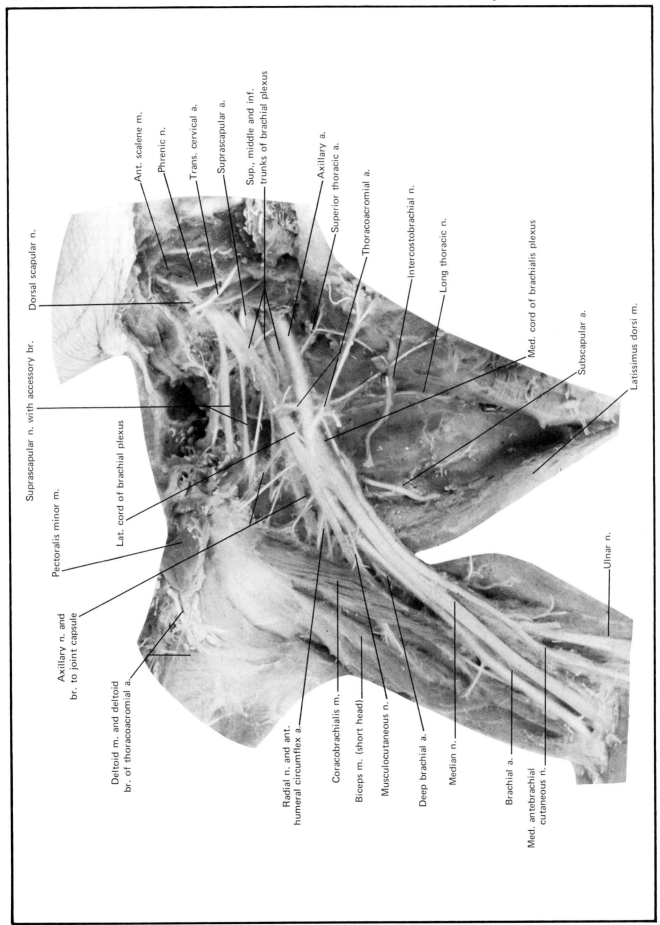

Dorsal scapular n.

Ant. scalene m.

Phrenic n.

Trans. cervical a.

Suprascapular a.

Sup., middle and inf. trunks of brachial plexus

Axillary a.

Superior thoracic a.

Thoracoacromial a.

Intercostobrachial n.

Long thoracic n.

Med. cord of brachialis plexus

Subscapular a.

Latissimus dorsi m.

Suprascapular n. with accessory br.

Pectoralis minor m.

Lat. cord of brachial plexus

Axillary n. and br. to joint capsule

Deltoid m. and deltoid br. of thoracoacromial a.

Radial n. and ant. humeral circumflex a.

Coracobrachialis m.

Biceps m. (short head)

Musculocutaneous n.

Deep brachial a.

Median n.

Brachial a.

Med. antebrachial cutaneous n.

Ulnar n.

ARTERIOGRAM OF THE LEFT SHOULDER REGION

The right and left subclavian arteries that are the source of the vasculature to the upper extremities may differ in their origins from the aortic arch, but with the commencement of their branches a single description suffices for both sides.

In this illustration the thoracic viscera have been removed so that the profuse vascularity of the lungs would not obscure the anastomotic relations of the shoulder. The segment of the *left subclavian* proximal to its first branch, the *left vertebral artery,* was sectioned and dissected out with the other mediastinal vessels. The remainder of the subclavian artery gives rise to the *thyrocervical* and *costocervical trunks.* The first is directly involved with the circulation of the shoulder through the *transverse scapular artery* and the *descending branch* of the *transverse cervical artery.* These supply blood to muscles of the dorsal scapular region and engage in numerous anastomotic unions with branches of the axillary artery.

At the external edge of the first rib, the origin of the small *superior thoracic artery* indicates the point where the subclavian artery becomes the *axillary artery.* Two larger vessels, the *thoracoacromial* and *lateral thoracic arteries,* arise in approximation to the midpoint of the axillary artery. The thoracoacromial conventionally divides into the *pectoral, subclavian, acromial* and *deltoid branches* which supply their named regions. The *lateral thoracic artery* descends along the external surface of the serratus anterior muscle, which it supplies by perforating branches that have fine anastomoses with the underlying intercostal arteries. The course of the *subscapular artery* approximates the axillary border of the scapula and gives origin to the *scapular circumflex artery.* This vessel enters the infraspinous fossa deep to the triangular space.

The *anterior* and *posterior humeral circumflex arteries,* which usually arise independently from the axillary artery, are here depicted as branches of a common origin from the subscapular artery. These vessels encircle the surgical neck of the humerus and supply numerous fine branches to the bone and joint capsule.

The last section of the axillary artery provides several branches to the immediate muscular regions of the upper brachium before the axillary artery becomes the *brachial artery.* This transition occurs where the artery passes anterior to the lateral edge of the teres major, a point that angiographically lies just proximal to the origin of the *deep brachial artery.*

Typically, the brachial artery is a single vessel throughout its course; but in the particular case shown here, the oft-found "split" brachial artery is illustrated. In this condition the median nerve usually passes between the arterial divisions.

In visualizing the circulation to the shoulder as a whole, it becomes apparent that should ligation of the axillary artery be required at some point proximal to the origin of the subscapular artery, the numerous anastomoses of branches around the scapular region would provide sufficient collateral circulation to maintain the viability of the limb.

Plate 13   Arteriogram of Left Shoulder Region   31

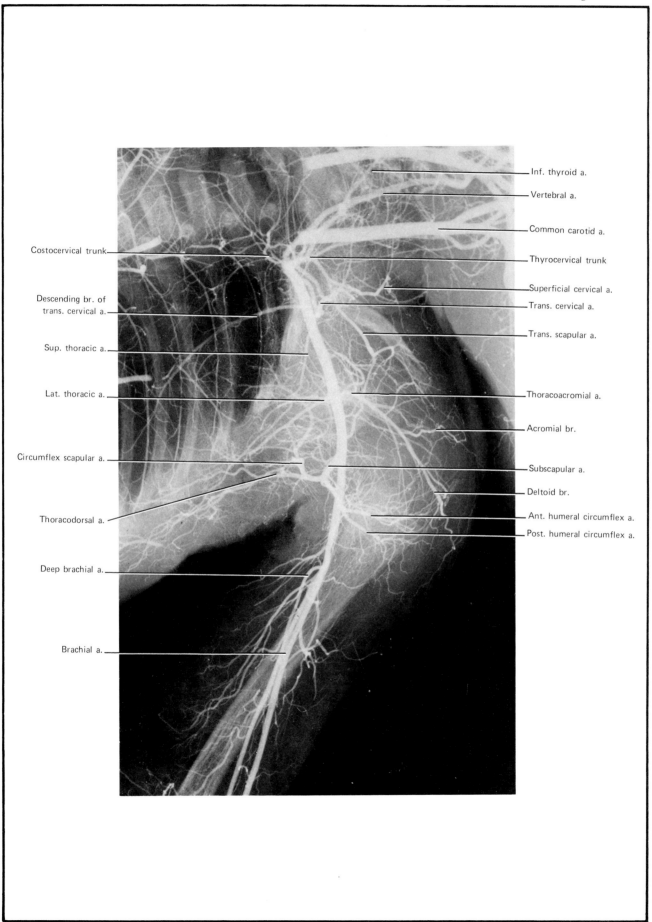

Costocervical trunk

Descending br. of
trans. cervical a.

Sup. thoracic a.

Lat. thoracic a.

Circumflex scapular a.

Thoracodorsal a.

Deep brachial a.

Brachial a.

Inf. thyroid a.

Vertebral a.

Common carotid a.

Thyrocervical trunk

Superficial cervical a.

Trans. cervical a.

Trans. scapular a.

Thoracoacromial a.

Acromial br.

Subscapular a.

Deltoid br.

Ant. humeral circumflex a.

Post. humeral circumflex a.

Frontal Section of the Shoulder Joint

This section shows that the articulating components of the fetal shoulder joint are nearly a perfect chondrous model of the definitive ossified articulation seen in the adult.

Note that the *glenoid fossa,* even when deepened by the connective tissue of the *labrum,* embraces less than one half of the spheroid formed by the *humeral head.* Obviously, a strong capsule and the combined action of all its activating muscles must provide the necessary joint stability. Here it is shown that the *deltoid* forms a thick muscular epaulet that helps to hold the articular surfaces firmly in apposition while abducting the *humerus.* The illustrated *teres major* and *subscapularis muscles* also enhance the apposition while adducting the humerus. The tendon of the *supraspinatus muscle,* the most superior of the muscles forming the rotator cuff, may be seen passing between the *acromion* and *coracoid processes* to insert on the highest facet of the *greater tuberosity.* The position of the acromion over the top of the joint indicates why upward dislocations of the joint are relatively rare and usually are accompanied by acromial fractures. On the other hand, downward subluxations require only stretching or laxity of the tendons and ligaments.

Plate 14   Frontal Section of Shoulder Joint   33

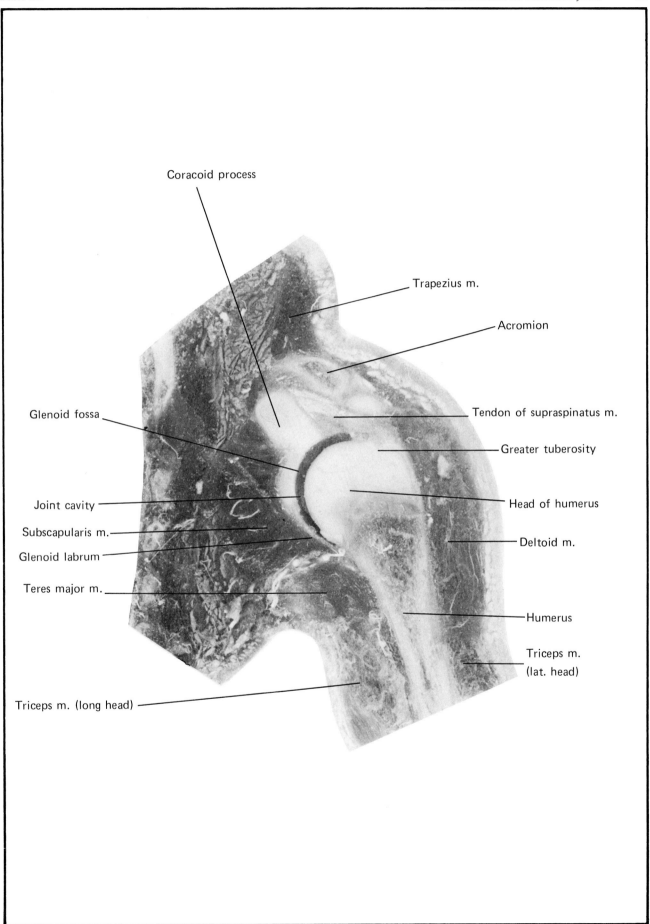

Coracoid process

Trapezius m.

Acromion

Tendon of supraspinatus m.

Glenoid fossa

Greater tuberosity

Joint cavity

Head of humerus

Subscapularis m.

Deltoid m.

Glenoid labrum

Teres major m.

Humerus

Triceps m.
(lat. head)

Triceps m. (long head)

CROSS SECTION THROUGH THE MIDDLE OF THE BRACHIUM

This is a photograph of the distal surface of a cut through the middle third of the arm. The relations of the *medial intermuscular septum* and its vascular and nervous contents to the flexors and extensors are well illustrated.

Note the *musculocutaneous nerve* and its muscular arterial branches coursing along the deep surface of the biceps.

The large *radial nerve*, in the process of giving branches to the *triceps*, can be seen in the company of the *deep brachial artery* as they wind posterolaterally around the extensor surface of the *humerus*.

The disproportionate amount of subcutaneous fat is characteristic of the term fetus.

Plate 15   Cross Section through Middle of Brachium   35

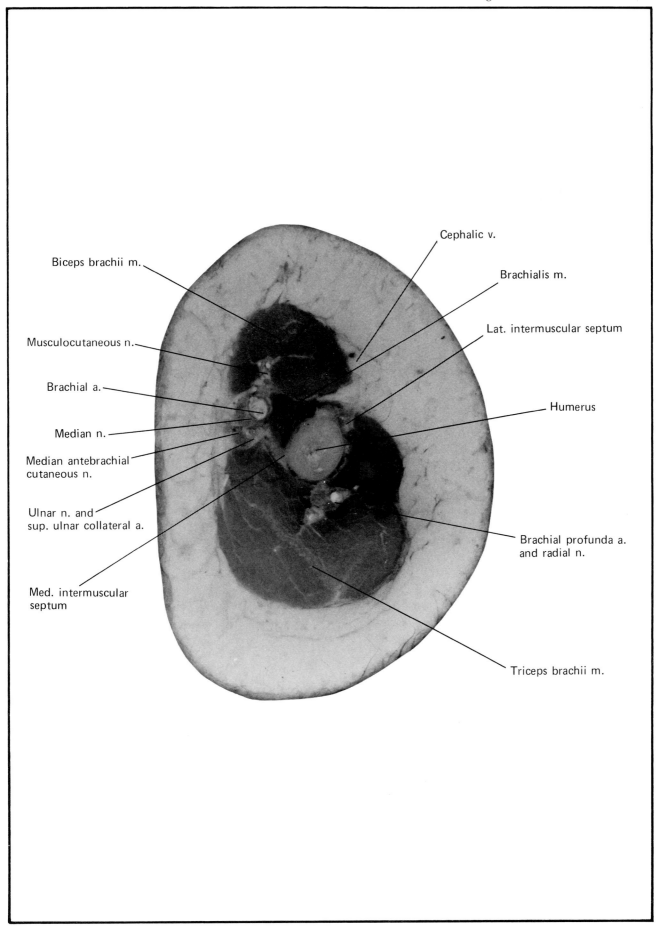

Cephalic v.

Biceps brachii m.

Brachialis m.

Musculocutaneous n.

Lat. intermuscular septum

Brachial a.

Humerus

Median n.

Median antebrachial
cutaneous n.

Ulnar n. and
sup. ulnar collateral a.

Brachial profunda a.
and radial n.

Med. intermuscular
septum

Triceps brachii m.

DISSECTION OF THE ANTEROMEDIAL ASPECT OF THE BRACHIUM

The axillary artery and its concurrent nerves course distally along the medial edge of the coracobrachialis muscle where, at a point marked by the lateral edge of the teres major, they enter the medial intermuscular septum. The designation *brachial artery* is here applied to the vessel.

The medial intermuscular septum is part of the deep investing fascia of the musculature that is attached to the medial surface of the humerus. In conjunction with the lateral intermuscular septum it forms a structural boundary that separates the flexors from the extensors. The *coracobrachialis muscle,* however, belongs to neither of these groups. It originates on the coracoid process and adducts the humerus through its insertion, which lies in the same plane as the intermuscular septum. Between the fibers of this muscle passes the *musculocutaneous nerve,* a derivative of the lateral cord of the brachial plexus. This nerve can be seen passing between the *biceps brachii* and the *brachialis,* where it provides both muscles with motor branches. Terminating on the skin of the forearm, it forms the lateral antebrachial cutaneous nerve.

The *median nerve,* formed from the lateral and medial cords of the brachial plexus, accompanies the brachial artery in its transit through the brachium. Both structures enter the forearm medial to the insertion of the biceps, but the nerve most often passes between the bifid head of the *pronator teres.* The median nerve supplies most of the motor branches to the flexors in the forearm and thenar compartment of the hand.

Three nerves that are derivatives of the medial cord of the brachial plexus leave the medial intermuscular septum in the midregion of the brachium. The most superficial, *the medial brachial cutaneous nerve,* provides sensory innervation to the skin on the medial surface of the brachium. The *medial antebrachial cutaneous nerve* performs the same function for the skin on the medial area of the flexor surface of the forearm. The conspicuous *ulnar nerve* courses along the medial fibers of the deep head of the *triceps* to pass through a dorsal groove on the *medial epicondyle* of the humerus to enter the forearm. It travels deep to the flexors that parallel the ulnar and continues into the hypothenar and deep compartments of the hand.

The short head of the biceps brachii is the most conspicuous component of that muscle seen in this view. Leaving its origin on the coracoid process, its fibers pass medial to the insertion of the *pectoralis major.* They blend with those of the long head in the midbrachial region, and their combined insertion on the bicipital tuberosity of the radius furnishes a powerful flexion and supination of the forearm. The brachialis muscle, lying deep to the biceps, originates on the anterior surface of the humerus and inserts on the coronoid process of the ulna. Activating the nonrotatory hinge of the ulnohumeral joint, it produces a pure flexion only.

Of the large venous systems of the brachium, the *cephalic vein* is the most superficial. It is formed by the subcutaneous cephalic plexus of the dorsolateral surface of the forearm and passes proximally along the lateral surface of the biceps brachii to where its proximal section is here visible between the insertions of the deltoid muscle and pectoralis major muscle. The deeper brachial veins form a plexus of several thin walled channels (venae commitantes) that entwine the brachial artery within the medial intermuscular septum. These vessels are formed by the deep veins of the forearm and the superficial basilic veins of the antebrachial flexor surface.

Plate 16   Anteromedial Aspect of Brachium   37

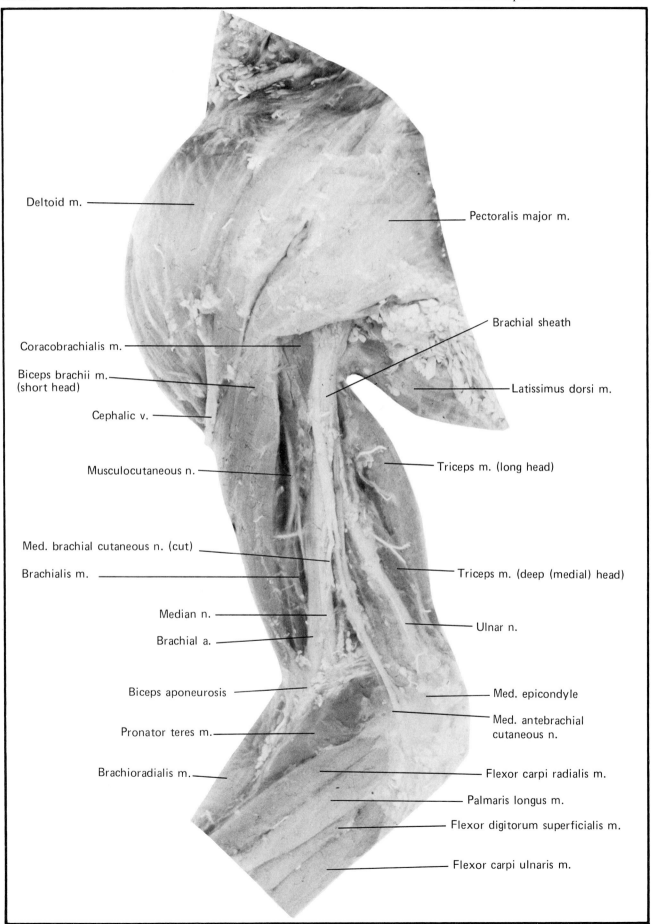

Deltoid m.

Pectoralis major m.

Brachial sheath

Coracobrachialis m.

Biceps brachii m.
(short head)

Latissimus dorsi m.

Cephalic v.

Musculocutaneous n.

Triceps m. (long head)

Med. brachial cutaneous n. (cut)

Brachialis m.

Triceps m. (deep (medial) head)

Median n.

Ulnar n.

Brachial a.

Biceps aponeurosis

Med. epicondyle

Med. antebrachial
cutaneous n.

Pronator teres m.

Brachioradialis m.

Flexor carpi radialis m.

Palmaris longus m.

Flexor digitorum superficialis m.

Flexor carpi ulnaris m.

SAGITTAL SECTION THROUGH THE ELBOW JOINT

As in the shoulder joint, the articular surfaces of the humeroulnar joint in the term fetus are generally radiolucent and entirely modeled in cartilage. The extent and limitation of the joint movements become apparent with the analysis of the joint structure. The medial articular condyle of the humerus shown here (the *trochlea*) is grooved like a pulley to receive the *semilunar notch* of the *ulna*. The fit of the two surfaces permits no rotation or sidewise deviation and limits the motion to pure flexion.

The insertion of the *brachialis muscle* to the ulnar region anterior to the *coronoid process* limits the action of this muscle to flexion. The passage of the *median nerve* and a muscular branch of the *brachial artery* between the two origins of the *pronator teres* is also well depicted.

Plate 17   Sagittal Section through Elbow Joint   39

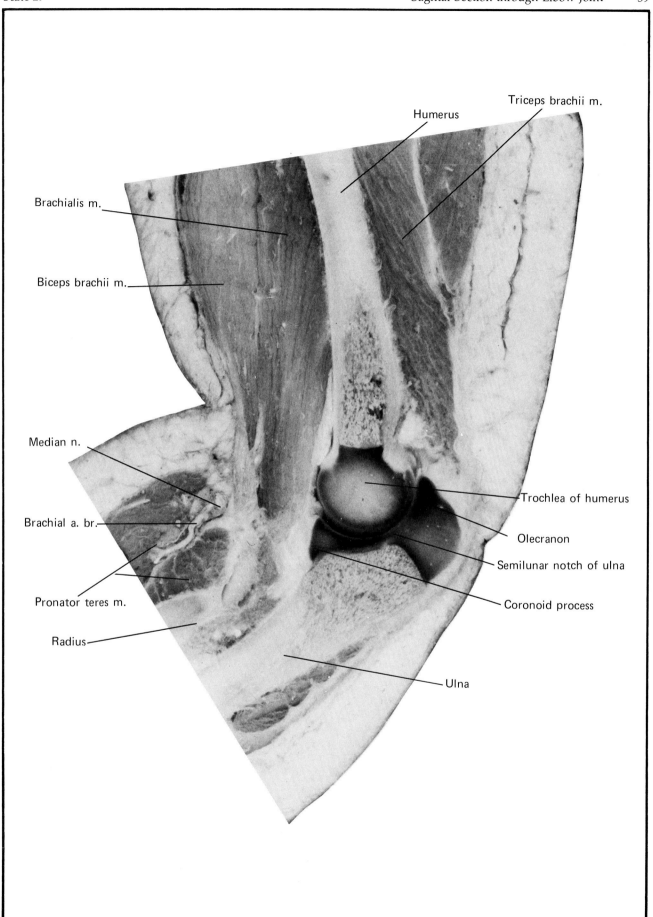

Humerus

Triceps brachii m.

Brachialis m.

Biceps brachii m.

Median n.

Brachial a. br.

Pronator teres m.

Radius

Trochlea of humerus

Olecranon

Semilunar notch of ulna

Coronoid process

Ulna

CROSS SECTION THROUGH THE MIDDLE OF THE RIGHT ANTEBRACHIUM

This section well illustrates the anterior flexor and dorsal extensor muscle masses that are separated by the *radius* and *ulna* and their intervening *interosseous membrane*.

In the flexor muscles, the plane indicated by a line that would connect the *ulnar artery* and *nerve* with the *median nerve* and the *radial artery* roughly separates the superficial and deep flexor groups.

Note that the ulnar nerve and artery course between the *flexor carpi ulnaris* and the *flexor digitorum superficialis* while the radial artery, unaccompanied by a nerve, runs more superficially. The median nerve is adherent to the deep surface of the flexor digitorum superficialis and is often associated with a conspicuous artery. The *anterior interosseous nerve* and *artery* travel along the interosseous membrane to supply deep flexors.

Lying external to the ulna and radius, the major *basilic* and *cephalic veins* course in the subcutaneous adipose tissue.

Plate 18   Cross Section through Middle of Right Antebrachium   41

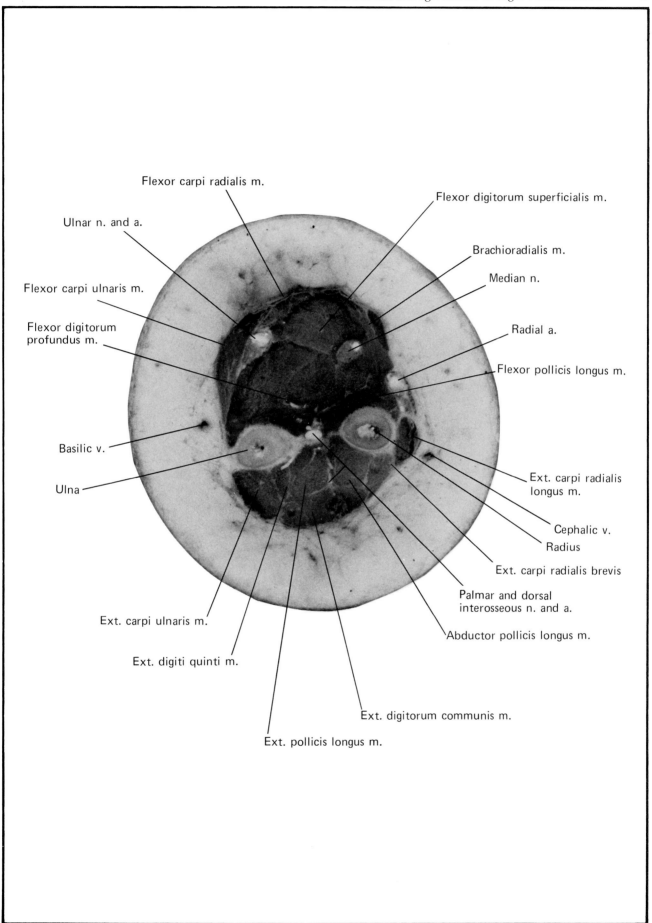

Flexor carpi radialis m.

Flexor digitorum superficialis m.

Ulnar n. and a.

Brachioradialis m.

Median n.

Flexor carpi ulnaris m.

Radial a.

Flexor digitorum
profundus m.

Flexor pollicis longus m.

Basilic v.

Ulna

Ext. carpi radialis
longus m.

Cephalic v.

Radius

Ext. carpi radialis brevis

Ext. carpi ulnaris m.

Palmar and dorsal
interosseous n. and a.

Ext. digiti quinti m.

Abductor pollicis longus m.

Ext. digitorum communis m.

Ext. pollicis longus m.

SUPERFICIAL DISSECTION OF THE PALMAR SURFACE OF THE HAND AND WRIST

The skin and investing fascia have been stripped from the forearm, hand and anterior surface of the thumb and two fingers. The palmar carpal ligament, a thickening of the antebrachial fascia that joins the dorsal extensor retinaculum in encircling the wrist, has been removed along with the palmar aponeurosis. (These features are well illustrated in Plate 11).

Commencing with the radial side, the *abductor pollicis longus* and *brachioradialis muscles* form the lateral border of the forearm. The first of these is an extensor muscle that wraps around the radius to abduct the first metacarpus. The brachioradialis, however, is a flexor and supinator of the wrist despite the fact that it originates on the lateral epicondyle and is innervated by the radial nerve. It inserts on the distal radius. The remainder of the superficial muscles seen here on the palmar side of the antebrachium primarily originate on the medial epicondyle and cross the wrist joint. The *flexor carpi radialis*, which inserts into the base of the second metacarpus, flexes and abducts the wrist.

The tendon of the *palmaris longus* and its insertion into the palmar aponeurosis have been removed to show the tendons of the *flexor digitorum superficialis*. In addition, the flexor retinaculum has been removed. This was a thick, fibrous band, bridging the carpal projections at the base of the thenar and hypothenar eminences. It thus roofed the carpal tunnel to prevent bowstringing of the tendons during flexion of the wrist.

The long flexors of the fingers are actually muscular complexes with four distinct digital insertions that exhibit a considerable independence in their actions. The flexor digitorum superficialis shows this division into separate components in the distal half of the forearm, and as the tendons pass through the carpal tunnel, the two to the index finger and little finger pass beneath the others. The median nerve travels along the deep surface of the flexor digitorum superficialis and enters the palm with its tendons.

The *flexor carpi ulnaris* is the most medial muscle of the antebrachium. Its tendon crosses the wrist at the base of the hypothenar eminence and inserts on the pisiform and hamulus to flex and adduct the wrist.

This figure shows the superficial thenar, hypothenar and midpalmar muscles of the palm of the hand. The *flexor pollicis brevis, abductor pollicis brevis, flexor digiti minimi* and *abductor digiti minimi* are intrinsic muscles of the thumb and little finger whose actions are self-explanatory.

In the midpalmar compartment, the digital distribution of the arteries, flexor tendons and nerves are apparent.

The *superficial palmar arterial arch* receives the major contribution of the *ulnar artery* to the hand. This artery is accompanied by the ulnar nerves as it passes lateral to the base of the hypothenar eminence. Because they are also superficial to the flexor retinaculum, both structures are more subject to injury at this point. The arterial arch, which is completed by the *superficial palmar branch* of the *radial artery*, supplies the major common digital arteries to the fingers on the ulnar side of the hand. Finer vessels supply the thumb and radial fingers. This is the reciprocal arrangement of the arterial distribution of the deep palmar arch shown in Plate 21.

Each *common digital artery* and its corresponding *nerve*, with the exception of those to the thumb and little finger, serves the interdigital aspects of adjacent fingers. This concept is best illustrated by the angiograph in Plate 24.

The sensory innervation of the palmar surface of the digits is inconsistently distributed between branches of the *median* and *ulnar nerves*. The most frequent pattern, however, shows a line of sensory demarcation that bisects the middle finger. Here the medial proper digital nerve and artery are derived from the ulnar nerve and primarily the ulnar artery, and the lateral counterparts are derived from the median nerve and deep radial artery.

The lumbricals are exposed in this dissection of the middle palmar compartment. They are spindle-shaped muscles that originate in the forks of the flexor digitorum superficialis tendons. They pass to the radial side of each finger and insert into the dorsal extensor assembly. There they serve to flex the metacarpophalangeal joint while extending the distal phalanges.

Plate 19   Hand and Wrist: Superficial Dissection of Palmar Surface   43

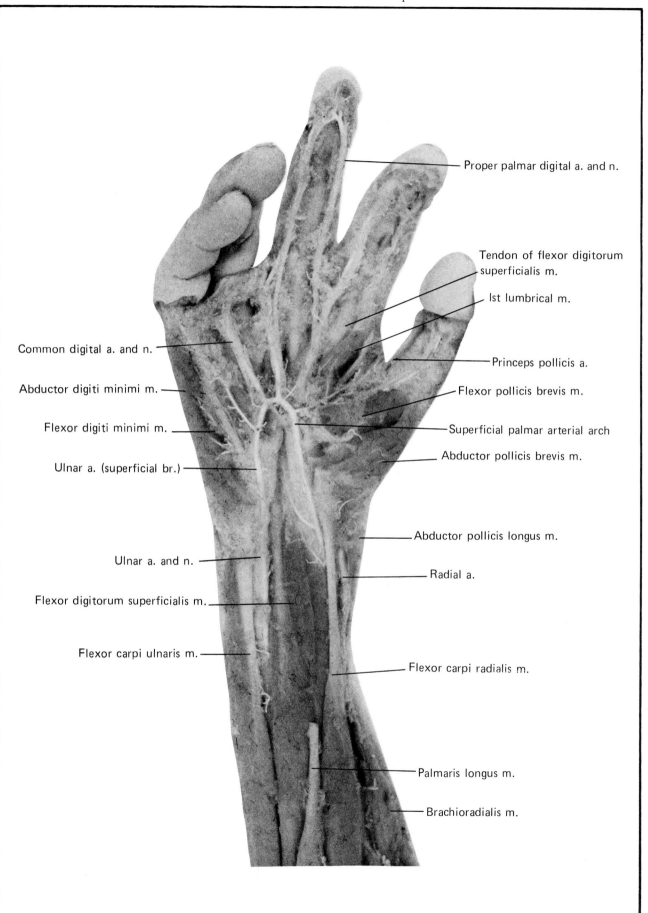

Proper palmar digital a. and n.

Tendon of flexor digitorum superficialis m.

Ist lumbrical m.

Common digital a. and n.

Princeps pollicis a.

Abductor digiti minimi m.

Flexor pollicis brevis m.

Flexor digiti minimi m.

Superficial palmar arterial arch

Ulnar a. (superficial br.)

Abductor pollicis brevis m.

Abductor pollicis longus m.

Ulnar a. and n.

Radial a.

Flexor digitorum superficialis m.

Flexor carpi ulnaris m.

Flexor carpi radialis m.

Palmaris longus m.

Brachioradialis m.

DEEP DISSECTION OF THE ANTEBRACHIUM

The tendons of the flexor carpi radialis and flexor digitorum superficialis have been divided at the wrist and reflected. The proximal reflection shows the *median nerve* still adherent to the fascia on the deep surface of the superficial flexor. Medial retraction of the *flexor carpi ulnaris* has separated the deep flexors to expose in greater detail the structures related to the interosseous membrane.

The *flexor digitorum profundus* arises on the ulna and sends four tendons through the carpal tunnel deep to those of the superficial flexor. Each tendon enters the flexor sheath of a finger and passes through the split tendons of the superficialis to insert onto the base of the terminal phalanx. In the same plane, the *flexor pollicis longus* originates primarily from the anterior surface of the radius and the adjacent part of the interosseous membrane. After passing through the carpal tunnel and between the adductors and short flexors of the thumb, it inserts onto the base of the terminal phalanx. The *pronator quadratus* is a short, flat muscle that arises on the lower anterior surface of the nonpivoting ulna. Its fibers run transversely across the

forearm, partly wrapping around the distal one fourth of the radius to insert on its lateral border. Contraction of this muscle assists the action of the pronator teres in rotating the radius into pronation. These muscles also stabilize the antebrachium against the strong supinating effect of the biceps and brachioradialis as they flex the forearm.

The *ulnar nerve* runs a course concurrent with the *ulnar artery* on the surface of the medial deep flexors. This nerve provides the motor supply of the flexor carpi ulnaris and the ulnar half of the flexor digitorum profundus. *The radial artery,* which branches from the brachial artery deep to the *pronator teres,* courses along the radius between the origin of the *flexor pollicis longus* and the insertion of the *brachioradialis.* It divides lateral to the wrist to send a large branch dorsal to the metacarpus of the thumb and a smaller branch ventral to the superficial palmar arch.

The anterior *interosseous artery* and *nerve* form a neurovascular bundle that runs along the anterior surface of the interosseous membrane. This artery is a derivative of the common interosseous branch of the ulnar artery that partly supplies the deep antebrachial muscles and extends branches to the anterior carpal region. The anterior interosseous nerve is a branch of the median nerve and sends a motor supply to the pronator quadratus and sensory fibers to the carpal joints.

Plate 20   Deep Dissection of Antebrachium   45

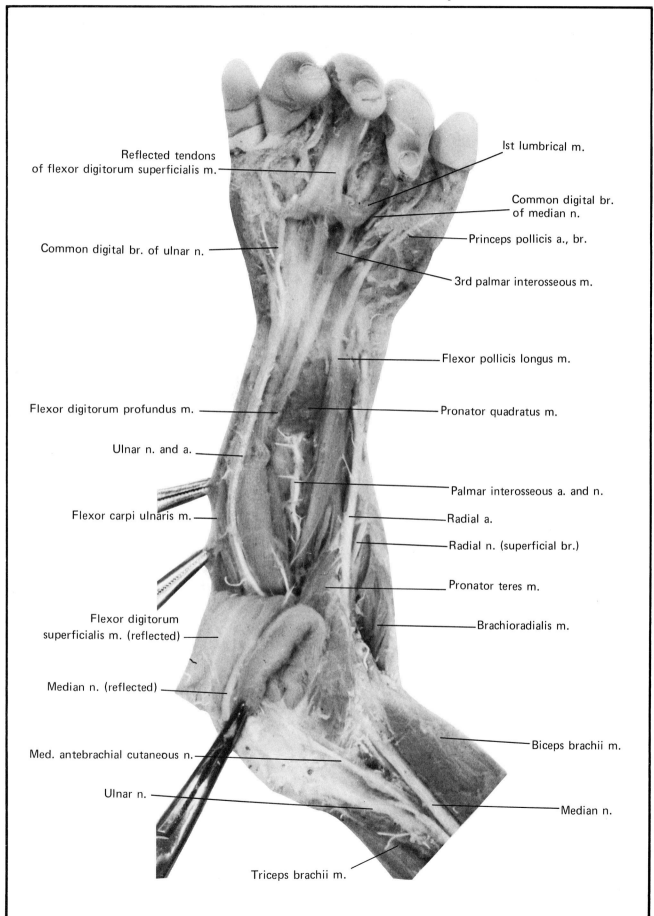

Reflected tendons
of flexor digitorum superficialis m.

Ist lumbrical m.

Common digital br.
of median n.

Princeps pollicis a., br.

Common digital br. of ulnar n.

3rd palmar interosseous m.

Flexor pollicis longus m.

Flexor digitorum profundus m.

Pronator quadratus m.

Ulnar n. and a.

Palmar interosseous a. and n.

Flexor carpi ulnaris m.

Radial a.

Radial n. (superficial br.)

Pronator teres m.

Flexor digitorum
superficialis m. (reflected)

Brachioradialis m.

Median n. (reflected)

Biceps brachii m.

Med. antebrachial cutaneous n.

Ulnar n.

Median n.

Triceps brachii m.

DEEP DISSECTION OF THE HAND

In this plate, both the superficial and deep antebrachial flexors of the fingers have been reflected, and muscles and arteries of the adductor interosseous compartment have been exposed.

The *deep palmar arterial arch* has a more proximal location than its superficial counterpart. Since its largest source is the dorsal branch of the *radial artery*, it provides the major arterial supply to the lateral digits of the hand. This is a situation that is reciprocal to the primarily ulnar distribution of the superficial arch branches.

The large *radialis indicis artery* can be seen emerging deep to the transverse head of the *adductor pollicis*. After supplying the thumb and first two fingers, the radial contribution to the arch becomes visible between the origins of the transverse and the oblique heads of the adductor pollicis where it anastomoses with the deep ulnar branches and gives off smaller digital vessels. The arterial supply to the carpals and their palmar ligaments is shown as central anastomotic branches of the deep arch and the anterior interosseous artery. The sectioned superficial ulnar branch of the superficial arch is still visible near the origin of the *opponens digiti minimi*.

Plate 21　　　　　　　　　　　　　　　　Deep Dissection of Hand　　47

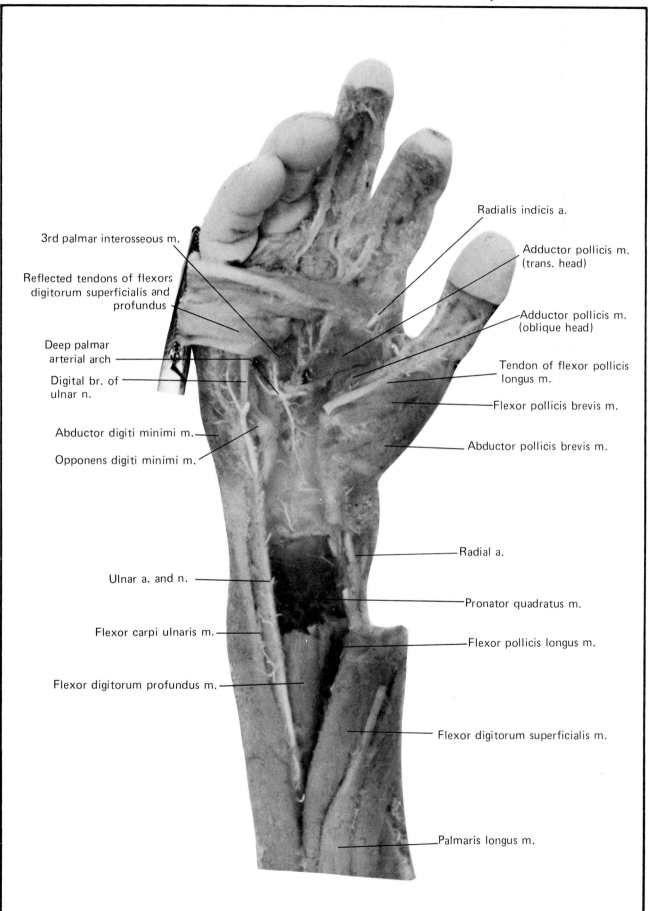

3rd palmar interosseous m.

Reflected tendons of flexors digitorum superficialis and profundus

Deep palmar arterial arch

Digital br. of ulnar n.

Abductor digiti minimi m.

Opponens digiti minimi m.

Ulnar a. and n.

Flexor carpi ulnaris m.

Flexor digitorum profundus m.

Radialis indicis a.

Adductor pollicis m. (trans. head)

Adductor pollicis m. (oblique head)

Tendon of flexor pollicis longus m.

Flexor pollicis brevis m.

Abductor pollicis brevis m.

Radial a.

Pronator quadratus m.

Flexor pollicis longus m.

Flexor digitorum superficialis m.

Palmaris longus m.

CROSS SECTION THROUGH THE LEFT CARPAL REGION

The crescentic trough of carpal bones that with the flexor retinaculum form the carpal tunnel is dramatically illustrated in this photograph. Unfortunately, this section is slightly proximal to the full extent of the retinaculum, but its manner of being slung between the tip of the *pisiform* and the *ridge of the trapezium* may be readily conceptualized.

The bundled arrangement of the long flexor tendons can be sorted into three layers. The deepest layer represents the tendons of the *flexor pollicis longus* and *flexor digitorum profundus*, and the more superficial two layers are tendons of the *flexor digitorum superficialis*.

The large *superficial branch* of the *ulnar artery* running with the *ulnar nerve* can be seen near the tip of the pisiform. The smaller *superficial palmar branch* of the *radial artery* enters the palm with the *median nerve*.

The deep branch of the radial artery passes lateral to the ridge of the trapezium.

The *dorsal ulnar carpal artery* can be noted running in the same plane as the *extensor tendons*.

Plate 22   Cross Section through Carpal Region   49

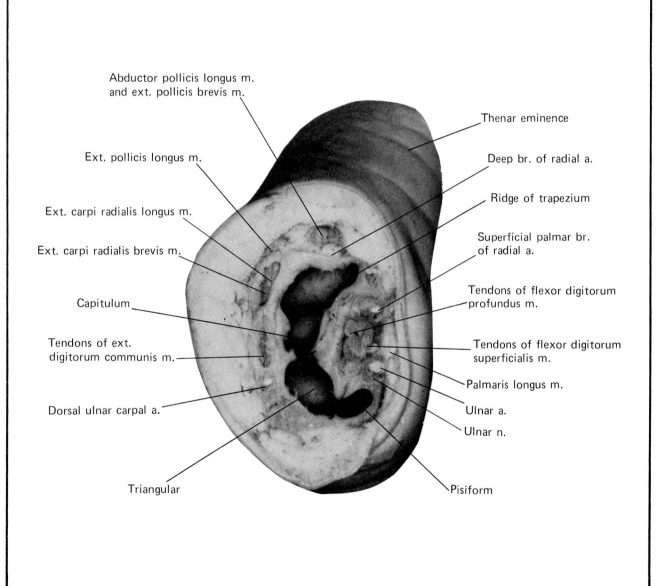

Abductor pollicis longus m.
and ext. pollicis brevis m.

Thenar eminence

Deep br. of radial a.

Ext. pollicis longus m.

Ridge of trapezium

Ext. carpi radialis longus m.

Superficial palmar br.
of radial a.

Ext. carpi radialis brevis m.

Tendons of flexor digitorum
profundus m.

Capitulum

Tendons of ext.
digitorum communis m.

Tendons of flexor digitorum
superficialis m.

Palmaris longus m.

Dorsal ulnar carpal a.

Ulnar a.

Ulnar n.

Triangular

Pisiform

FRONTAL SECTION THROUGH THE CARPALS OF THE LEFT WRIST

In contrast to the radiographically vacant carpal region of fetal x-rays, this figure shows that the wrist joint complex is beautifully preformed in cartilage. All of the carpals except the sesamoid pisiform of the palmar surface can be identified according to their positions and definitive shapes.

Particularly well shown is the intricate system of intercarpal ligaments that carry nutritive vessels. This function is in addition to their structural role.

Plate 23   Frontal Section through Carpals   51

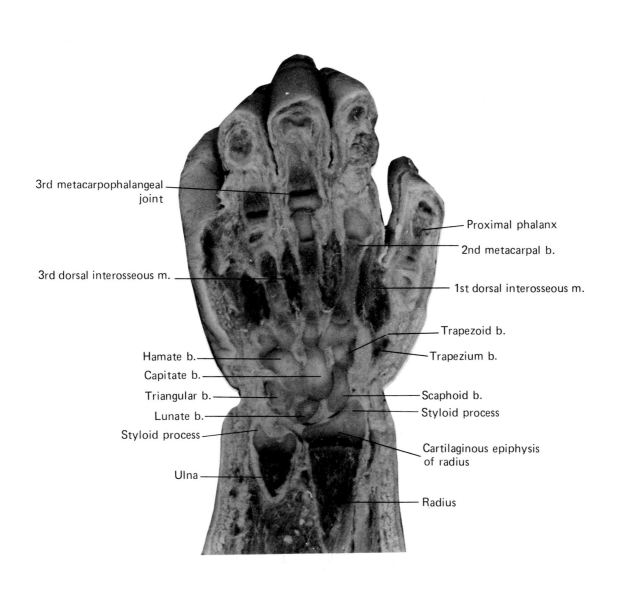

3rd metacarpophalangeal —
joint

Proximal phalanx

2nd metacarpal b.

3rd dorsal interosseous m. —

1st dorsal interosseous m.

Trapezoid b.

Hamate b.—

Trapezium b.

Capitate b.—

Triangular b. —

Scaphoid b.

Lunate b.—

Styloid process

Styloid process —

Cartilaginous epiphysis
of radius

Ulna —

Radius

ARTERIOGRAM OF THE HAND AND WRIST

This plate well illustrates the reciprocal patterns of origin and distribution of the arteries associated with the two palmar arches. By following the *ulnar artery* distally into the palmar region, its termination as two branches may be discerned. The largest and most superficial of these is the major contribution to the *superficial palmar arch,* and the smaller division abruptly penetrates to its adductor interosseous compartment to anastomose with the *deep palmar arch.*

The superficial arch is completed by joining the *superficial palmar branch* of the *radial artery.* Since this is much smaller than the ulnar half of the arch, its derivatives are also smaller. Hence the larger *common palmar digital arteries* to the medial (ulnar) side of the hand come from the superficial arch whereas those of the lateral (radial) side are from the deep arch.

The large termination of the radial artery may be traced dorsal to the metacarpus of the thumb, where it enters the deep palmar compartment between the adductor pollicis and the first interosseous muscle. Here it gives off the *princips pollicis* and *radial indicis arteries.* It then continues across the deep compartment where it anastomoses with the ulnar branch to complete the arch. Prior to entering the hand the radial artery sends the *dorsal carpal artery* to the back of the wrist. This vessel has numerous anastomoses with the dorsal branch of the *anterior interosseous artery* to supply the carpals and their dorsal ligaments. A corresponding *dorsal carpal branch* of the ulnar artery may be noted.

A series of fine *common dorsal digital arteries* arise by the union of dorsal perforators from the deep palmar arch and metacarpal branches of the dorsal carpal arteries, and they mimic the distribution of their palmar common digitals.

The larger common palmar digital arteries can be traced to the metacarpophalangeal joints where they form the *proper digital arteries.* The two palmar proper digital arteries of each finger reunite in an anastomotic arch around the terminal phalanx. A profuse spray of branches from these arches form the *digital arterial tufts* that feed numerous arteriovenous anastomoses. Thermoregulation in the extremities is the most obvious function of the arterial tufts.

Plate 24   Arteriogram of Hand and Wrist   53

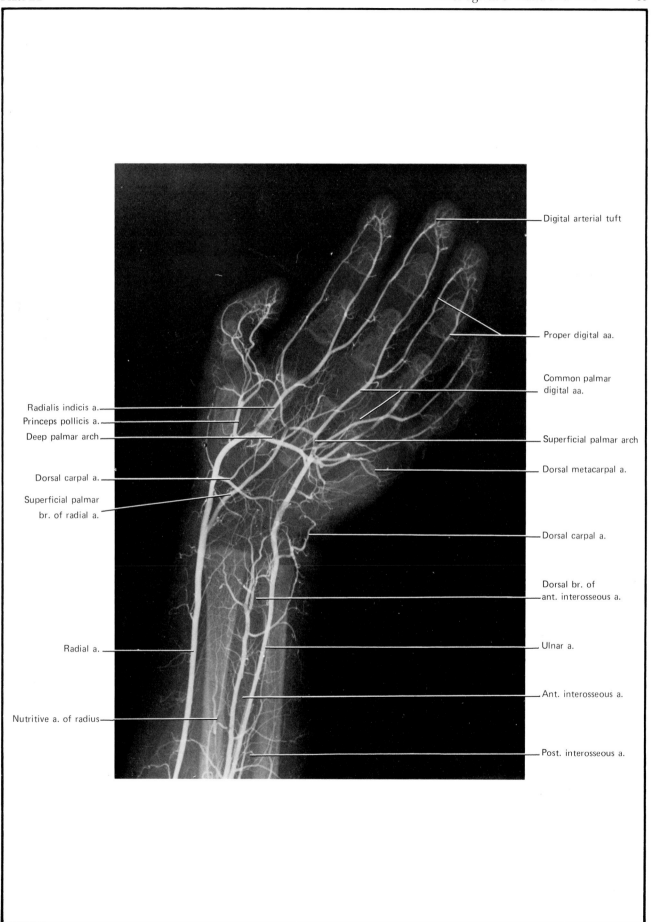

Digital arterial tuft

Proper digital aa.

Common palmar
digital aa.

Radialis indicis a.

Princeps pollicis a.

Deep palmar arch

Superficial palmar arch

Dorsal carpal a.

Dorsal metacarpal a.

Superficial palmar
br. of radial a.

Dorsal carpal a.

Dorsal br. of
ant. interosseous a.

Radial a.

Ulnar a.

Ant. interosseous a.

Nutritive a. of radius

Post. interosseous a.

CROSS SECTION THROUGH THE MIDDLE OF THE LEFT PALM

The division of the hand into three muscular compartments and a midpalmar space is best illustrated in cross section.

The thenar compartment underlies the thenar eminence and contains the intrinsic flexors of the thumb and the opponens pollicis. *The median nerve* enters the palm with the *tendons of the long flexors* to supply motor fibers to the first and frequently second lumbricals and to the thenar muscles by a recurrent branch. All of the other intrinsic muscles of the hand are innervated by the *ulnar nerve.*

The tendon of the *flexor pollicis longus* separates the thenar muscles from those of the adductor interosseous compartment. This compartment includes both the transverse and oblique heads of the *adductor pollicis* and all of the interrosseous muscles. There are three *palmar interossei,* which are so situated that they adduct the first, third and fourth fingers inward toward the second finger. As the axial digit of the hand, the second finger receives no insertions of the palmar interossei.

There are four *dorsal interossei.* The middle two insert on their respective proximal sides of the first phalanx of the second finger and thus alternately deviate this finger laterally and medially. The first and fourth dorsal interossei abduct the first and third fingers away from the second finger. Thus the *abductor digiti quinti* is functionally a fifth dorsal interosseous muscle.

The remaining hypothenar muscles, the *opponens digiti quinti* and the *flexor digiti quinti brevis,* create the hypothenar eminence.

Plate 25   Cross Section through Middle of Palm   55

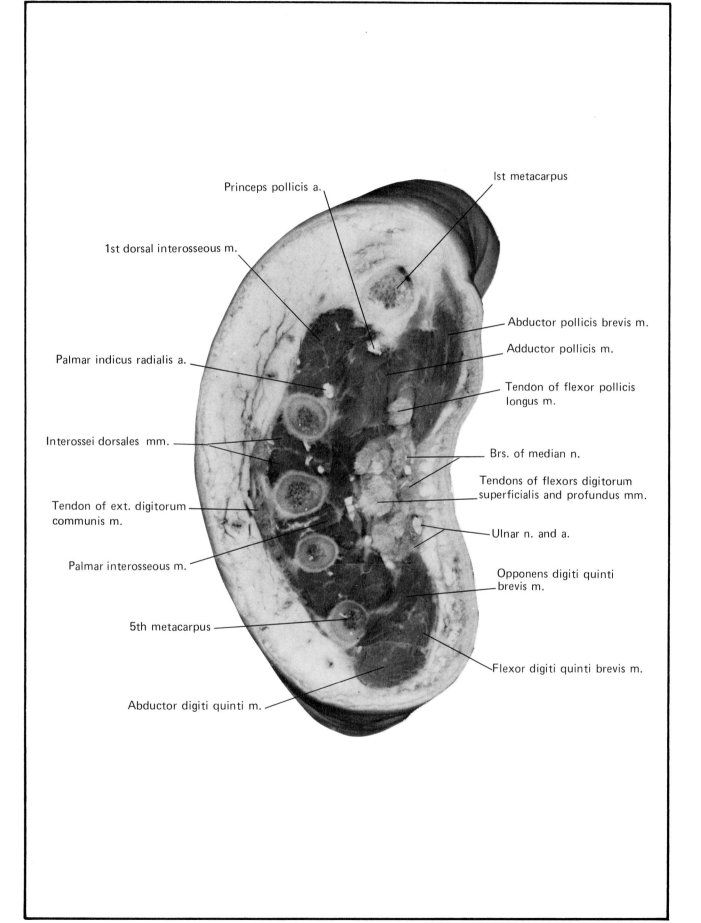

Princeps pollicis a.

1st metacarpus

1st dorsal interosseous m.

Abductor pollicis brevis m.

Adductor pollicis m.

Palmar indicus radialis a.

Tendon of flexor pollicis longus m.

Brs. of median n.

Interossei dorsales mm.

Tendons of flexors digitorum superficialis and profundus mm.

Tendon of ext. digitorum communis m.

Ulnar n. and a.

Palmar interosseous m.

Opponens digiti quinti brevis m.

5th metacarpus

Flexor digiti quinti brevis m.

Abductor digiti quinti m.

CROSS SECTION THROUGH THE PROXIMAL PHALANGES

The structural organization of the *flexor sheath* as an osseoaponeurotic tunnel is illustrated in these sections, and the more simply constructed *extensor assemblies* may be discerned as a dark strap of connective tissue dorsal to the shaft of the phalanx. The double set of *proper digital arteries* coursing dorsal to their respective *digital nerves* brackets each flexor sheath.

Plate 26   Cross Section of Proximal Phalanges   57

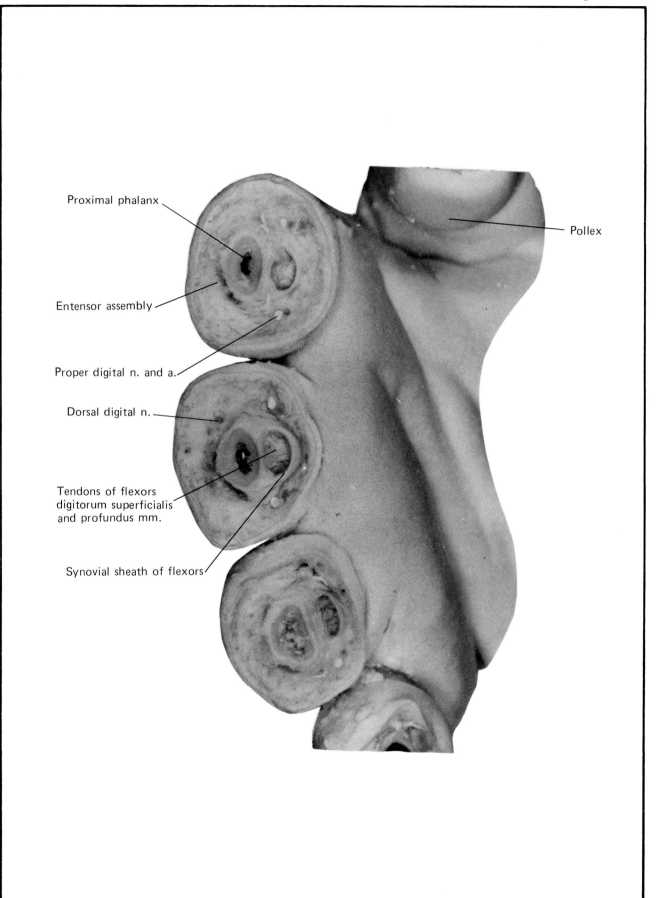

Proximal phalanx

Pollex

Entensor assembly

Proper digital n. and a.

Dorsal digital n.

Tendons of flexors
digitorum superficialis
and profundus mm.

Synovial sheath of flexors

FLEXOR ASSEMBLY OF THE FINGERS

The ring finger and little finger have been amputated and the flexor sheath opened to better display the arrangement of the flexor tendons to the second finger.

Note that the tendon of the *flexor digitorum superficialis,* which has been elevated by the clamp, commences to split anterior to the shaft of the proximal phalanx. Its two divisions continue distally to insert on the sides of the middle phalanx. The tendon of the *flexor digitorum profundus* passes through the interval produced by the split to insert on the base of the terminal phalanx.

Plate 27   Flexor Assembly of Fingers   59

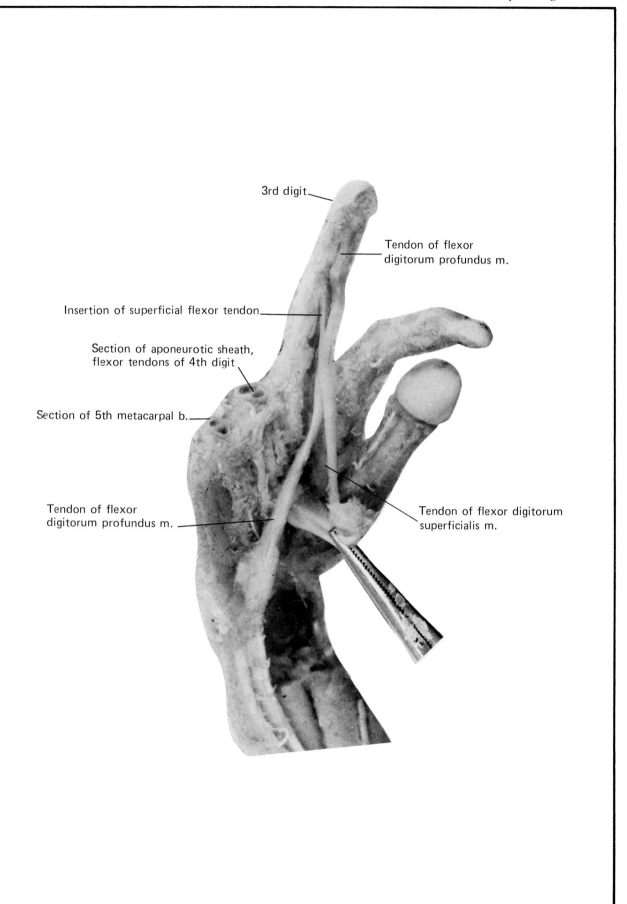

3rd digit

Tendon of flexor
digitorum profundus m.

Insertion of superficial flexor tendon

Section of aponeurotic sheath,
flexor tendons of 4th digit

Section of 5th metacarpal b.

Tendon of flexor
digitorum profundus m.

Tendon of flexor digitorum
superficialis m.

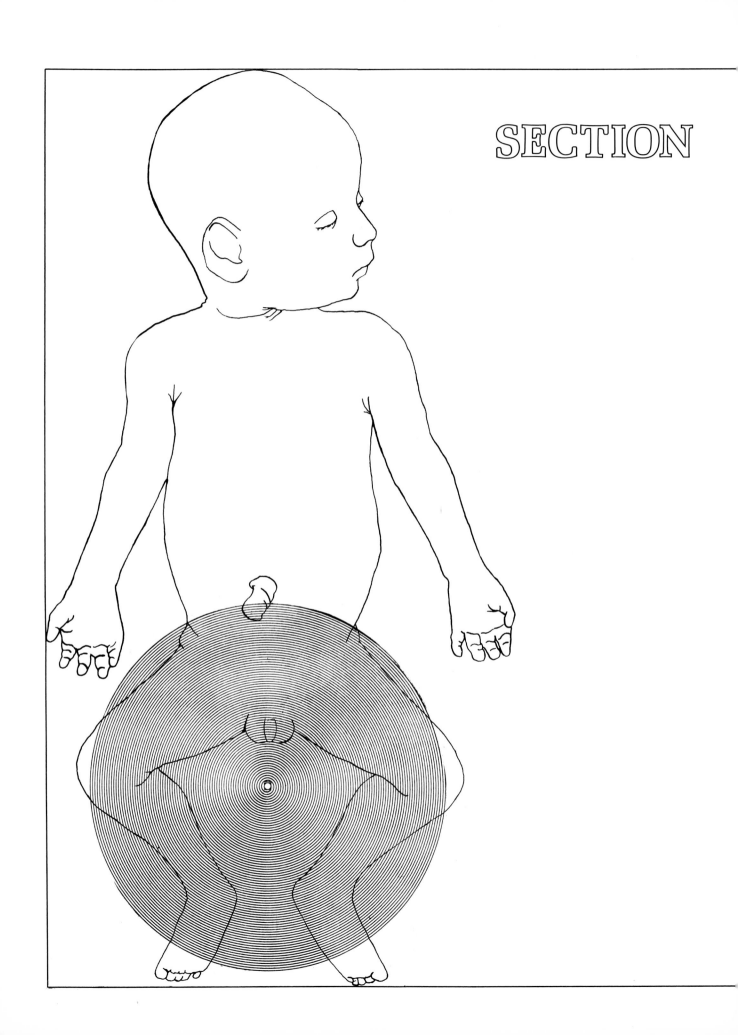

SECTION

THREE

LOWER EXTREMITY

X-RAY: OSTEOLOGY OF THE LOWER EXTREMITY

In contrast to the upper extremity, it will be noted that the leg is directly attached to the axial skeleton through the sacroiliac joint. As in all fetal joints, the actual articulation is formed by cartilage and is radiolucent, but its site is readily discernible where the ossified ala of the ilium approximates the upper sacral vertebrae. Between the bodies of the vertebrae and the ilium small spherical centers indicate the ossification of the sacral costal process. As the name implies, this fused homologue of true ribs will bear the sacral articular surface of the sacroiliac joint.

The hip bone shows its tripartite origin in the radiologically visible parts of the *ilium, ischium* and *pubis.* Each of these ossifications is suspended in a cartilaginous matrix that approximates the definitive adult shape, and all contribute in nearly equal proportions to form the deep socket of the *acetabulum* that receives the spherical head of the femur. Sexual differences in the shape of the pelvis do not appear until puberty.

The shaft of the *femur* is well represented in calcified bone, but the greater trochanter, neck and head of the femur are cartilaginous. The shape of the head is identical to that of the adult, although the fetal neck forms less of an angle with the shaft than it does in the definitive femur. A distinct medial protuberance indicates the position of the lesser trochanter.

A radiolucent spot at the midpoint of the femoral shaft marks the main nutritional foramen of the diaphysis. The artery and veins passing through this aperture are derivatives of the deep femoral vessels.

Unlike the arm the fetal lower extremity shows secondary centers of ossification prior to term. The indicated center in the *distal femoral epiphysis* appears at the onset of the 7th month of gestation and has been used as a medicolegal indication of fetal viability.

The shafts of the *tibia* and *fibula* are shown in their proper relative proportions, and the small ossification center of the *proximal tibial epiphysis* that appears just before or after full term is indicated.

The ossification of the larger tarsals precedes that of the carpal bones, so that the calcified centers of the *talus* and *calcaneus* are well defined before birth. The developmental state of the metatarsals and phalanges is equivalent to that of their homologues in the upper extremity at term.

Plate 28   X-Ray: Osteology of Lower Extremity   63

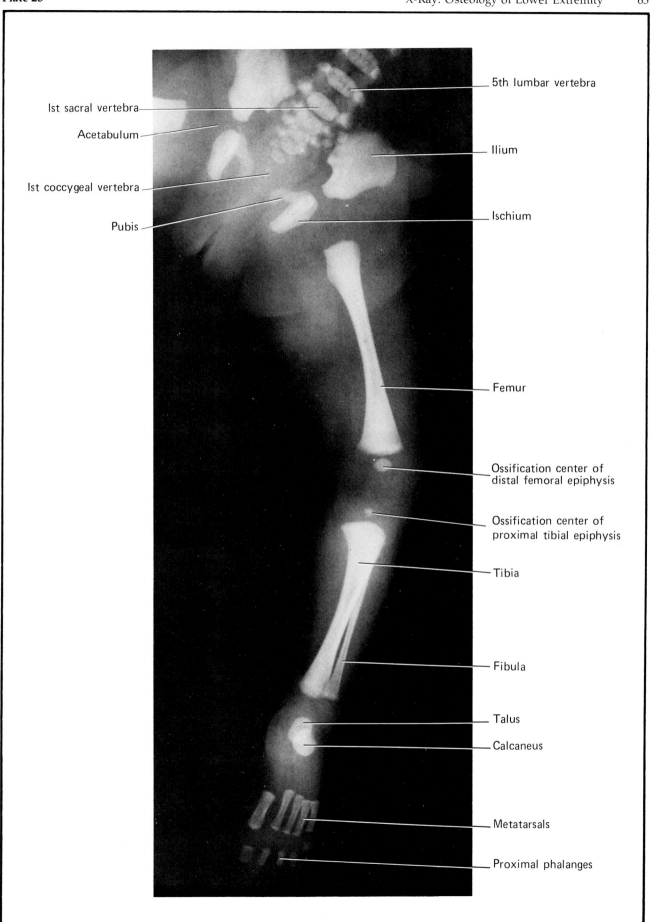

5th lumbar vertebra

Ist sacral vertebra

Acetabulum

Ilium

Ist coccygeal vertebra

Ischium

Pubis

Femur

Ossification center of
distal femoral epiphysis

Ossification center of
proximal tibial epiphysis

Tibia

Fibula

Talus

Calcaneus

Metatarsals

Proximal phalanges

ARTERIOGRAM OF THE LOWER EXTREMITY

The common iliac artery is the source of arterial distribution to the lower limb. In the lumbosacral region this vessel divides into a medial *hypogastric* (internal iliac) and a lateral *external iliac artery*. The first of these descends into the pelvis to supply the pelvic viscera and pudendal structures in addition to the internal and external pelvic musculature that activates the hip joint. The *superior* and *inferior gluteal arteries* and the *obturator artery* are the major muscular branches of the hypogastric, and their distribution is detailed in Plate 35. The obturator artery supplies the adductor region of the thigh, and its extensive anastomosis with other femoral vessels is well shown in this illustration.

As in the arm a single major arterial stem courses through the proximal half of the limb before dividing into two or more vessels in the distal half. The stem artery is designated as the *external iliac, femoral* or *popliteal artery* according to the region traversed. The external iliac originates in the lower lumbar region and enters the leg by passing deep to the inguinal ligament, at which point it becomes the femoral artery. Just before leaving the iliac region it provides vessels to the abdominal and pelvic walls.

Just after entering the femoral triangle (see Plate 36), the femoral artery gives rise to the *medial* and to the *lateral circumflex arteries* and the deep femoral artery. Both circumflex arteries freely anastomose with the obturator and gluteal arteries around the region of the hip joint. A large descending branch of the lateral circumflex artery provides branches to the quadriceps muscles.

The course of the deep femoral artery parallels that of the femoral but runs closer to the shaft of the femur. Because the posterior femoral region lacks any conspicuous longitudinal artery, this vessel provides its muscles with several perforating branches.

The femoral artery runs a progressively deeper course as it descends the limb until, in the distal one fourth of the thigh, it penetrates the adductor magnus muscle. At this point it enters the region behind the knee where it is known as the *popliteal artery*.

Through a set of *superior* and *inferior geniculate* branches the popliteal artery furnishes collateral circulation to the knee before it divides into the *anterior* and *posterior tibial arteries* (see Plate 40). The anterior tibial artery passes between the tibia and fibula to enter the anterior extensor compartment of the leg. It descends to the ankle, where at the level of the talotibial articulation it becomes the *dorsalis pedis artery*.

The posterior tibial artery descends in the flexor compartment of the leg and enters the foot beneath the medial malleolus; here it divides into the medial and lateral plantar arteries.

The *peroneal artery*, a lateral branch of the posterior tibial, descends in the lateral (peroneal) compartment of the leg to terminate in the collateral network of the ankle. A prominent *perforating branch* passes between the tibia and fibula to supply the lateral malleolus and dorsum of the foot.

The *dorsal* and *plantar arcuate vessels* bear a reciprocal relationship to each other and their digital distributions resemble the palmar vascularity (see Plate 45).

Plate 29   Arteriogram of Lower Extremity   65

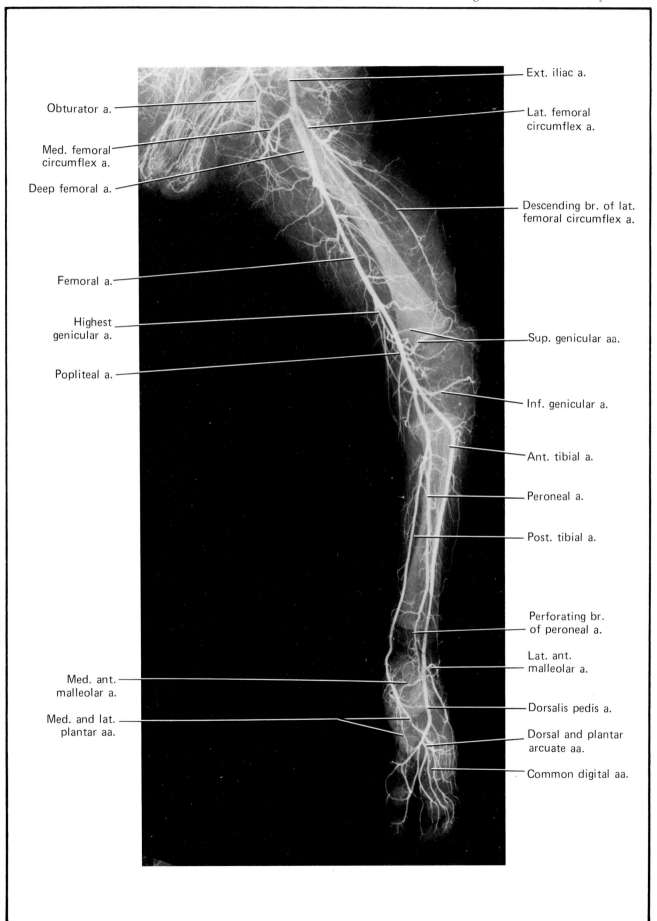

Obturator a.

Med. femoral
circumflex a.

Deep femoral a.

Femoral a.

Highest
genicular a.

Popliteal a.

Med. ant.
malleolar a.

Med. and lat.
plantar aa.

Ext. iliac a.

Lat. femoral
circumflex a.

Descending br. of lat.
femoral circumflex a.

Sup. genicular aa.

Inf. genicular a.

Ant. tibial a.

Peroneal a.

Post. tibial a.

Perforating br.
of peroneal a.

Lat. ant.
malleolar a.

Dorsalis pedis a.

Dorsal and plantar
arcuate aa.

Common digital aa.

SUPERFICIAL LATERAL ASPECT OF THE LOWER EXTREMITY

In this illustration the skin, superficial fascia and some of the investing fascia have been removed to provide an overview of the lower limb musculature.

The origin of the broad *gluteus maximus* may be traced from the dorsal sacral and iliac regions across the aponeurotic fascia that covers the *gluteus medius* muscle. From this expanse its superior fibers converge upon the fascia lata covering the greater trochanter. The more inferior fibers follow the contour of the buttock to insert on the upper posterior part of the femur. The direction of these fibers indicates the action of the maximus in extending and abducting the thigh. Between the *iliac crest* and the upper border of the gluteus maximus, the thick gluteal aponeurosis has been removed to reveal the fibers of the gluteus medius that are directed toward the *greater trochanter*.

The projection inferior to the maximus is the fetal perineum. Its components and their essential relationships are identical to those in the adult except that the conical shape of the muscular sling of the *levator ani* is greatly exaggerated. This causes the pelvic diaphragm to protrude much lower than its relative level in the adult, in whom it lies medial to the ischial tuberosities. Because the fetal pelvic outlet is also relatively narrower, the lateral extent of the fat-filled *ischiorectal fossa* is more restricted.

The muscles of both the thigh and the leg are sheathed in tough stockings of investing fascia called the fascia lata and the crural fascia, respectively. Invaginations of these fasciae that attach to the bones form the various intermuscular septae that separate the muscular compartments.

The thickness of the fascia lata is not uniform, being heaviest over the lateral thigh. In one area it is quite aponeurotic and forms the *iliotibial tract*. This is actually the tendon of insertion of the *tensor fasciae latae muscle*. In this picture most of the fascia lata has been dissected away, leaving primarily the fascial insertion of the gluteus maximus and the iliotibial tract.

The large extensor muscle group on the anterior thigh is collectively called the quadriceps femoris. It is comprised of the *vastus medialis, vastus intermedius, vastus lateralis* and the *rectus femoris*; only the last two are visible in this view. The three vasti originate on the shaft of the femur, and the rectus originates on the rim of the acetabulum and the anteroinferior iliac spine. The quadriceps tendon inserts on the patella and, acting through the inferior patellar tendon, extends the leg.

The most lateral of the posterior thigh muscles, the *biceps femoris,* has two heads. The *long head* originates on the ischial tuberosity and the *short head* originates on the posterior lower half of the femur. Their combined tendon forms the lateral hamstring of the thigh and inserts on the upper fibula to produce flexion and lateral rotation of the leg.

The medial flexors, the *semimembranosus* and *semitendinosus* muscles, originate on the ischial tuberosity in common with the long head of the biceps. In this lateral view only their tendons are visible as they form the medial hamstring. The semimembranosus inserts behind the medial tibial condyle and the semitendinosus on the upper anteromedial surface of the tibia. Both muscles flex and medially rotate the leg and, in crossing the hip joint, extend the thigh.

The crural fascia has been removed from the leg and all three muscular compartments are demonstrable in this lateral view. The posterior flexor compartment shows the bellied *gastrocnemius* overlying the *soleus* muscle. The former arises from posterior attachments just above both condyles of the femur and, crossing the knee, assists in the flexion of the leg. The soleus arises from the posterior surfaces of the tibia and fibula and combines with the fibers of the gastrocnemius to form a common insertion, the *tendo calcaneus,* that strongly flexes the foot. The deep flexor muscles are displayed in Plate 41.

The lateral (peroneal) compartment contains the *peroneus longus* and *brevis* muscles. Both of these arise on the lateral surface of the fibula and insert on the foot through tendons that pass behind the lateral malleolus. The tendon of the brevis inserts on the tuberosity of the fifth metatarsal, and the longus turns under the foot to insert on the plantar surface of the medial tarsals. In combination, these muscles flex and evert (pronate) the foot to counteract the inversion (supination) produced by most of the other flexors and extensors. The foot in this photograph has been inverted to show more of the dorsal surface.

Of the three major muscles in the anterior crural compartment, only the *tibialis anterior* and *extensor digitorum longus* are visible in the view presented here. The first descends to the medial aspect of the foot to insert on the first cuneiform and the base of the first metatarsal, and therefore may act as a strong inverter and extensor of the foot.

The extensor digitorum longus crosses the ankle more laterally and sends individual tendons to the four lateral toes. Each of these tendons is joined by a contribution from the *extensor digitorum brevis* that originates on the calcaneus just below the lateral malleolus.

The tendon of the *extensor hallucis longus* runs deep between the other extensors but becomes visible here on the dorsum of the first metatarsal. It also is joined by a tendon of the extensor digitorum brevis.

Plate 30   Superficial Lateral Aspect   67

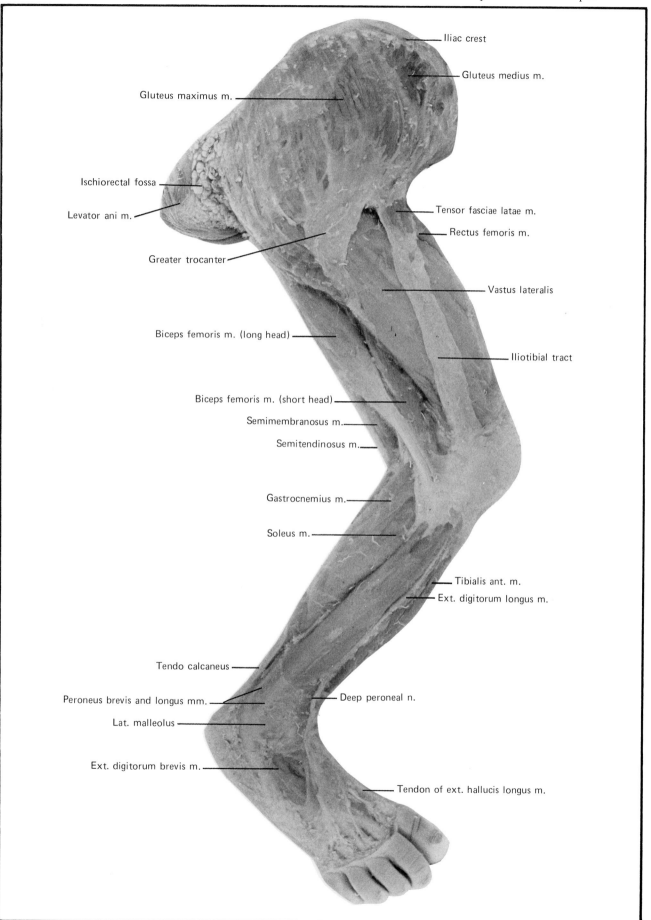

Iliac crest

Gluteus medius m.

Gluteus maximus m.

Ischiorectal fossa

Levator ani m.

Tensor fasciae latae m.

Rectus femoris m.

Greater trocanter

Vastus lateralis

Biceps femoris m. (long head)

Iliotibial tract

Biceps femoris m. (short head)

Semimembranosus m.

Semitendinosus m.

Gastrocnemius m.

Soleus m.

Tibialis ant. m.

Ext. digitorum longus m.

Tendo calcaneus

Peroneus brevis and longus mm.

Deep peroneal n.

Lat. malleolus

Ext. digitorum brevis m.

Tendon of ext. hallucis longus m.

POSTERIOR ASPECT OF THE SUPERFICIAL MUSCULATURE OF THE LOWER EXTREMITY

With the exception of the *adductor magnus* and *gracilis,* all of the muscles displayed in this view of the lower limb have been described in the previous example. Nevertheless, this discussion serves to enhance the comprehension of the relationships of the posterior thigh and leg muscles.

The lower edge of the *gluteus maximus* covers the common origin of the long muscles of the medial and lateral hamstrings, but their divergence to each side of the leg from the ischial tuberosity is obvious. In the lower posterior thigh their separation exposes the deep popliteal fossa that conveys the nerves, arteries and deep veins to the leg.

As the large sciatic nerve descends in the deeper posterior thigh it is crossed by the long head of the *biceps femoris.* Under this muscle it splits into the large *tibial nerve,* which is the superficial central structure seen in the popliteal fossa, and the lateral *common peroneal nerve* that descends along the posterior border of the biceps femoris tendon.

The lateral and medial heads of the *gastrocnemius* show their individual origins from the posterior femur just above its distal condyles. The merging of the two heads with the underlying soleus to form the tendo calcaneus explains why this combination of muscles has been called the triceps surae.

Plate 31   Posterior Aspect of Superficial Musculature   69

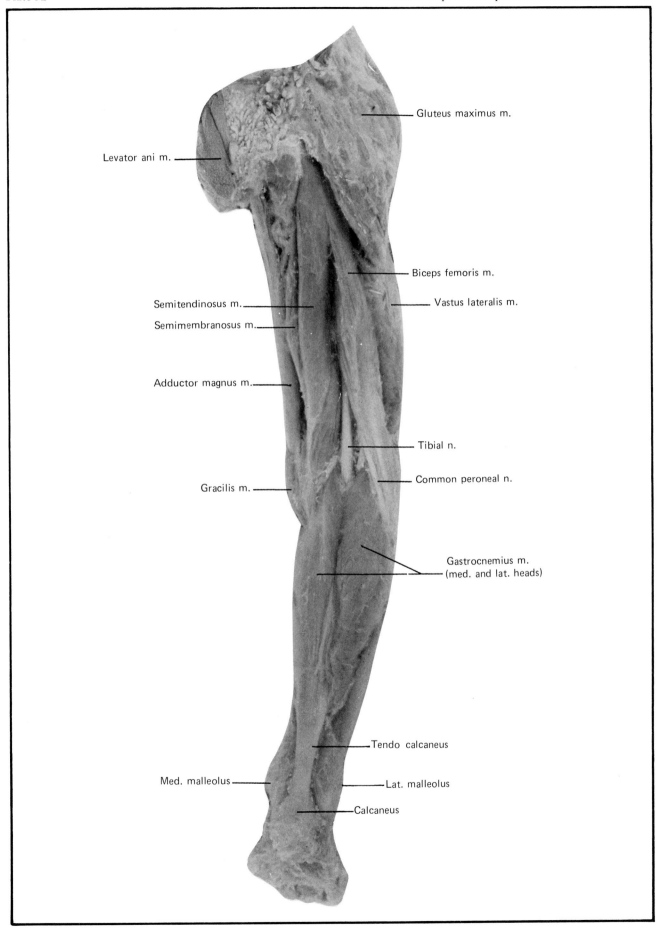

Gluteus maximus m.

Levator ani m.

Biceps femoris m.

Semitendinosus m.

Vastus lateralis m.

Semimembranosus m.

Adductor magnus m.

Tibial n.

Common peroneal n.

Gracilis m.

Gastrocnemius m.
(med. and lat. heads)

Tendo calcaneus

Med. malleolus

Lat. malleolus

Calcaneus

DISSECTION OF THE GLUTEAL REGION I

Here the *gluteus maximus* has been sectioned from its femoral insertions and the accessory origins along the surface of the gluteus medius, and it has been reflected posteriorly. Adherent to its deep surface, the vessels and nerves supplying the maximus and the superficial posterior femoral region are well delineated. Superiorly, a small branch of the *superior gluteal artery* is seen emerging above the *sciatic nerve*. From the nerve itself, the branches of the *inferior gluteal nerve* that innervates the maximus course with derivatives of the *inferior gluteal artery*. Just lateral to the ischial tuberosity, between the sciatic nerve and the origin of the *long head* of the *biceps*, the *posterior femoral cutaneous nerve* runs toward the inferior gluteal margin, from where it provides sensory innervation to the skin of the posterior thigh.

The *gluteus medius* converges to insert on the *greater trochanter* that is seen here covered by a lightly colored vascular membrane. A corresponding light area is found on the deep surface of the reflected gluteus maximus. These synovial membranes mark the site of the bursa which permits the maximus to freely slide over the trochanter.

The size and relations of the sciatic nerve emerging below the *piriformis* muscle are indicated. As the largest nerve of the body it requires a conspicuous vasa vasorum that, in this region, are provided by the *arteria comitans of the sciatic nerve*. This vessel is derived from a branch of the inferior gluteal artery that also supplies the hip joint. The arteria comitans penetrates the sciatic nerve and may be exposed a considerable distance from its source by dividing the nerve bundle.

Plate 32   Gluteal Region: Dissection I   71

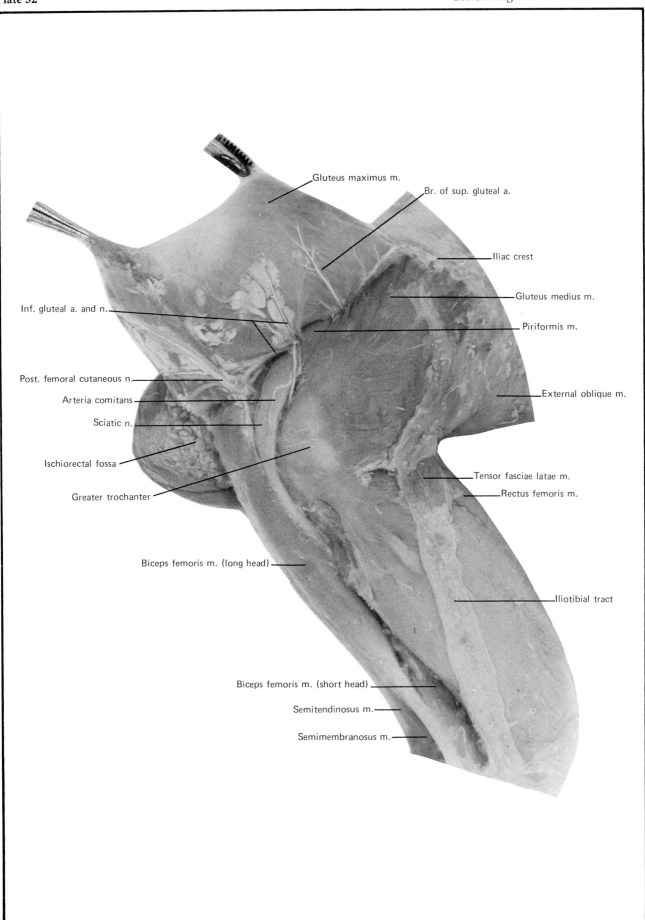

Gluteus maximus m.

Br. of sup. gluteal a.

Iliac crest

Gluteus medius m.

Piriformis m.

Inf. gluteal a. and n.

Post. femoral cutaneous n.

Arteria comitans

Sciatic n.

Ischiorectal fossa

Greater trochanter

External oblique m.

Tensor fasciae latae m.

Rectus femoris m.

Biceps femoris m. (long head)

Iliotibial tract

Biceps femoris m. (short head)

Semitendinosus m.

Semimembranosus m.

DISSECTION OF THE GLUTEAL REGION II

This plate shows the continued dissection of the same specimen presented in the previous illustration.

The *gluteus medius* has been separated from its insertion on the *greater trochanter* and reflected superiorly to expose the *gluteus minimus*. The sciatic nerve has been removed to reveal the insertions of the complex system of small muscles that rotate the hip laterally.

Topographically, the key structure in this region is the *piriformis muscle* because it separates the *superior* and *inferior gluteal nerves* and *vessels*. Originating on the anterior sacral surface, the piriformis leaves the pelvis through the greater sciatic foramen to insert on the superior border of the greater trochanter. It occupies most of the foramen but still leaves a small aperture above it and a larger one below for the egress of pelvic nerves and vessels.

Above the piriformis the branches of the superior gluteal nerve emerge to innervate both the gluteus medius and gluteus minimus muscles. They form neurovascular bundles with some branches of the superior gluteal artery, which distributes vessels to all three gluteal muscles.

Through the large lower aperture, located between the inferior border of the piriformis and the sacrospinous ligament, pass the inferior gluteal artery and nerve, the *posterior femoral cutaneous nerve* and the large sciatic nerve (here removed). The inferior gluteal nerve provides the exclusive motor innervation of the maximus, and the artery sends branches to all regional structures and extensively anastomoses with derivatives of the femoral artery.

Inferior to the piriformis, the combination of the *superior* and *inferior gemelli* and the *obturator internus* forms the tripartite muscle. The structure can be seen blending its insertion on the greater trochanter with that of the piriformis. The obturator internus arises within the pelvis on its lateral wall and exits through the lesser sciatic foramen between the sacrotuberous and sacrospinous ligaments. Here its tendon makes a very acute turn around the sciatic notch. The two gemelli arise from the upper and lower borders of the notch and accompany the obturator tendon to its insertion.

The *quadratus femoris* arises from the lateral surface of the superior ramus of the ischium and inserts on the intertrochanteric crest behind the greater trochanter.

In the adult these lateral rotators are usually exposed when the leg is in extension, and they show a more horizontal disposition in relation to the conventional anatomic position. In the fetus, however, the hip is normally flexed. This, in combination with the slightly different proportions of the pelvis, causes the lateral rotators to display a more oblique course, particularly in the case of the quadratus femoris.

Plate 33   Gluteal Region: Dissection II   73

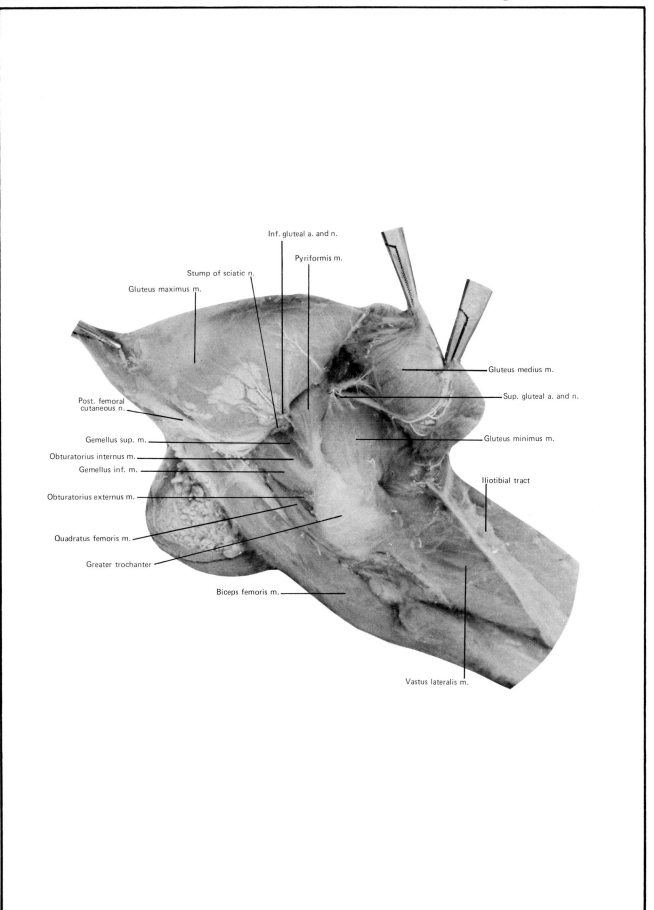

Inf. gluteal a. and n.

Pyriformis m.

Stump of sciatic n.

Gluteus maximus m.

Gluteus medius m.

Sup. gluteal a. and n.

Post. femoral
cutaneous n.

Gemellus sup. m.

Obturatorius internus m.

Gemellus inf. m.

Gluteus minimus m.

Obturatorius externus m.

Iliotibial tract

Quadratus femoris m.

Greater trochanter

Biceps femoris m.

Vastus lateralis m.

DEEP DISSECTION OF THE POSTERIOR FEMORAL REGION

In this view the *gluteus maximus* and *medius* have been reflected to expose the posterior aspect of the hip joint capsule and its relations to the posterior structures of the thigh. At the point where the long head of the *biceps femoris* crosses the *sciatic nerve*, it has been divided and retracted laterally to display the entire course of the sciatic nerve within the thigh.

Note that the sciatic nerve descends medial to the *greater trochanter* immediately posterior to the neck of the femur. The articular branch of the *inferior gluteal artery* that supplies vascularity to the hip joint can be seen giving fine branches to the joint capsule and the synovial membrane of the subgluteal bursa of the greater trochanter. It also supplies the *arteria comitans of the sciatic nerve*.

The division between the *medial tibial* and *lateral peroneal* parts of the sciatic nerve may be observed to commence in the upper femoral region, and it is not unusual to find the sciatic to be divided as high as the pelvis.

Where the long head of the biceps was sectioned as it crossed the sciatic nerve, a branch of the tibial division may be seen giving motor branches to it and to the *semitendinosus* and *semimembranosus* muscles. The peroneal division supplies no thigh muscles except the short head of the biceps. The profusion of muscular arteries penetrating the hamstrings are derivatives of *perforating branches of the deep femoral artery*.

Medial to the tibial nerve in the distal femoral region, the large *popliteal artery* may be noted entering the popliteal fossa through the adductor canal.

Plate 34   Deep Dissection of Posterior Femoral Region   75

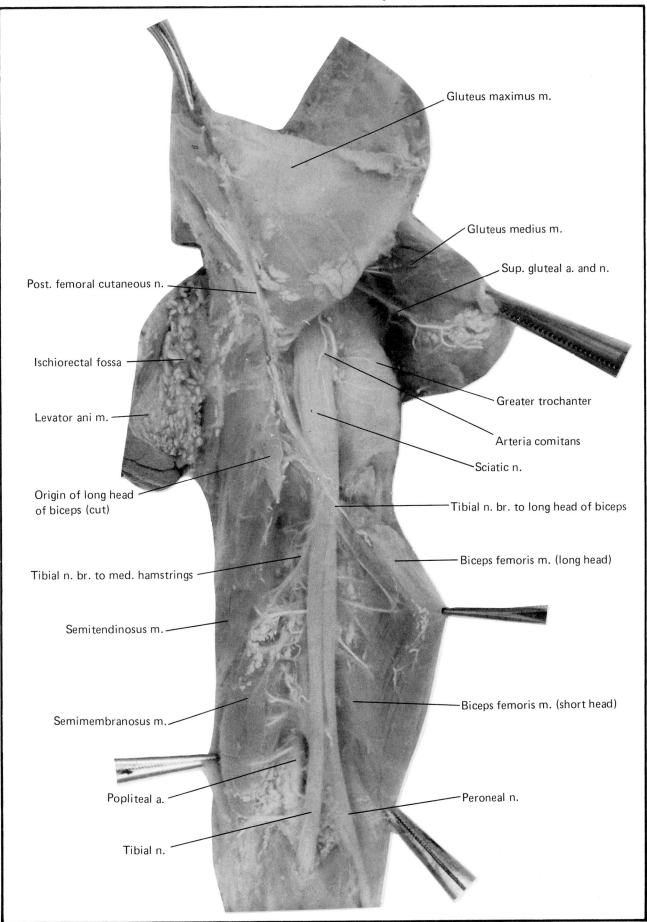

Gluteus maximus m.

Gluteus medius m.

Sup. gluteal a. and n.

Post. femoral cutaneous n.

Ischiorectal fossa

Levator ani m.

Greater trochanter

Arteria comitans

Sciatic n.

Origin of long head
of biceps (cut)

Tibial n. br. to long head of biceps

Biceps femoris m. (long head)

Tibial n. br. to med. hamstrings

Semitendinosus m.

Semimembranosus m.

Biceps femoris m. (short head)

Popliteal a.

Peroneal n.

Tibial n.

ARTERIOGRAM OF THE PELVIC AND FEMORAL REGIONS OF THE LOWER EXTREMITY

This is an anterior-posterior (A-P) view of the arteries of the left pelvis and thigh in a female fetus approximately 30 weeks old. The abdominal aorta and its dependent visceral branches have been removed to give a less obstructed view of the pelvic circulation.

The *common iliac arteries* that have been sectioned here just below their bifurcation from the aorta arise in the posterior abdominal wall and shortly divide into the *external iliac* and *hypogastric* (internal iliac) arteries. Because the *umbilical arteries* are derivatives of the hypogastric division, this artery is relatively massive during intrauterine life. However, after parturition it is the external iliac that becomes the larger artery.

The hypogastric artery plays a dual role and supplies branches to the pelvic viscera as well as the lumbar, gluteal and medial femoral regions. Only those branches involved with the lower extremity are of concern in this section, and the visceral vessels will be presented in a different view and discussed in the areas devoted to that subject.

After sending arteries to the sacral and lumbar regions, the hypogastric artery provides the greater blood supply to all of the gluteal muscles through the *superior gluteal artery,* which here is well illustrated radiographically.

Just before the major stem of the hypogastric turns forward and upward to become the umbilical artery, it sends a branch inferiorly that, in this specimen, is a common source of the *internal pudendal, obturator* and *inferior gluteal arteries.* In different cases considerable variation is found in both the site and sequence of the origins of these vessels, but eventually they can be identified by their area of distribution.

Smaller and less constant in caliber than its superior counterpart, the *inferior gluteal artery* is seen here passing laterally behind the hip joint.

The *obturator artery* leaves the pelvis through the obturator foramen. It gives muscular branches to the adductors of the femur and collateral anastomoses to the *medial femoral circumflex artery.*

The external iliac artery has no consequential branches within the pelvis until it is about to pass under the inguinal ligament. Here it sends the *inferior epigastric artery* up the anterior abdominal wall and gives off the *deep circumflex iliac artery* laterally.

Upon entering the femoral triangle, the external iliac becomes the *femoral artery* and almost immediately gives three major branches to various regions of the thigh. The *medial femoral circumflex* gives muscular branches to the adductors and forms collateral connections with the obturator. The *lateral femoral circumflex* artery embraces the region below the greater trochanter, and through a large descending branch it supplies much of the anterior and lateral regions of the quadriceps.

The *deep femoral artery,* that in this view is partially obscured by superimposition of the femoral artery, courses in the septum betwen the adductor and extensor compartments and supplies the lower adductor region and hamstrings through a series (usually 4 or 5) of perforating branches. As the deep femoral artery approaches the shaft of the femur near the middle of the thigh, a conspicuous *femoral nutritional artery* is sent into the bone to provide its medullary cavity with ascending and descending branches.

The deeper course of the deep femoral artery can be appreciated better by comparing this A-P view with that of the whole pelvic region in which the thigh is more flexed and laterally rotated.

In its descent through the adductor canal of the thigh, the femoral artery gives off a number of muscular branches before piercing the adductor magnus to become the *popliteal artery.*

There is an abundance of collateral connections between both gluteals, the obturator and the three large proximal branches of the femoral artery. Thus the external iliac may be ligated without critically compromising the vascular nutrition of the lower limb.

Plate 35   Arteriogram of Pelvic and Femoral Regions   77

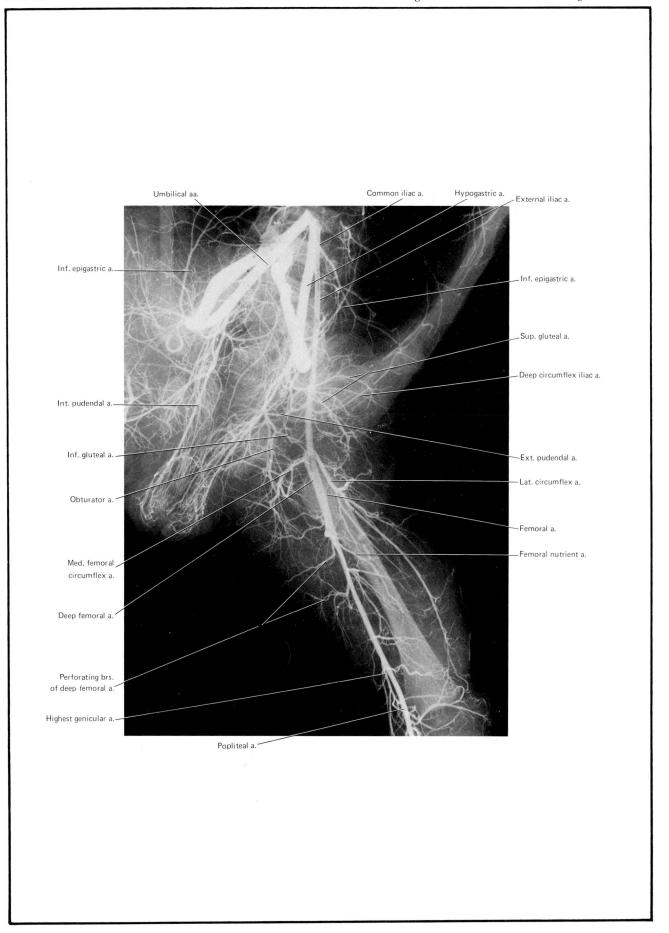

Umbilical aa.

Common iliac a.

Hypogastric a.

External iliac a.

Inf. epigastric a.

Inf. epigastric a.

Sup. gluteal a.

Deep circumflex iliac a.

Int. pudendal a.

Inf. gluteal a.

Ext. pudendal a.

Obturator a.

Lat. circumflex a.

Femoral a.

Femoral nutrient a.

Med. femoral
circumflex a.

Deep femoral a.

Perforating brs.
of deep femoral a.

Highest genicular a.

Popliteal a.

DISSECTION OF THE FEMORAL TRIANGLE

When the vessels and nerves that pass under the *inguinal ligament* first enter the lower extremity, they occupy an interval between the anterior and medial muscles of the thigh known as the femoral triangle. The inguinal ligament serves as the base of the triangle, and the lateral and medial sides are formed by the *sartorius* and *adductor longus* muscles, respectively. The *iliopsoas* and *pectineus* muscles provide the floor. Before dissection the space is covered by the fascia lata that is perforated near the base of the triangle to admit the great saphenous vein. In addition to the vessels and nerves, the space contains fat and the inguinal lymph nodes.

In the illustration the *femoral nerve* is seen as the most lateral large structure descending anterior to the iliopsoas. The Neoprene-injected *femoral artery* is shown giving rise to the *lateral* and *medial circumflex* and *deep femoral arteries*. As the *inferior epigastric artery* arises from the most distal part of the *external iliac artery*, its origin beneath the inguinal ligament locates the point of transition between the iliac and femoral arteries.

Crossed by the medial femoral circumflex artery, the thin walled *femoral vein* ascends the thigh alongside the femoral artery and receives the great saphenous vein at a point approximating the origins of the circumflex arteries. It becomes the external iliac vein upon passing beneath the ligament.

Plate 36　　　　　　　　　　　　　　　　　　　　　　Dissection of Femoral Triangle　　79

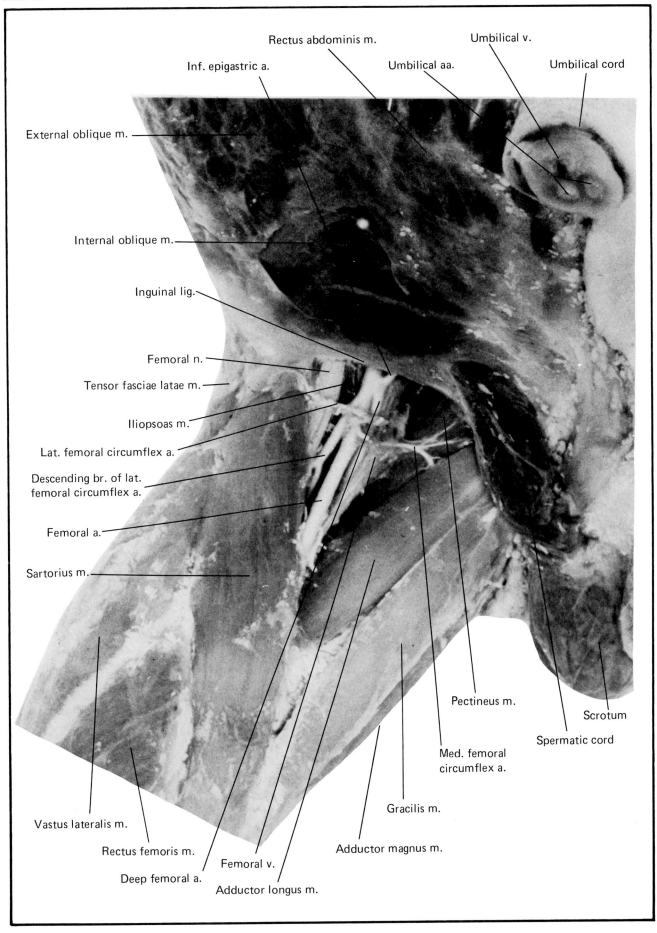

Rectus abdominis m.

Inf. epigastric a.

Umbilical v.

Umbilical aa.

Umbilical cord

External oblique m.

Internal oblique m.

Inguinal lig.

Femoral n.

Tensor fasciae latae m.

Iliopsoas m.

Lat. femoral circumflex a.

Descending br. of lat. femoral circumflex a.

Femoral a.

Sartorius m.

Pectineus m.

Scrotum

Spermatic cord

Med. femoral circumflex a.

Gracilis m.

Vastus lateralis m.

Rectus femoris m.

Adductor magnus m.

Femoral v.

Deep femoral a.

Adductor longus m.

DISSECTION OF THE ANTEROMEDIAL ASPECT OF THE THIGH

In this view the *sartorius* and *gracilis* muscles have been divided in the midthigh region and reflected to expose the adductors and reveal the contents of the femoral canal. The insertions of both of these muscles are combined with that of the *semitendinosus* to attach to the anteromedial surface of the proximal tibia. All of them serve to medially rotate the flexed leg, but flexion and adduction of the thigh are additional individual actions of the sartorius and gracilis, respectively.

The adductor muscles occupy the medial compartment of the thigh. The smallest member of this group, the *pectineus*, may be seen in the floor of the femoral triangle as it extends from the superior ramus of the pubis to insert on the femur below the lesser trochanter. Just medial to the pectineus, the *adductor longus* arises on the pubic symphysis and extends down the thigh to insert on the upper half of the linea aspera, a ridge that runs down the posterior surface of the femur.

Posterior to the longus the *adductor brevis* also arises from the symphysis and inserts with the longus on the linea aspera.

The *adductor magnus* has an extensive origin from the inferior rami of the pubis and ischium, and its attachment to the femur runs almost the whole length of the linea aspera just lateral to that of the other adductors.

Its most medial fibers extend to the medial epicondyle of the femur where they insert as a tendon.

All of the adductors are innervated by the obturator nerve, and they adduct, flex and medially rotate the thigh. Exceptions are that the femoral nerve may innervate part of the pectineus and the longest fibers of the magnus that extend and laterally rotate the femur are innervated by the sciatic nerve.

The *obturator nerve* divides into anterior and posterior branches that are separated by the adductor brevis. Here a branch of the anterior division may be seen entering the upper reflected part of the gracilis.

When the vascular structures enter the leg, a sleeve of connective tissue is derived from the inguinal ligament which wraps the femoral veins and artery in a common investment called the femoral sheath. At the apex of the femoral triangle the femoral sheath passes deep to the sartorius and continues down the thigh in a subsartorial tunnel called the adductor canal. This terminates when the vessels pierce the adductor magnus and enter the popliteal fossa.

In this illustration the femoral veins have been dissected away, and the course of the artery and its concurrent branch of the nerve have been exposed by the reflection of the sartorius.

The *femoral nerve* travels a short distance with the artery before it divides into muscular branches to the quadriceps and the sartorius. However, the *saphenous nerve*, a large sensory branch of cutaneous distribution to the anteromedial crural region, accompanies the *femoral artery* throughout the canal but does not pierce the magnus. It is seen here passing deep to the distal sartorius to gain access to the leg.

Plate 37   Anteromedial Aspect of Thigh   81

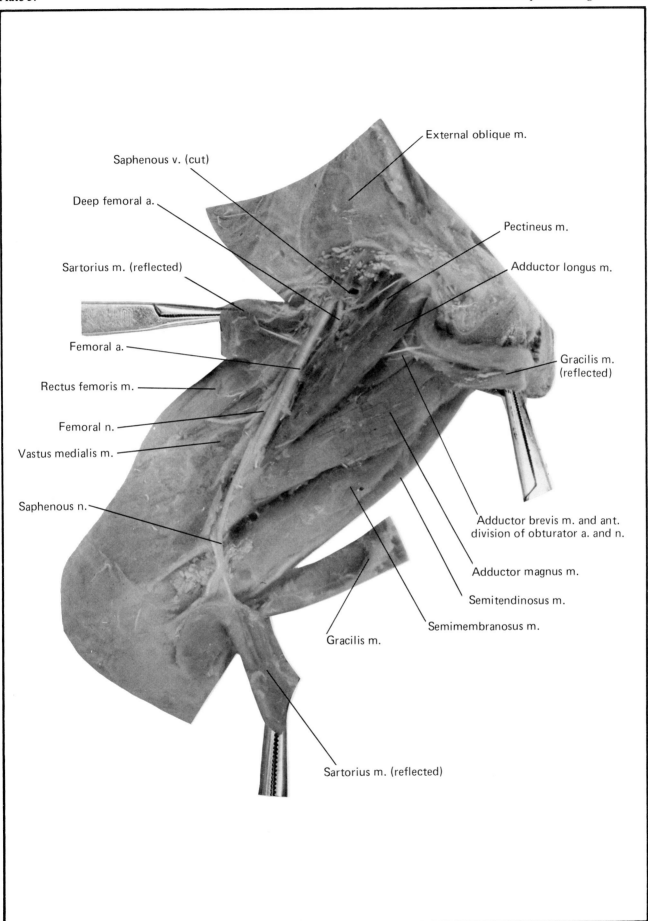

Saphenous v. (cut)

Deep femoral a.

Sartorius m. (reflected)

Femoral a.

Rectus femoris m.

Femoral n.

Vastus medialis m.

Saphenous n.

External oblique m.

Pectineus m.

Adductor longus m.

Gracilis m. (reflected)

Adductor brevis m. and ant. division of obturator a. and n.

Adductor magnus m.

Semitendinosus m.

Semimembranosus m.

Gracilis m.

Sartorius m. (reflected)

CROSS SECTION THROUGH THE MIDDLE OF THE THIGH

In this section of the midregion of the right thigh it is apparent that the shaft of the *femur* is almost entirely enveloped by the quadriceps. Only at the pronounced posterior ridge, the *linea aspera*, do the intermuscular septa and the other muscles have attachment to the bone. Within the individual muscles comprising the quadriceps group, one or two sizable motor branches of the femoral nerve accompanied by an artery may be noted.

The relations of the adductor canal to the *vastus medialis*, adductors and the overlying *sartorius* are easily appreciated in this view. The *femoral vein* is subdivided into several channels (venae comitantes) that weave around the *femoral artery* within the femoral sheath.

At the level of this section the large nerve seen running posterior to the artery is the *saphenous branch* of the *femoral nerve*.

The *deep femoral artery*, which arises in the femoral triangle, can be noted here running close to the femur in the medial *intermuscular septum*.

Of the *adductor* muscles, only the *longus* and *magnus* reach this level and are inserted on the linea aspera medial to the origin of the *short head* of the *biceps*.

The long hamstrings are clearly defined as they embrace the *sciatic nerve* in its descent down the posterior thigh.

Plate 38   Cross Section through Middle of Thigh   83

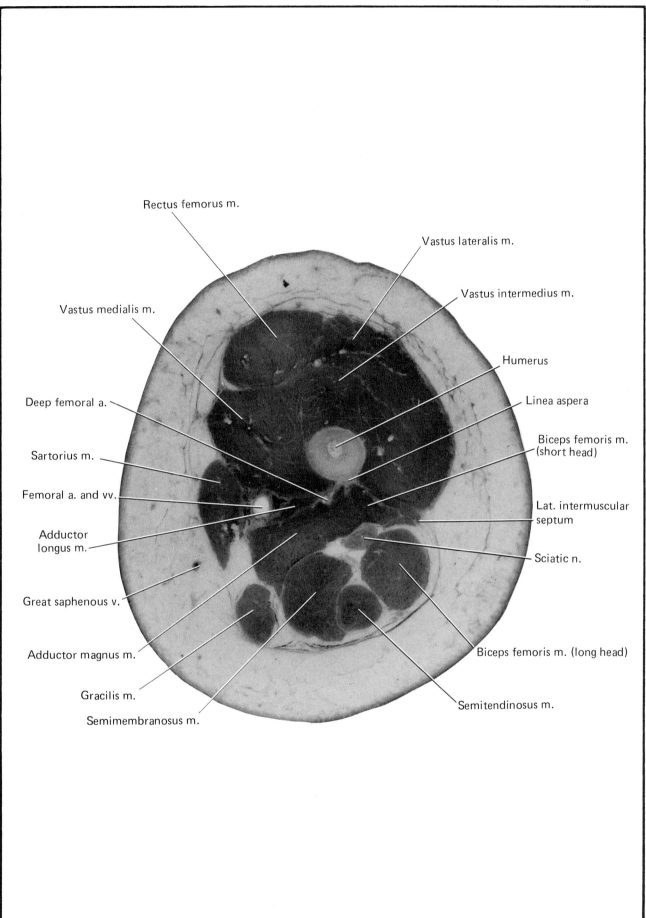

Rectus femorus m.

Vastus lateralis m.

Vastus intermedius m.

Vastus medialis m.

Humerus

Deep femoral a.

Linea aspera

Sartorius m.

Biceps femoris m.
(short head)

Femoral a. and vv.

Lat. intermuscular
septum

Adductor
longus m.

Sciatic n.

Great saphenous v.

Adductor magnus m.

Biceps femoris m. (long head)

Gracilis m.

Semitendinosus m.

Semimembranosus m.

SAGITTAL SECTION OF THE KNEE

In this illustration the mutually articulating ends of the *femur* and *tibia* have been divided precisely in half so that the plane of section passes through the *intercondyloid fossa* of the femur and the cartilaginous precursor of the intercondylar eminence of the tibia. Thus both the *anterior* and *posterior cruciate ligaments* have been exposed. Both of these thick bands of collagenous fibers arise between the tibial condyles and cross with the posterior ligament medial to the anterior to attach to the inner aspects of the femoral condyles. They restrict any forward or backward overriding of the femur when the joint is activated.

Well depicted is the blending of the deep and superficial components of the femoral extensors to form the *quadriceps tendon* that, acting through the *patella* and the *patellar tendon*, extends the leg.

In the popliteal fossa the median course of both the *popliteal artery* and the *tibial nerve* is shown.

In the upper posterior crural compartment the disposition of the *popliteus* and the small belly of the *plantaris* muscle is revealed. The first is analogous to the supinator of the forearm while the second sends a long thin tendon to the calcaneus and resembles the palmaris longus.

Plate 39   Sagittal Section of Knee   85

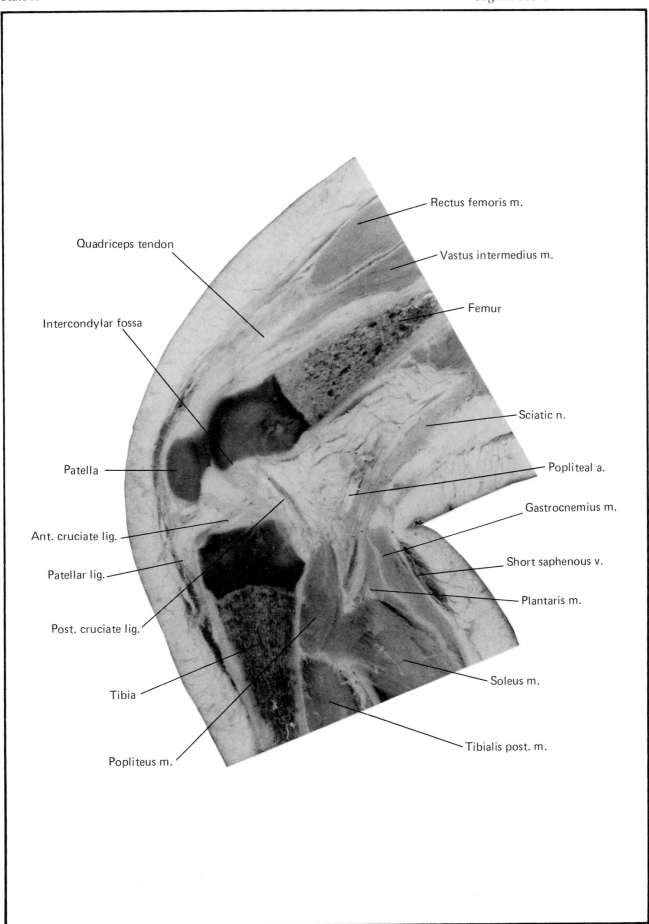

Quadriceps tendon

Intercondylar fossa

Patella

Ant. cruciate lig.

Patellar lig.

Post. cruciate lig.

Tibia

Popliteus m.

Rectus femoris m.

Vastus intermedius m.

Femur

Sciatic n.

Popliteal a.

Gastrocnemius m.

Short saphenous v.

Plantaris m.

Soleus m.

Tibialis post. m.

ARTERIOGRAM OF THE KNEE REGION

The periarticular tissues of the knee, like those of most large joints, are well supplied by a number of articular vessels that have many collateral connections with other proximal and distal arteries in the limb. In this arteriogram of the anteromedial view of the fetal knee, the terminal course of the *deep femoral artery* may be discerned by the cumulative density despite the superimposition of the *femoral artery*.

Shortly below the level of the last perforating branch of the deep femoral artery, the femoral artery passes through the adductor magnus and enters the popliteal fossa as the *popliteal artery*. Here it gives off the *highest genicular* branch that is the common origin of the *superior* and *inferior lateral genicular arteries*. The *medial superior* and *inferior geniculate arteries* arise directly from the *popliteal artery* before it divides into the tibial branches.

The *descending branch* of the *lateral femoral circumflex artery* provides numerous anastomoses with both of the superior geniculate arteries just above the patella. This collateral network also receives contributions from the upper muscular branches of the popliteal artery.

A *middle genicular artery* sends branches into the intercondyloid fossa and assists in the supply of the cruciate ligaments.

The proximal sections of both the *anterior* and *posterior tibial arteries* can be seen giving a number of recurrent branches to the knee, but the most prominent of these is the *anterior tibial recurrent artery* that turns upward just after the anterior tibial artery pierces the interosseous membrane to enter the anterior crural compartment.

Plate 40 Arteriogram of Knee Region 87

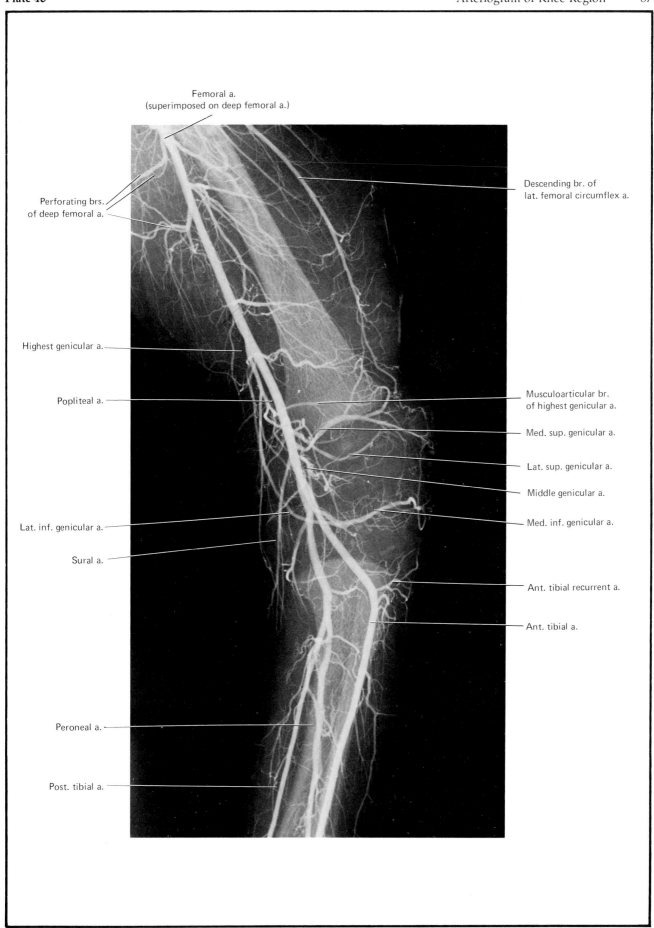

Femoral a.
(superimposed on deep femoral a.)

Perforating brs.
of deep femoral a.

Highest genicular a.

Popliteal a.

Lat. inf. genicular a.

Sural a.

Peroneal a.

Post. tibial a.

Descending br. of
lat. femoral circumflex a.

Musculoarticular br.
of highest genicular a.

Med. sup. genicular a.

Lat. sup. genicular a.

Middle genicular a.

Med. inf. genicular a.

Ant. tibial recurrent a.

Ant. tibial a.

DISSECTION OF THE POPLITEAL AND POSTERIOR CRURAL REGIONS

Removal of the gastrocnemius and the sectioning of the tibial origin of the soleus to permit its lateral retraction has exposed the deeper structures of the popliteal and posterior crural regions.

Behind the knee the *popliteal artery* runs deep to the tibial nerve as it sends off muscular and geniculate branches. Both structures descend between the sectioned heads of the *gastrocnemius*, which marks the origins of this muscle above each femoral condyle, and pass superficial to the *popliteus*.

A flat triangular muscle, the popliteus, has a tendinous origin just below the lateral epicondyle of the femur. Inserting as a broad expansion on the upper posterior surface of the tibia, it flexes and medially rotates the leg.

The *flexor digitorum longus* can be seen as the most medial of the deep crural flexors, and the *tibialis posterior* lies deep to the *posterior tibial nerve* and *artery*, as seen in the upper part of the leg in this illustration. However, as these muscles descend the leg their tendons reverse position and that of the tibialis becomes anterior to the flexor digitorum and passes immediately posterior to the *medial malleolus* to attach to the plantar surfaces of the navicular and first cuneiform. The flexor digitorum longus enters the foot behind the medial malleolus between the tibialis posterior tendon and the posterior tibial artery and nerve and eventually inserts on the terminal phalanges of the four lateral digits. The flexor digitorum flexes the foot and digits and produces a slight inversion, whereas the tibialis flexes and strongly inverts the foot.

The *flexor hallucis longus* is the conspicuous muscle arising on the posterior aspect of the fibula and descending behind the medial malleolus deep to the posterior tibial artery and nerve. Its tendon, too deep to be visible here, travels under the sustenaculum tali, a grooved projection of the calcaneus, and crosses the medial plantar surface of the foot to insert on the terminal phalanx of the great toe.

Posterior to the tibial condyles, the anterior tibial artery branches from the popliteal, and passing between the tibia and fibula it penetrates the interosseus membrane to enter the anterior crural compartment. At the level of the popliteus the popliteal artery becomes the posterior tibial. Deep to the tibial origin of the *soleus*, the tibial artery laterally gives rise to the peroneal artery that runs very close to the posterior surface of the fibula under the flexor hallucis longus. This artery supplies the lateral compartment of the leg and ends in a perforating branch to the dorsum of the foot and anastomotic connections around the lateral malleolus.

The posterior tibial artery and nerve are well shown in this figure as they course in the fascial plane that separates the soleus from the underlying tibialis posterior. Accompanying the Neoprene-injected artery, a channel of the posterior tibial venous plexus may be noted. Both the artery and the nerve enter the foot between the tendons of the flexors digitorum longus and hallucis longus, where they form medial and lateral plantar branches.

All of the posterior crural and the plantar muscles receive their motor innervation from the posterior tibial nerve.

Splitting from the sciatic nerve in the thigh, the *common peroneal nerve* obliquely crosses the popliteal fossa along the medial border of the *biceps femoris*. It descends lateral to the neck of the fibula (where it is prone to injury) and enters the peroneus longus. Here the nerve divides into the superficial and deep peroneal nerves. The first provides motor branches to the peroneal muscles and sensory fibers to the foot while the second is the motor nerve of the anterior crural and dorsal foot muscles.

Plate 41   Popliteal and Posterior Crural Regions   89

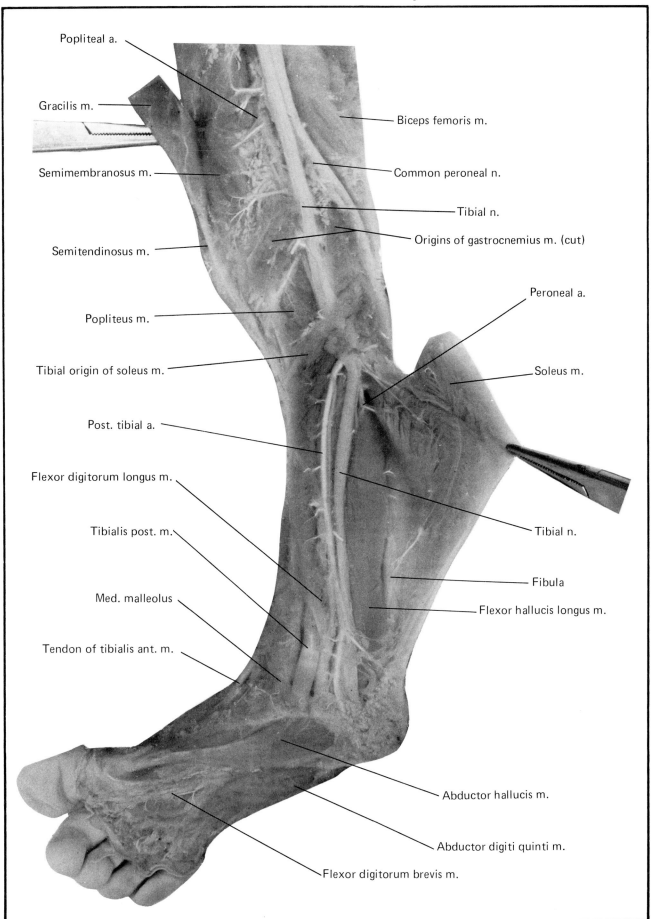

Popliteal a.

Gracilis m.

Semimembranosus m.

Semitendinosus m.

Popliteus m.

Tibial origin of soleus m.

Post. tibial a.

Flexor digitorum longus m.

Tibialis post. m.

Med. malleolus

Tendon of tibialis ant. m.

Biceps femoris m.

Common peroneal n.

Tibial n.

Origins of gastrocnemius m. (cut)

Peroneal a.

Soleus m.

Tibial n.

Fibula

Flexor hallucis longus m.

Abductor hallucis m.

Abductor digiti quinti m.

Flexor digitorum brevis m.

DISSECTION OF THE ANTERIOR AND LATERAL CRURAL COMPARTMENTS

The fascial septum separating the *tibialis anterior* and the *extensor digitorum longus* muscles has been split to expose the deep structures of the extensor compartment.

The tibialis muscle, which here has been reflected medially, arises on the anterolateral surface of the tibia and the fascial plane it shares in common with the extensor digitorum longus. The thick tibialis tendon passes to the medial side of the foot to insert on the plantar surfaces of the first cuneiform and the base of the first metatarsal where it produces extension (dorsiflexion) and strong inversion of the foot.

The *extensor hallucis longus* arises from the anterior surface of the fibula medial to the extensor digitorum and from the interosseous membrane. It is not visible without the reflection of the tibialis anterior, and its tendon is not readily discerned until it surfaces on the dorsum of the first metatarsal. The extensor hallucis extends the foot and the great toe, on which it eventually inserts as a typical digital extensor assembly.

The extensor digitorum longus arises from the upper anterior surface of the fibula and descends to the dorsum of the foot where it divides into four tendons, one for each of the four lesser toes. These extend the toes through the extensor assemblies on the back of each digit, and the more lateral tendons may also evert the foot.

Lateral to the extensor digitorum an inconstant muscle, the *peroneus tertius*, arises from the lower anterior surface of the fibula and inserts on the fifth metatarsal to assist in extension and eversion of the foot.

The *extensor digitorum brevis* is an intrinsic muscle of the foot. Arising on the lateral surface of the calcaneus below the malleolus, it divides into five fleshy extensors whose short tendons join the extensor assemblies to enhance the digital action of the long extensors. The distinct medial slip of this muscle may be called the *extensor hallucis brevis*.

The lateral crural compartment is separated from the flexor and extensor regions, respectively, by the posterior and anterior peroneal septa, and contains the peroneal muscles. The *peroneus longus* originates on the upper lateral surface of the fibula and becomes superficial and posterior to the brevis in the lower leg. Its tendon lies medial to that of the brevis as it passes posterior to the lateral malleolus. Just behind the tuberosity of the fifth metatarsal it is directed obliquely across the deep plantar region to insert on the heads of the medial metatarsals and the third cuneiform.

The *peroneus brevis* arises from the lower two thirds of the fibula, from where it sends its tendon around the lateral malleolus to insert on the prominent tuberosity of the fifth metatarsal. Both peroneal muscles flex and evert the foot, with the peroneus brevis being a very important counteraction to the inversion produced by most other crural muscles. In addition, the tendon of the longus helps to support the transverse metatarsal arch.

The muscles of the anterior and lateral compartments receive motor innervation from the deep and superficial branches of the common peroneal nerve. The deep branch courses between the *anterior tibial artery* and the extensor hallucis longus and enters the foot behind the hallucis tendon. It sends a motor branch to the extensor brevis and terminates as sensory branches to the medial toes.

After the *superficial peroneal nerve* innervates the peroneal muscles, it leaves the anterior peroneal septum to provide cutaneous innervation to the dorsum of the foot, as can be seen here.

Two straps of the crural fascia form retinaculae which bind the extensor tendons to the ankle and prevent their bowstringing under tension. The first, the *transverse crural ligament*, encircles the ankle above the malleoli. The second leaves the lateral malleolus and extends medially by splitting into a Y-shaped band around the medial malleolus. This *cruciate crural ligament* is the more distinct member of the pair in this illustration.

Plate 42   Anterior and Lateral Crural Compartments   91

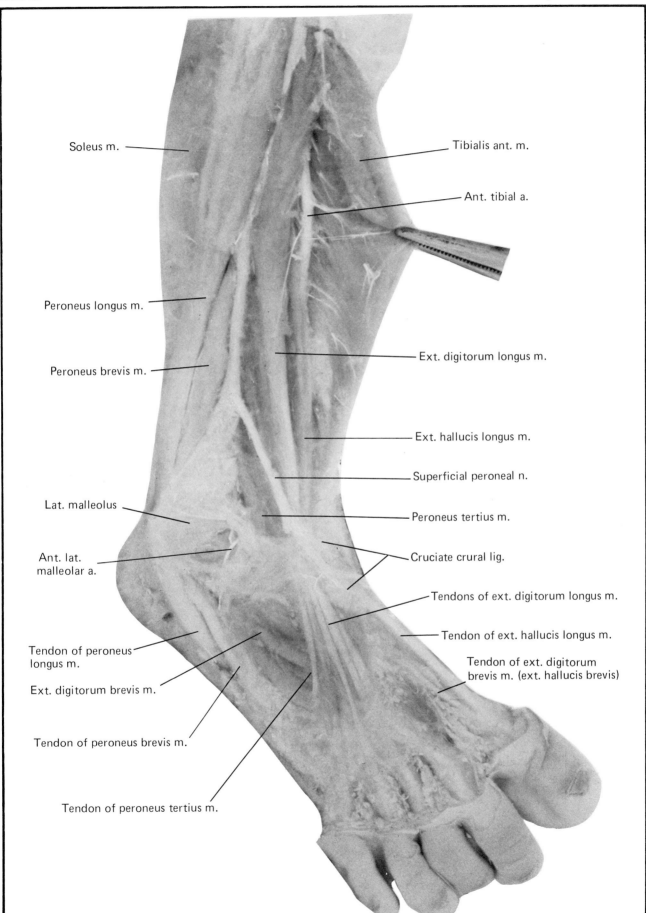

Soleus m.

Tibialis ant. m.

Ant. tibial a.

Peroneus longus m.

Ext. digitorum longus m.

Peroneus brevis m.

Ext. hallucis longus m.

Superficial peroneal n.

Lat. malleolus

Peroneus tertius m.

Ant. lat.
malleolar a.

Cruciate crural lig.

Tendons of ext. digitorum longus m.

Tendon of ext. hallucis longus m.

Tendon of peroneus
longus m.

Tendon of ext. digitorum
brevis m. (ext. hallucis brevis)

Ext. digitorum brevis m.

Tendon of peroneus brevis m.

Tendon of peroneus tertius m.

SUPERFICIAL DISSECTION OF THE PLANTAR REGION

In this view the sole of the foot and most of the plantar aponeurosis have been removed to reveal the superficial plantar muscles.

The *abductor hallucis* arises on the medial tuberosity of the *calcaneus* and associated ligaments and extends along the medial border of the foot. Near its origin it covers the tendons, vessels and nerves that enter the foot behind the medial malleolus, and its insertion combines with the medial head of the flexor hallucis brevis to attach to the medial base of the proximal phalanx of the great toe.

The *flexor digitorum brevis* occupies the center of the plantar region, arising by a tendon from the tuberosity of the calcaneus and from the plantar aponeurosis, which sends penetrating septa between the brevis and adjacent muscles. It inserts by four tendons into the lesser digits. These short, thin tendons split to form tunnels for the deep flexor tendons and then reunite and redivide to attach to the sides of the middle phalanx.

The *abductor digiti quinti* is the most lateral superficial muscle of the foot, arising from the lateral and inferior aspects of the calcaneus and from the lateral septum of the plantar aponeurosis. It inserts with the underlying tendon of the flexor digiti quinti brevis onto the lateral base of the phalanx, which it abducts.

Plate 43   Superficial Dissection of Plantar Region   93

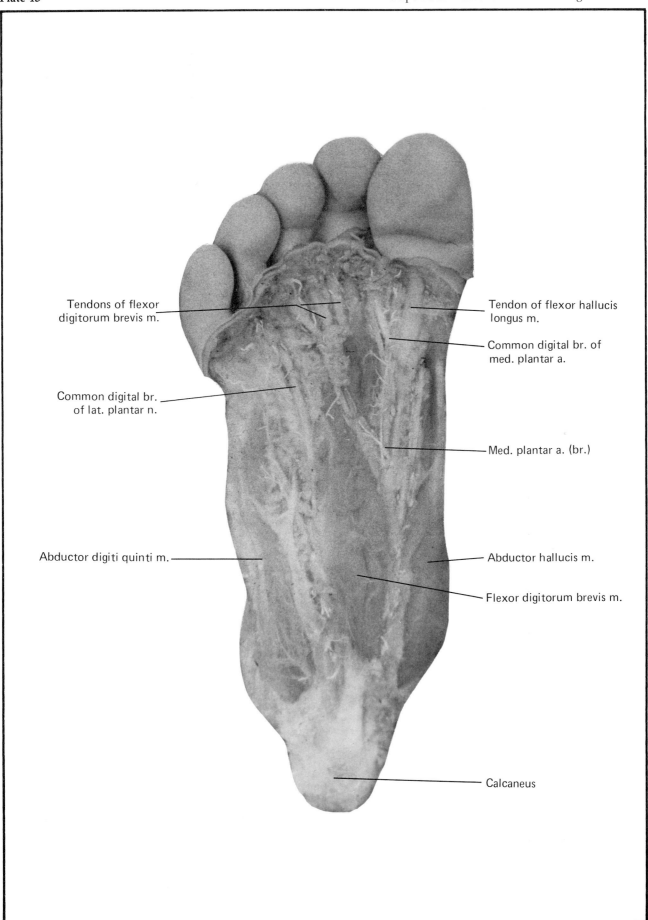

Tendons of flexor
digitorum brevis m.

Tendon of flexor hallucis
longus m.

Common digital br. of
med. plantar a.

Common digital br.
of lat. plantar n.

Med. plantar a. (br.)

Abductor digiti quinti m.

Abductor hallucis m.

Flexor digitorum brevis m.

Calcaneus

DEEP DISSECTION OF THE PLANTAR REGION

The flexor digitorum brevis and the tendons of the *flexor digitorum longus* have been severed and reflected forward to expose the underlying structures. Examination of the reflected tendons reveals a *lumbrical muscle* arising and coursing on the medial side of each tendon toward its proper digit, where it passes to the medial side of the base of the phalanx and inserts on the extensor assembly. The actions, mode of insertion and mutual relationships of the plantar digital flexors and their lumbricals are very similar to those in the hand.

Further dissection of the medial border of the foot has exposed the *flexor hallucis brevis*, a short bifid muscle that originates on the ligamentous coverings of the cuboid and inserts by medial and lateral heads into the sides of the base of the proximal phalanx of the great toe. Each tendon incorporates one of the two sesamoids associated with the first metatarsophalangeal joint, and their combined action flexes the toe.

The groove formed between the sesamoids transmits the tendon of the *flexor hallucis longus* that can be seen entering the foot lateral to the plantar nerve. This tendon passes beneath the *medial plantar nerve* to insert on the terminal phalanx of the great toe. It is very important in flexing the medial side of the foot while striding and in supporting the medial longitudinal arch.

In the middle area, corresponding to the adductor-interosseous compartment of the hand, the transverse and oblique heads of the *adductor hallucis* muscle are well displayed. The oblique head arises from the bases of the middle metatarsals and from the sheath of the *peroneus longus* tendon, and the transverse head originates from the plantar ligaments of the metatarsophalangeal joints. The combined insertion joins the tendon of the lateral head of the flexor hallucis brevis to adduct the great toe.

Laterally, the *flexor digiti quinti brevis* has been exposed. It arises from the plantar base of the fifth metatarsal and the sheath of the peroneus longus to insert on the lateral base of the proximal phalanx of the little toe.

Because of the necessary reflection of the long flexor tendons, a short accessory flexor muscle, the *quadratus plantae*, was sacrificed. This muscle arose from the medial tuberosity of the calcaneus deep to the origin of the flexor digitorum brevis and inserted onto the lateral side of the flexor digitorum longus tendon as it entered the plantar region. It assists in digital flexion.

The innervation of the plantar muscles is by the *medial* and *lateral plantar nerves*. The distribution of these divisions of the posterior tibial nerve is nearly identical to that of the median and ulnar nerves in the hand. The flexor digitorum brevis, abductor hallucis and flexor hallucis brevis (medial half) are innervated by the medial plantar nerve, the abductor and flexor digiti quinti with the adductor hallucis and all interossei by the lateral plantar nerve. Again as in the hand, the lumbricals are inconsistently divided between the two.

The lateral plantar nerve and artery and the long plantar ligament have been divided to expose the tendon of the peroneus longus.

Plate 44   Deep Dissection of Plantar Region   95

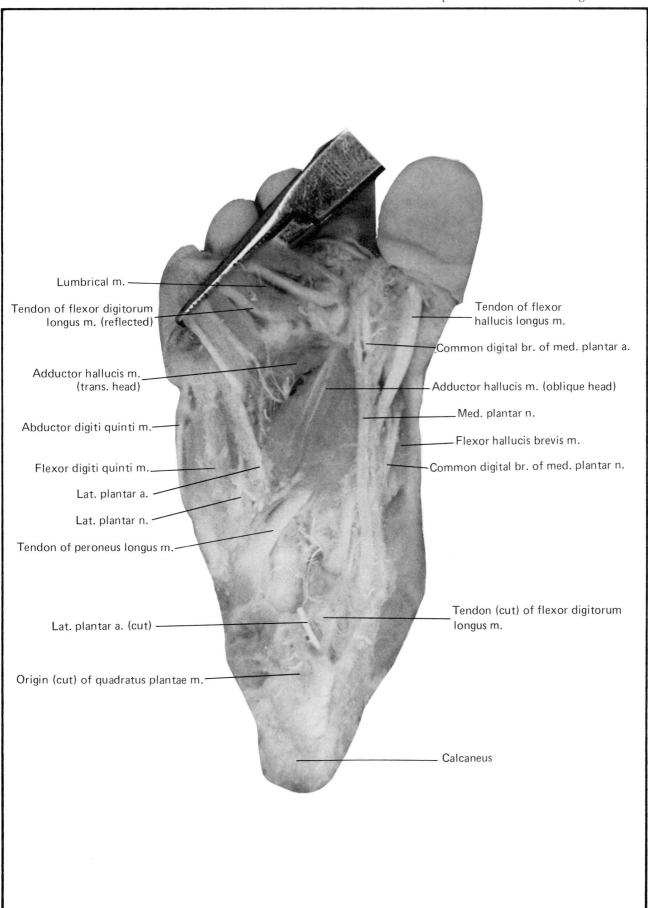

Lumbrical m.

Tendon of flexor digitorum
longus m. (reflected)

Adductor hallucis m.
(trans. head)

Abductor digiti quinti m.

Flexor digiti quinti m.

Lat. plantar a.

Lat. plantar n.

Tendon of peroneus longus m.

Lat. plantar a. (cut)

Origin (cut) of quadratus plantae m.

Tendon of flexor
hallucis longus m.

Common digital br. of med. plantar a.

Adductor hallucis m. (oblique head)

Med. plantar n.

Flexor hallucis brevis m.

Common digital br. of med. plantar n.

Tendon (cut) of flexor digitorum
longus m.

Calcaneus

ARTERIOGRAM OF THE LEFT ANKLE AND FOOT

This plate shows a slightly medial oblique view of the arterial distribution in the ankle and foot. The *anterior tibial artery* here is the largest vessel in the lower crural region. It descends along the lateral surface of the tibia deep to the tibialis anterior. An artifactitious constriction just above the ankle marks where it is obliquely crossed by the tendon of the extensor hallucis longus. At the distal end of the tibia it enters the foot as the *dorsalis pedis artery* and runs between the tendons of the extensor digitorum longus and extensor hallucis longus to terminate as the *dorsal arcuate artery*. A *lateral tarsal branch*, derived below the ankle, supplies collaterals to the malleolar region and sends a branch distally to complete the arch of the arcuate artery.

Resembling the palmar arterial arches, the arcuate arteries of the foot give origin to the common digital arteries. The dorsal arcuate is the larger, and like the deep palmar arch it receives its greatest contribution on its preaxial side. The reciprocal version of this arrangement (as in the superficial palmar arch) is noted in the plantar arcuate artery where the postaxial contribution (lateral plantar artery) is larger.

The *peroneal artery* is seen here traveling in the lateral flexor compartment near the fibula. Just above the ankle, at a point marked by an abrupt change in the direction of the artery, it penetrates the interosseous membrane and becomes the perforating branch that supplies collaterals to the dorsum of the foot and the lateral malleolar regions.

The *posterior tibial artery* descends along the surface of the tibialis posterior muscle and enters the plantar region between the long digital flexor tendons behind the medial malleolus. It divides into a small *medial plantar artery* and a much larger *lateral plantar artery*. The proximal sections of these vessels course in the same plane as the plantar tendons of the long flexors, but distally they penetrate more deeply to form the arcuate vessel (which is incomplete in this specimen) and its digital branches that lie adjacent to the interosseous muscles.

A network of numerous anastomotic branches derived from all three of the major vessels supplies the periarticular tissue of the ankle and the carpal bones.

Plate 45   Arteriogram of Left Ankle and Foot   97

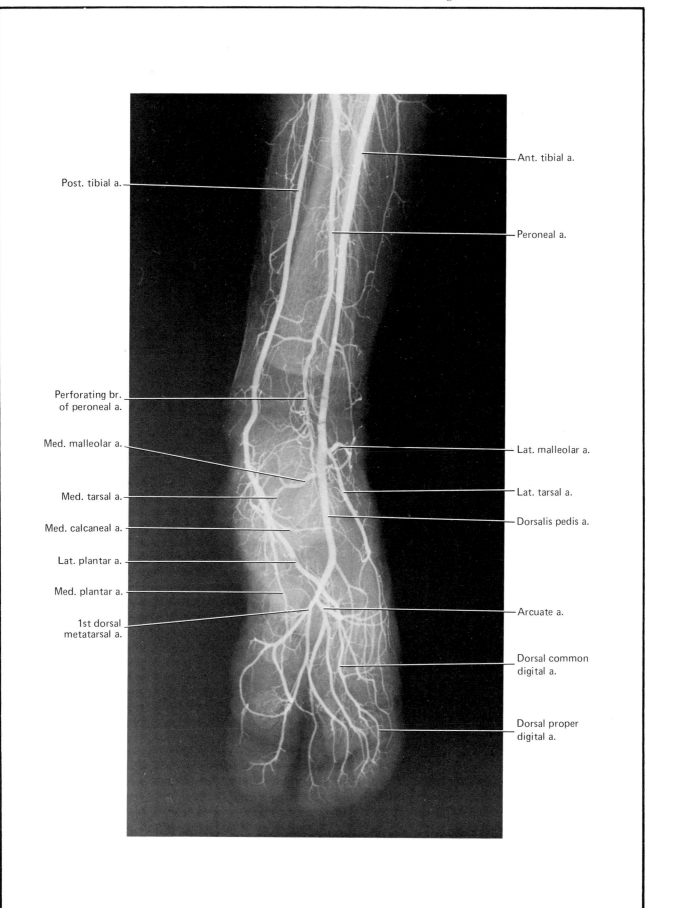

Post. tibial a.

Perforating br.
of peroneal a.

Med. malleolar a.

Med. tarsal a.

Med. calcaneal a.

Lat. plantar a.

Med. plantar a.

1st dorsal
metatarsal a.

Ant. tibial a.

Peroneal a.

Lat. malleolar a.

Lat. tarsal a.

Dorsalis pedis a.

Arcuate a.

Dorsal common
digital a.

Dorsal proper
digital a.

CROSS SECTION THROUGH THE MIDDLE OF THE RIGHT LEG

This section clearly shows that the anteromedial surface of the *tibia* is without muscular covering and therefore is subcutaneous. At this level, however, the *fibula* is entirely sheathed in muscle, yet it is still attached to the lateral border of the tibia by the *interosseous membrane*. Connecting the lateral surface of the fibula with the crural fascia, the marked *posterior peroneal (crural) septum* and less distinct *anterior peroneal septum* separate the lateral compartment from the anterior extensor and posterior flexor compartments.

In the posterior compartment the combination of the two heads of the *gastrocnemius* with the *soleus* to form the triceps cruri is apparent. In the fascial plane between these muscles and the deep flexors, the relative positions of the *posterior tibial nerve* and *artery* and the *peroneal artery* are illustrated.

The *anterior tibial artery* and *deep peroneal nerve* are quite conspicuous deep to the *tibialis anterior* and the long extensors, and a small artery in the peroneal compartment marks the position of the *superficial peroneal nerve.*

Note the superficial veins in the subcutaneous fat.

Plate 46   Cross Section through Middle of Leg   99

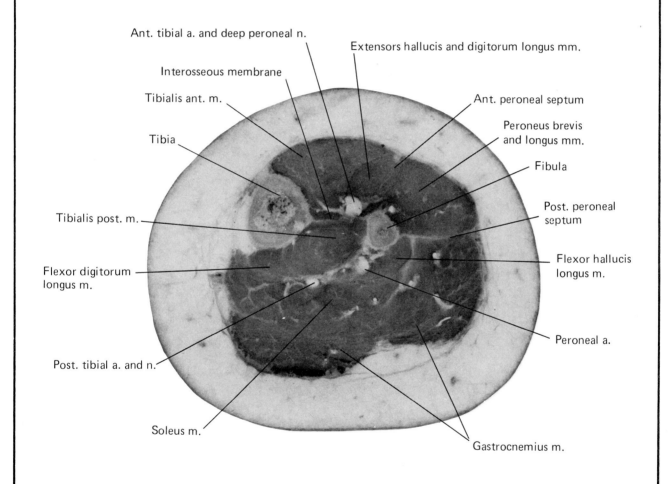

Ant. tibial a. and deep peroneal n.

Interosseous membrane

Tibialis ant. m.

Tibia

Tibialis post. m.

Flexor digitorum longus m.

Post. tibial a. and n.

Soleus m.

Extensors hallucis and digitorum longus mm.

Ant. peroneal septum

Peroneus brevis and longus mm.

Fibula

Post. peroneal septum

Flexor hallucis longus m.

Peroneal a.

Gastrocnemius m.

CROSS SECTION THROUGH THE RIGHT ANKLE JOINT

Sectioned at the level of the malleoli, this specimen provides visualization of the spatial relations of the flexor, extensor and peroneal tendons just before they enter the foot.

On the anterior aspect of the ankle, the superficial tendons of the *tibialis anterior* and the commencement of the four divisions of the *extensor digitorum longus* can be seen. The deeper *flexor hallucis longus* tendon is shown in close relation to the *anterior tibial* (dorsalis pedis) *artery*. The *cruciate crural ligament* that binds these tendons to the ankle is well shown in this view.

The arrangement of the tendons of the posterior flexor and lateral peroneal muscles and their respective relationships to the medial and lateral malleoli are clearly defined. Note the position of the *posterior tibial artery* and *nerve* with reference to the long flexor tendons.

Plate 47   Cross Section through Ankle Joint   101

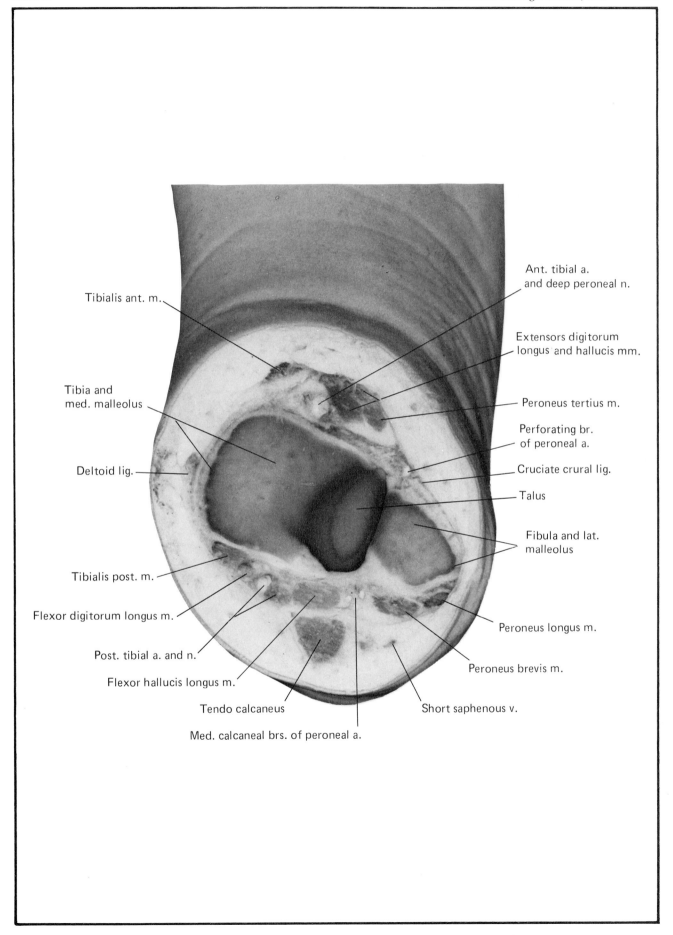

Tibialis ant. m.

Tibia and
med. malleolus

Deltoid lig.

Tibialis post. m.

Flexor digitorum longus m.

Post. tibial a. and n.

Flexor hallucis longus m.

Tendo calcaneus

Med. calcaneal brs. of peroneal a.

Ant. tibial a.
and deep peroneal n.

Extensors digitorum
longus and hallucis mm.

Peroneus tertius m.

Perforating br.
of peroneal a.

Cruciate crural lig.

Talus

Fibula and lat.
malleolus

Peroneus longus m.

Peroneus brevis m.

Short saphenous v.

FRONTAL SECTION THROUGH THE ANKLE JOINT

The articular relationship between the distal tibiofibular unit and the talus is best illustrated in the frontal section. Here it can be observed that the distal ends of the *tibia* and *fibula* are bonded together by the stout tibiofibular ligament, and the inferior ends of both *malleoli* extend beyond a recessed articular surface to bracket the talus on each side. This mortise and tenon configuration permits the trochlea of the *talus* to slide back and forth but greatly restricts lateral motion. Thus, inversion and eversion of the foot must be permitted mostly by the intertarsal joints.

The plantar muscles that have their origins on the lateral, middle and medial tuberosities of the *calcaneus* are well shown here, as is the relationship of the flexor tendons. The position of the *sustenaculum tali*, a projecting shelf of the calcaneus that partly supports the talus, is indicated. This structure is also grooved on its inferior surface to pass the tendon of the *flexor hallucis longus*, which can be seen lying lateral to the *posterior tibial artery* and *nerve*.

Plate 48   Frontal Section through Ankle Joint   103

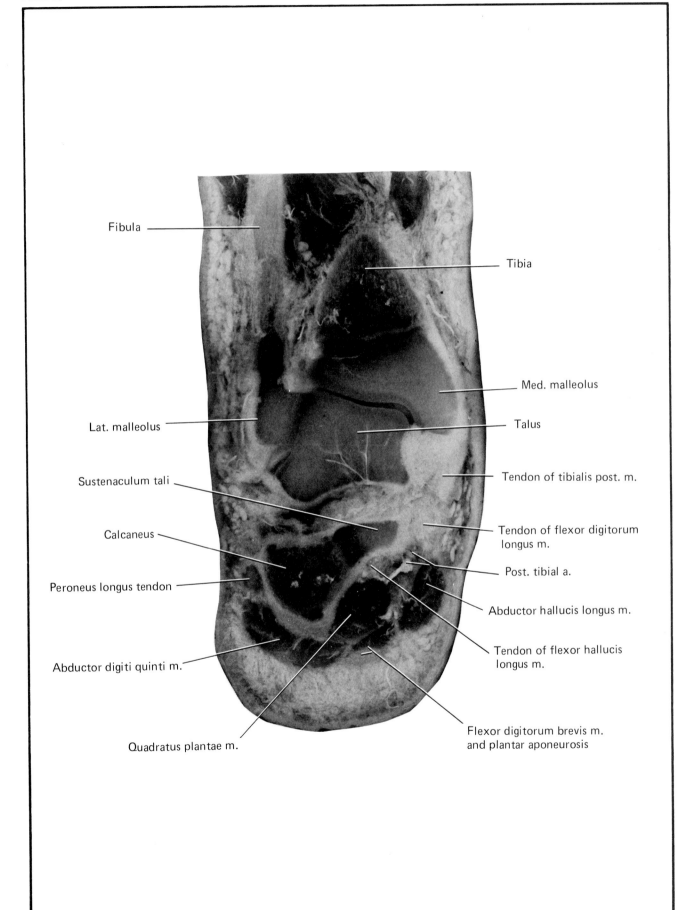

Fibula

Tibia

Med. malleolus

Lat. malleolus

Talus

Tendon of tibialis post. m.

Sustenaculum tali

Tendon of flexor digitorum
longus m.

Calcaneus

Post. tibial a.

Peroneus longus tendon

Abductor hallucis longus m.

Tendon of flexor hallucis
longus m.

Abductor digiti quinti m.

Quadratus plantae m.

Flexor digitorum brevis m.
and plantar aponeurosis

SAGITTAL SECTION THROUGH THE RIGHT FOOT

The specimen here has been sectioned through the sagittal plane of the second digit that constitutes the axis of the foot. Comparing this view with the frontal section, the type and range of motion permitted by the ankle joint is easily comprehended.

Despite the fact that the fetus and young child appear flatfooted, the skeletal structure of the tarsus and metatarsus (collective terms for the tarsal and metatarsal bones) resembles that of the adult in both the total conformation and the relative shape and size of the individual components.

In the tarsal section, the *calcaneus, talus, navicular* and *first cuneiform* may be identified sequentially. Together with the first and *second metatarsals* they form the medial longitudinal arch of the foot.

Dorsal to the first cuneiform and the head of the second metatarsal, a segment of the Neoprene-injected *dorsalis pedis artery* shows the relation of this structure to the underlying skeleton.

In the plantar area the layers of the intrinsic plantar muscles are well displayed, and the role of the long flexor tendons in the support of the medial arch becomes obvious.

Plate 49   Sagittal Section through Foot   105

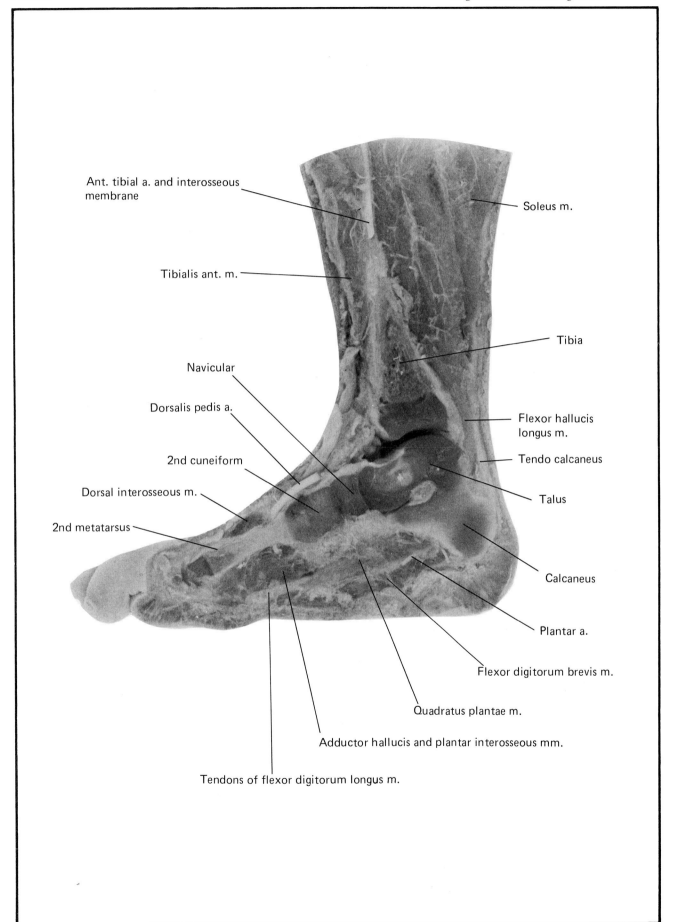

Ant. tibial a. and interosseous membrane

Tibialis ant. m.

Navicular

Dorsalis pedis a.

2nd cuneiform

Dorsal interosseous m.

2nd metatarsus

Soleus m.

Tibia

Flexor hallucis longus m.

Tendo calcaneus

Talus

Calcaneus

Plantar a.

Flexor digitorum brevis m.

Quadratus plantae m.

Adductor hallucis and plantar interosseous mm.

Tendons of flexor digitorum longus m.

HORIZONTAL SECTION THROUGH THE FOOT

The wishbone configuration formed by the *calcaneus* and the shafts of the *first* and *fifth metatarsals* in this section illustrates the medial and lateral arches of the foot.

The low tripod formed by the calcaneus and the distal ends of these metatarsals functions in weight bearing when standing, but striding requires a shift of stresses toward the medial longitudinal arch and great toe.

The form of the transverse metatarsal arch is indicated by the fact that the shafts of the first and last metatarsals lie in the plane of section whereas only the distal ends of the middle metatarsals have been cut. Their proximal ends provide a curved roof for the revealed *adductor-interosseous* muscles.

Plate 50   Horizontal Section through Foot   107

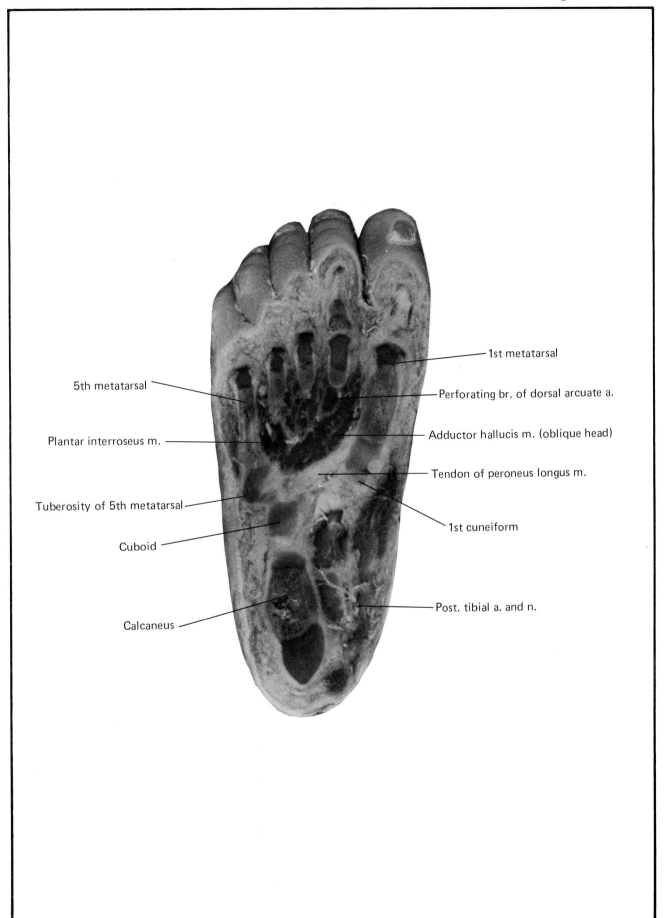

5th metatarsal

Plantar interroseus m.

Tuberosity of 5th metatarsal

Cuboid

Calcaneus

1st metatarsal

Perforating br. of dorsal arcuate a.

Adductor hallucis m. (oblique head)

Tendon of peroneus longus m.

1st cuneiform

Post. tibial a. and n.

CROSS SECTION OF THE FOOT THROUGH THE METATARSAL REGION

This section illustrates how the vault of the transverse metatarsal arch houses intrinsic plantar muscles.

The disposition of the *plantar* and *dorsal interossei* differs from that of the hand because the second toe is the axial digit. In the hand the second finger (third digit) is the axial digit, and the adduction-abduction performed, respectively, by the palmar and dorsal interossei is toward and away from this finger. In the foot the corresponding muscles are arranged to perform the same function with reference to the second digit.

Inferior to the adductor-interosseous group the tendons of the *flexor hallucis longus* and the *flexor digitorum longus* with the corresponding *lumbricals* can be seen. The small tendons of the *flexor digitorum brevis* lie inferolateral to those of their associated long flexors.

The large *deep plantar artery* is usually a perforating branch from the dorsal rather than plantar arcuate artery. It serves as the common digital vessel to the first and second toes.

Plate 51   Cross Section through Metatarsal Region   109

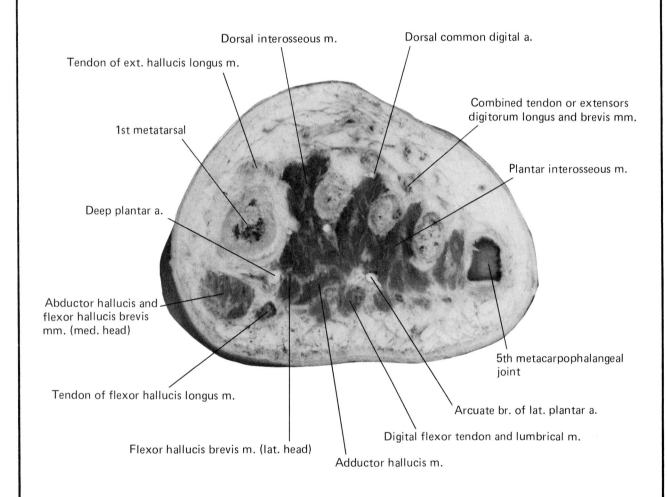

Dorsal interosseous m.

Dorsal common digital a.

Tendon of ext. hallucis longus m.

Combined tendon or extensors
digitorum longus and brevis mm.

1st metatarsal

Plantar interosseous m.

Deep plantar a.

Abductor hallucis and
flexor hallucis brevis
mm. (med. head)

5th metacarpophalangeal
joint

Tendon of flexor hallucis longus m.

Arcuate br. of lat. plantar a.

Digital flexor tendon and lumbrical m.

Flexor hallucis brevis m. (lat. head)

Adductor hallucis m.

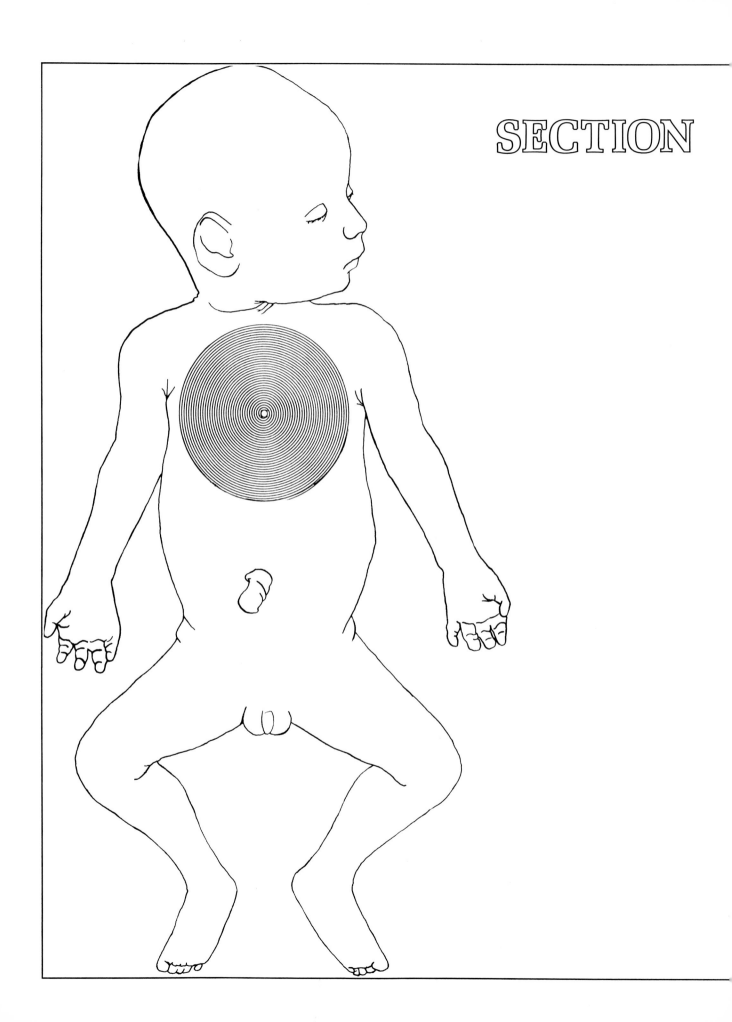

SECTION

FOUR
THORAX

ENLARGED POSITIVE ARTERIOGRAM OF THE FETAL THORAX

Plate 52   Arteriogram of Fetal Thorax   113

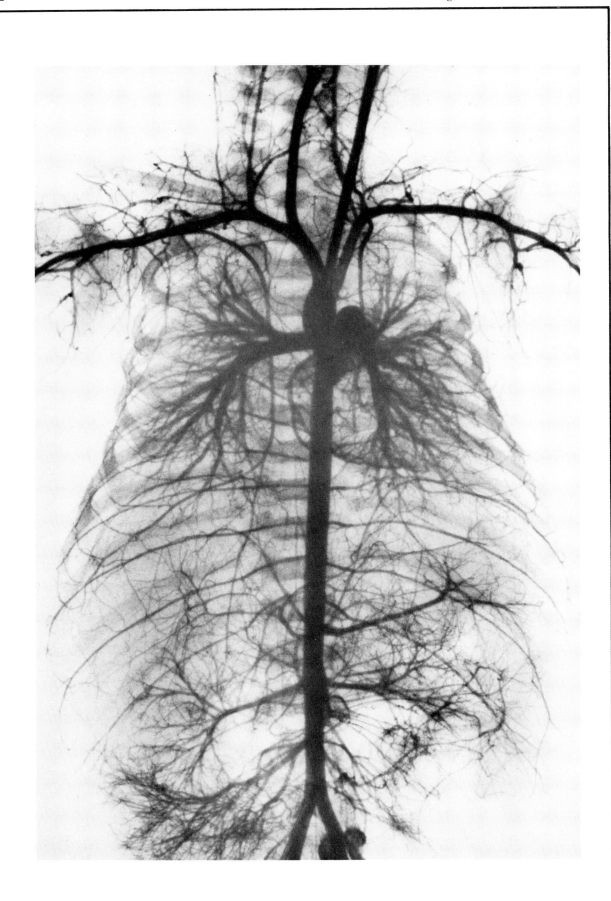

THE THORACOABDOMINAL SITUS

The removal of the entire anterior body wall here presents an overview of the thoracoabdominal situs and reveals the relative dimensions and positions of the *pleural, pericardial* and *peritoneal cavities.*

Because a considerable freedom of motion is a functional requirement of the viscera in all three coelomic cavities, both the outer surfaces of the organs and the inner surfaces of the cavities are lined with a single continuous sheet of serous membrane. This smooth, wet layer of tissue provides a slippery contact between the viscera and their containers. It is called the *parietal layer* where it lines the walls of a coelom and the *visceral layer* where it has been reflected over the organ surface. The area of transition between the parietal and visceral surfaces most frequently ensheaths the structures that enter and leave the organ and usually forms an elongated supportive *ligament* or *mesentery.*

Although the character and function of the opposing layers of serous membrane are virtually identical in all areas, they are specifically referred to as the pleura, the pericardium and the peritoneum in their respective body cavities.

The *mediastinum* is the central compartment of the thorax that is situated between the two pleural cavities. Here it can be seen containing the *thymus* in its anterior subdivision and the pericardial cavity which comprises the middle mediastinum. The deeper posterior and superior mediastinal regions contain numerous other structures that will be discussed with subsequent illustrations.

The lateral mediastinal walls are shown here covered with parietal pleura that has been cut along the lines where it was reflected onto the anterior thoracic wall. The leftward protrusion of the cardiac ventricles produces the major eccentricity of the mediastinum that results in a corresponding asymmetry of the lungs.

The pericardial cavity, which here remains unopened, is partially adherent to the diaphragm and sternum and contains only the heart and its proximal segments of the great vessels.

The muscular *diaphragm* separates the pleural and peritoneal cavities so that the greater part of its superior surface is covered by parietal (phrenic) pleura and much of the inferior surface is covered by parietal peritoneum.

The largest coelom is the abdominal cavity which contains the stomach, intestines and the associated digestive glands. It is continuous with its inferior subdivision, the pelvic cavity, where internal urogenital organs and the rectum are found.

The massive fetal *liver* is suspended from the inferior surface of the diaphragm by its peritoneal reflection, the coronary ligament. This organ occupies more than one third of the fetal abdominal cavity and extends to the umbilical region at term. Upon maturation, however, the liver will occupy approximately one fifth of the abdominal cavity, and its asymmetry will be more pronounced because of a relative attenuation of the left lobe.

In this anterior view of the undisturbed situs, much of the *small intestine* may be identified in the lower right quadrant, and the amount of the *large intestine* visible is dependent upon the extent of its distension by the accumulation of fetal fecal material (meconium).

The veil-like *greater omentum* is a redundancy of the dorsal mesentery of the stomach that hangs over the transverse portion of the large intestine.

Inferior reflection of the lower half of the anterior abdominal wall has exposed the fundus of the *uterus,* the *bladder* and the large *umbilical arteries.*

Plate 53   Thoracoabdominal Situs   115

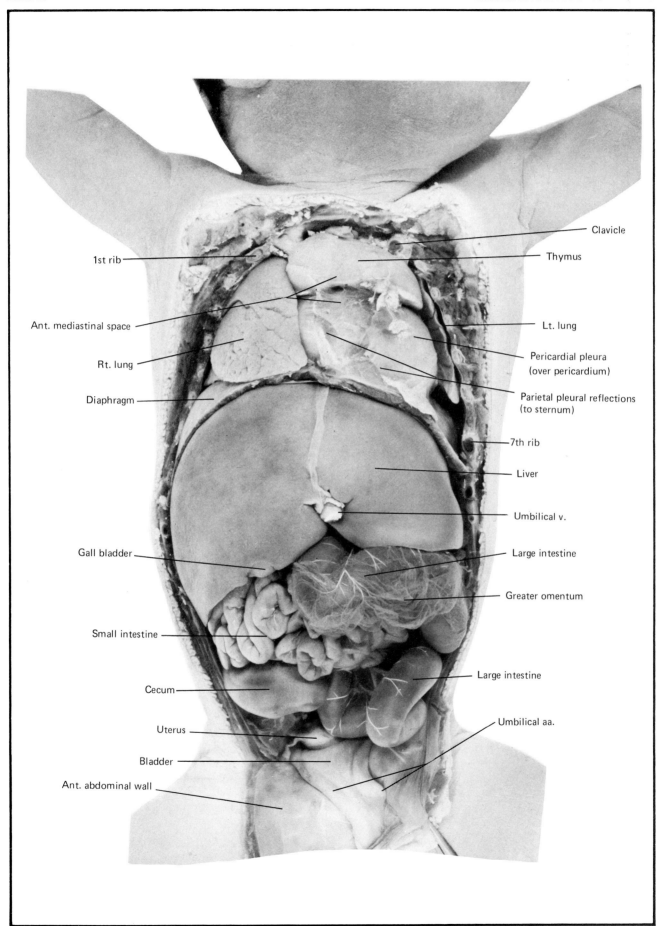

1st rib

Ant. mediastinal space

Rt. lung

Diaphragm

Gall bladder

Small intestine

Cecum

Uterus

Bladder

Ant. abdominal wall

Clavicle

Thymus

Lt. lung

Pericardial pleura
(over pericardium)

Parietal pleural reflections
(to sternum)

7th rib

Liver

Umbilical v.

Large intestine

Greater omentum

Large intestine

Umbilical aa.

INTERNAL ASPECT OF THE ANTERIOR THORACIC WALL

In this illustration the structure of the thoracic cage and its anterior relations to the *parietal pleura* and *diaphragm* may be discerned.

The wall of the thorax is supported by 12 pairs of costae (ribs plus their anterior cartilaginous extensions) that articulate with the vertebral column and the sternum. Since the 11th and 12th ribs are found only in the back and have no anterior articulation, the 10th rib is the most inferior member of the series to contribute to the anterior thoracic wall.

Although the thorax presents a rigid wall against external pressures, the muscular interval between the ribs both permits and assists the "bucket handle," raising and lowering the paired costae to increase and decrease the thoracic volume.

The intercostal muscles are disposed in three layers that are homologous to the layers of the abdominal musculature. Through the transparent and adherent parietal pleura, the oblique fibers of the *internal intercostal* muscles can be seen in each space, and branches of the *intercostal nerves* and *anterior intercostal vessels* can be noted. The fanlike disposition of the *transversus thoracis* muscle, a derivative of the most internal (third) intercostal layer, covers the descending *internal thoracic* vessels that give origin to the *anterior intercostal, musculophrenic* and *superior epigastric arteries*.

Parasternal lymph nodes are arrayed in the intercostal spaces along the internal thoracic vessels.

The lines of the mediastinal reflections of the *costal pleura* and its continuations upon the diaphragm to form the *phrenic pleura* can be traced.

Plate 54

Internal Aspect of Anterior Thoracic Wall   117

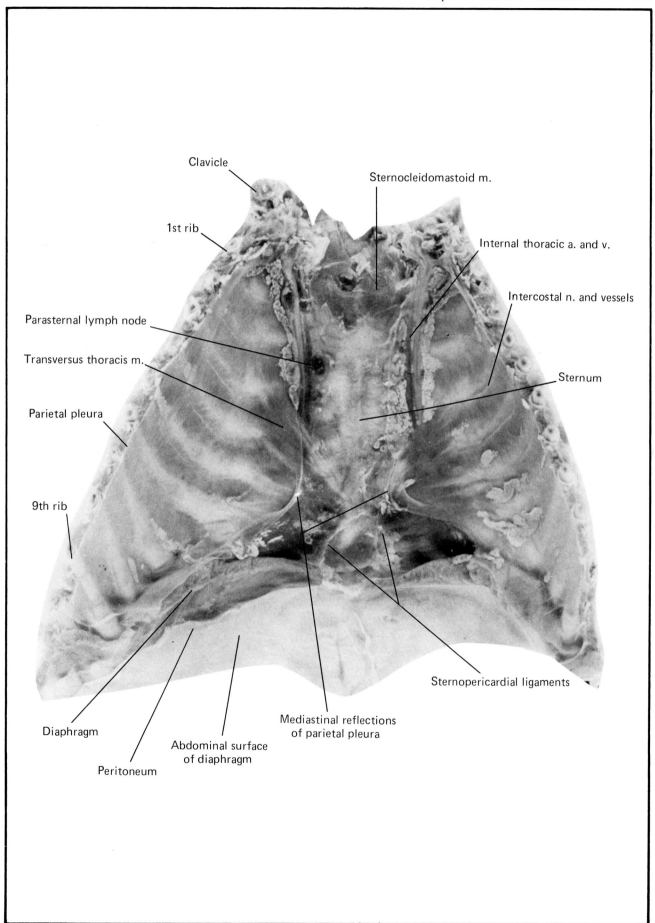

Clavicle

Sternocleidomastoid m.

1st rib

Internal thoracic a. and v.

Intercostal n. and vessels

Parasternal lymph node

Transversus thoracis m.

Sternum

Parietal pleura

9th rib

Sternopericardial ligaments

Diaphragm

Mediastinal reflections
of parietal pleura

Abdominal surface
of diaphragm

Peritoneum

THE THORACIC SITUS

In addition to the removal of the anterior thoracic wall, the anterior half of the pericardial sac has been excised in this exposure, and the topographic relations of the two ventricles and the right atrium are revealed. Note that the anterior (sternocostal) surface of the heart is formed mostly by the *right ventricle* and the *right atrium*. Here the right auricular appendage of the atrium is much distended by the white Neoprene injection mass, and the right border of the heart, which is formed exclusively by the right atrium, is concealed by the anterior borders of the superior and middle lobes of the right lung. The sharp margin of the right ventricle approximates the *diaphragm,* and the apex and *left ventricle* lie in relation to the anterior border and *lingula* of the *superior lobe* of the left lung.

It should be realized that these fetal lungs have not been inflated to show the extent of their eventual relationship to the pleural cavities. Nevertheless, the anterior borders of the functional neonatal lungs still do not extend as far foward toward the sternum as they do in the adult. Hence, in the fetus, the anterior mediastinum shows a much greater relative width that accommodates the bulk of the thymus.

The *thymus* is the only organ (except lymph nodes) to occupy the anterior mediastinum. It lies on the anterosuperior surface of the pericardium anterior to the great vessels of the upper thorax. Because its greatest functional importance as an immunologic organ is achieved shortly after birth, it is of considerable size in the late fetus and may be as large as the heart itself.

The marked domed shape of the diaphragm indicates its functional relationship to the two pleural cavities. Contraction of its muscular fasciculae tends to flatten the domes and produce the descent of the central portion. This enlarges the pleural cavities, draws the mediastinum downward and depresses the abdominal organs.

Because of the convexity of the diaphragm, its attachment to the lower costal wall forms an acute angle into which the costal pleura descends before it is reflected onto the phrenic surface. The resulting pleural recess, the *phrenicocostal sinus,* is never completely filled by the descent of the lung margin and tends to accumulate pleural effusions, particularly at its deepest part in the dorsal region.

Unfortunately, costal movement in the newborn does not produce the same degrees of respiratory assistance that it does in the adult, and early respiration is almost exclusively diaphragmatic. When, in addition, it is realized that the large size of the mediastinum reduces the relative volume of the pleural cavities and the massiveness of the liver tends to resist the excursions of the diaphragm, it becomes apparent that respiratory problems may be quite critical in the early months of life.

Plate 55   Thoracic Situs   119

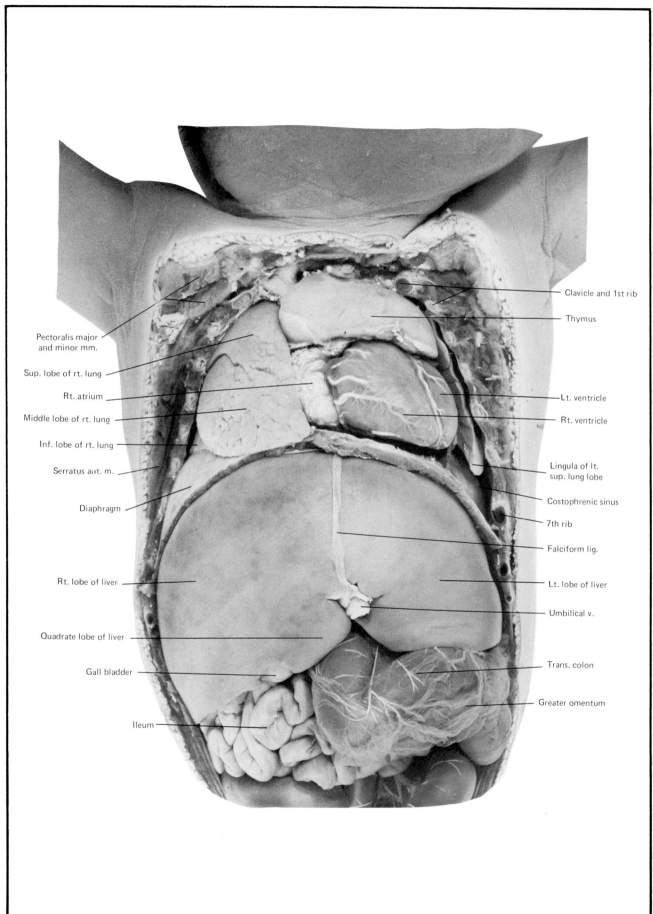

Clavicle and 1st rib

Thymus

Pectoralis major
and minor mm.

Sup. lobe of rt. lung

Rt. atrium

Middle lobe of rt. lung

Inf. lobe of rt. lung

Serratus ant. m.

Diaphragm

Lt. ventricle

Rt. ventricle

Lingula of lt.
sup. lung lobe

Costophrenic sinus

7th rib

Falciform lig.

Rt. lobe of liver

Quadrate lobe of liver

Gall bladder

Ileum

Lt. lobe of liver

Umbilical v.

Trans. colon

Greater omentum

ANTEROPOSTERIOR ARTERIOGRAM OF THE THORAX

Because of their confluence through the *ductus arteriosus,* both the pulmonary and the systemic circulations of the fetus may be outlined by a single umbilical injection of a radiopaque medium. Although the pulmonary and coronary arterial systems serve here to show the relative size and position of the largest organs of the thorax, the details of their finer ramifications are presented in following sections on pulmonary and cardiac anatomy.

The primary function of this illustration is to provide an overview of the great arteries of the thorax with their major somatic and visceral derivations.

The patterns of distribution of the *right* and *left carotid* and *subclavian arteries* are symmetrical, but the two sides differ in the manner of their origin from the *aortic arch.* On the right side the vasculature to the head, neck and arm arise from a common trunk, the *brachiocephalic artery,* that is the first derivative of the aortic arch, whereas the *left common carotid* and subclavian arteries arise independently from the middle and posterior parts of the arch.

In addition to supplying the upper extremity, the subclavian artery also gives branches to the thoracic wall primarily by way of the *internal thoracic artery.* This artery usually originates on the last section of the subclavian near the lateral border of the first rib (as on the left side here), but it may also branch from the adjacent proximal sections of the axillary (as shown on the right side).

The internal thoracic artery descends on the inner surface of the anterior thoracic wall lateral to the sternum. At each intercostal space it gives off an *anterior intercostal artery* that passes laterally below each rib to anastomose with its corresponding *posterior intercostal artery.* Inferior to the sixth costosternal articulation, the internal thoracic artery divides into the *musculophrenic artery,* which laterally follows the inferior margin of the thoracic cage, and the *superior epigastric artery,* which descends on the anterior abdominal wall. At each intercostal space the internal thoracic artery also sends a perforating branch superficially to contribute to the vasculature of the pectoral muscles and skin.

Just below the juncture of the ductus arteriosus and the posterior part of the aortic arch, the *thoracic aorta* descends along the left sides of the 5th to 12th thoracic vertebrae and provides segmental posterior intercostal arteries to all but the first two intercostal spaces. The first four pairs of these arteries initially pass obliquely upward to reach their proper intercostal levels. The two most superior spaces receive their arteries from the *costocervical artery,* a posterior branch of the subclavian that cannot readily be identified in this view. Each of the posterior intercostals sends perforating branches to the musculature and skin covering the posterior and lateral walls of the thorax.

The thoracic aorta also supplies the lungs, esophagus and posterior pericardium with a number of small but important ventral branches that are obscured here by the aortic shadow.

Because the concavity of the diaphragm accommodates the upper abdominal organs and affords them the protection of the thoracic wall, their vasculature is necessarily included in this illustration. The division between the pleural and abdominal cavities can be identified by the level of the *inferior phrenic arteries.* These are the first branches of the *abdominal aorta* and may be seen arching upward and laterally under the domes of the diaphragm.

Plate 56 Anteroposterior Arteriogram of Thorax 121

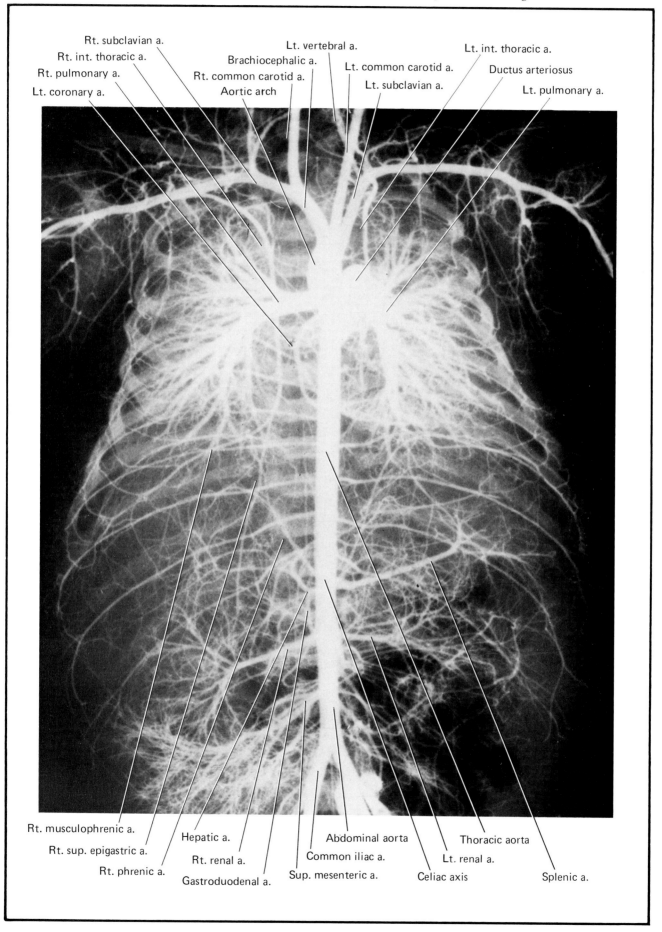

Rt. subclavian a.
Rt. int. thoracic a.
Rt. pulmonary a.
Lt. coronary a.
Rt. common carotid a.
Brachiocephalic a.
Aortic arch
Lt. vertebral a.
Lt. common carotid a.
Lt. subclavian a.
Lt. int. thoracic a.
Ductus arteriosus
Lt. pulmonary a.

Rt. musculophrenic a.
Rt. sup. epigastric a.
Rt. phrenic a.
Hepatic a.
Rt. renal a.
Gastroduodenal a.
Sup. mesenteric a.
Abdominal aorta
Common iliac a.
Celiac axis
Lt. renal a.
Thoracic aorta
Splenic a.

LATERAL ARTERIOGRAM OF THE THORAX

This view furnishes the perspective necessary to envision the three dimensional relationships of the arteries shown in the previous figure. However, certain aspects of the vasculature that are particularly clear in this illustration should be noted.

The coronary system that encircles the atrioventricular sulcus of the heart arises from the right and left aortic sinuses as the first branches of the aorta. At the apex of the *aortic arch*, the *brachiocephalic* and *left common carotid arteries* arise in close succession while the *left subclavian* is situated more posteriorly.

The relations of the *pulmonary trunk* and *ductus arteriosus* become clearer in this view. Although the pulmonary sinuses are obscured by the shadow of the ascending aorta, the course of the pulmonary trunk and its continuation as the ductus arteriosus may be discerned beneath the arch of the aorta.

The *thoracic aorta* commences its descent on the left side of the vertebral column, but as it approaches the diaphragm it turns slightly anteriorly and medially until it becomes centrally located directly anterior to the upper lumbar vertebrae. The final point of this transition may be detected by the slight bend produced at the level of the *celiac axis*.

Plate 57

Lateral Arteriogram of Thorax   123

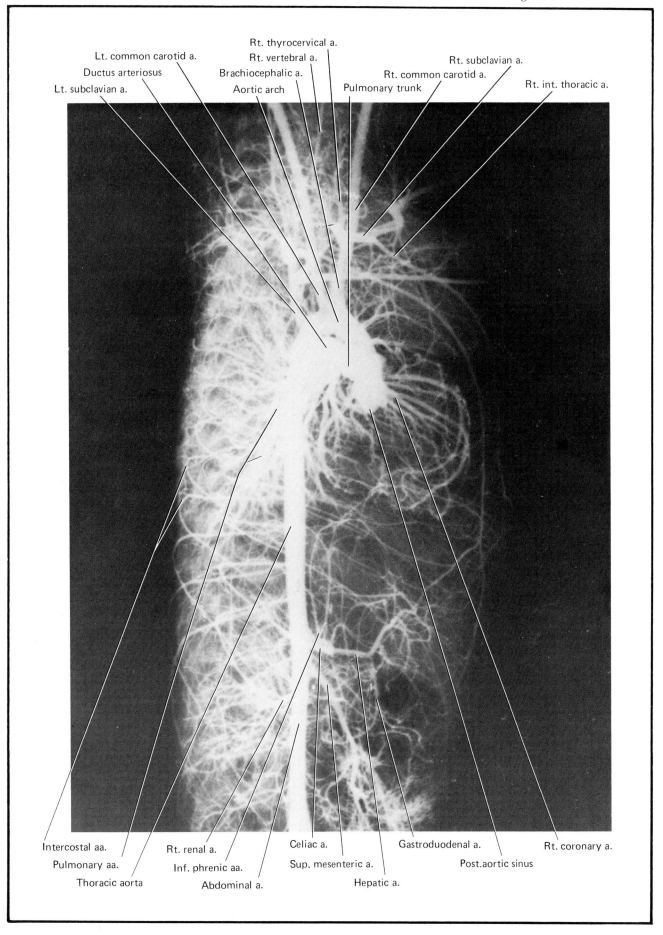

Rt. thyrocervical a.

Lt. common carotid a.   Rt. vertebral a.   Rt. subclavian a.

Ductus arteriosus   Brachiocephalic a.   Rt. common carotid a.

Lt. subclavian a.   Aortic arch   Pulmonary trunk   Rt. int. thoracic a.

Intercostal aa.   Rt. renal a.   Celiac a.   Gastroduodenal a.   Rt. coronary a.

Pulmonary aa.   Inf. phrenic aa.   Sup. mesenteric a.   Post.aortic sinus

Thoracic aorta   Abdominal a.   Hepatic a.

RIGHT LATERAL ASPECT OF THE MEDIASTINUM

One of the salient advantages in the use of the fetus as an anatomic subject is that the serous membranes are remarkably transparent. In the adult the thickness of the mediastinal pleura and its supporting fascia, plus the greater accumulation of subserous fat, necessitate the removal of these layers before the underlying structures may be identified visually. In the view presented here the lateral costal wall and the lung have been removed, but the serous membrane has been left intact over the remainder of the pleural cavity. Small accumulations of fat are obvious only beneath the pericardial pleura and in the superior mediastinum.

The mediastinum is conventionally subdivided into a superior, an anterior, a middle and a posterior region. In the fetus the *anterior mediastinum* is quite large, as it is occupied by the *thymus*, but in the adult this space is much reduced to contain only the lymphoid remnants of that structure. The *middle mediastinum* is coextensive with the *pericardial sac* and contains the heart, its proximal great vessels and the *phrenic nerve*. The remaining regions of the mediastinum are designated as the *superior* above the fourth intervertebral disc or the *posterior* below that level.

Because the thymus lies anterosuperior to the heart, it conceals the great arteries, and only venous structures can be discerned here without further dissection.

Superiorly, the *right brachiocephalic vein* flows into the *superior vena cava*. At the point of the juncture, they are joined by the *azygos vein* that arches over the root of the lung. The azygos leaves the lumbar region and courses up the right side of the vertebral column in the posterior mediastinum, where it collects intercostal tributaries that drain the back.

A short section of the *inferior vena cava* rises above the *diaphragm* and immediately enters the right atrium.

Note that the *right phrenic nerve* follows the great veins from the neck and eventually enters the diaphragm through the caval hiatus. In the middle mediastinum it courses between the fibrous pericardium and the pleura. The *phrenicopericardiac artery,* a branch of the inferior phrenic, travels upward from the diaphragm along the phrenic nerve to supply it and the pericardium.

The white Neoprene injection mass marks the position of the *pulmonary arteries* to be superior and posterior to the branches in the sectioned stump of the lung root, whereas the dark mass in the veins indicates their position as ventral and inferior.

The *right sympathetic trunk* runs a subpleural course on the posterior costal wall anterior to the heads of the ribs. Its segmental ganglia can be identified as a series of swellings of the trunk that roughly correspond to the intercostal spaces. In the lower thoracic region several large anterior derivatives of the trunk coalesce to form the *greater splanchnic nerve* that penetrates the diaphragmatic crura to reach the celiac ganglia of the abdomen.

Plate 58 Mediastinum: Right Lateral Aspect 125

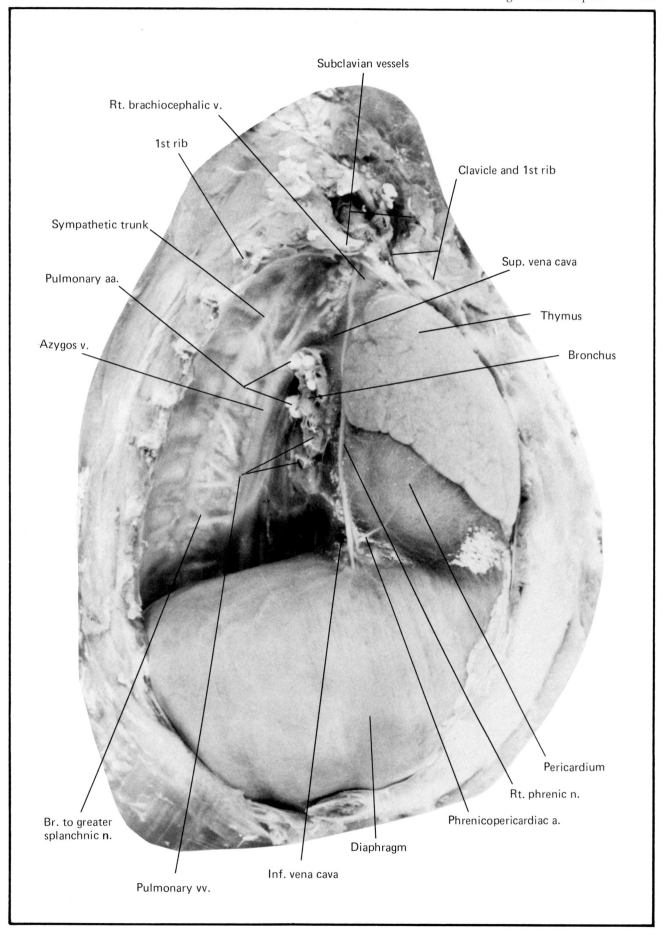

Subclavian vessels

Rt. brachiocephalic v.

1st rib

Clavicle and 1st rib

Sympathetic trunk

Sup. vena cava

Pulmonary aa.

Thymus

Azygos v.

Bronchus

Pericardium

Rt. phrenic n.

Br. to greater
splanchnic n.

Phrenicopericardiac a.

Diaphragm

Inf. vena cava

Pulmonary vv.

LEFT LATERAL ASPECT OF THE MEDIASTINUM

Here again the massiveness of the *thymus* can be appreciated as it covers the anterior parts of the aortic arch and the *ductus arteriosus* as well as the anterosuperior surface of the *pericardium*. Inferior to the thymus the left wall of the pericardium shows an anterior bulge indicating the ventricular apex and a posterior bulge that shows the position of the left atrium. Between these two landmarks, the *left phrenic nerve* descends to penetrate the *diaphragm* through a small hiatus it shares with the *left phrenicopericardiac artery*.

Although partially obscured by fat, the path of the *left subclavian artery* may be noted through the wall of the superior mediastinum. Leaving the posterior part of the aortic arch, it ascends to the base of the neck where it is bracketed by the *subclavian vein* and the trunks of the *brachial plexus*.

Just above the ductus arteriosus that arches directly over the root of the lung, the *left superior intercostal vein* collects tributaries from the upper three intercostal spaces and courses anteriorly to reach the left brachiocephalic vein. The lower intercostal veins drain into the azygos system.

The sectioned root of the left lung shows the white Neoprene-injected *pulmonary arteries* lying superior to the bronchial stump and the veins situated inferiorly where they directly enter the left atrium.

Anteromedial to the *aorta*, the *esophagus* may be seen descending between the posterior surface of the *pericardium* and the vertebral column with the *left vagus nerve* closely applied to its wall.

Through the *parietal pleura* of the posterior costal wall, the *left sympathetic trunk* and its contribution to the *greater splanchnic nerve* may be identified.

Note that one or two *lymph nodes* are apparent in each intercostal space near the heads of the ribs. These are the regional nodes of the intercostal lymphatics that drain medially into the *thoracic duct*.

Plate 59   Mediastinum: Left Lateral Aspect   127

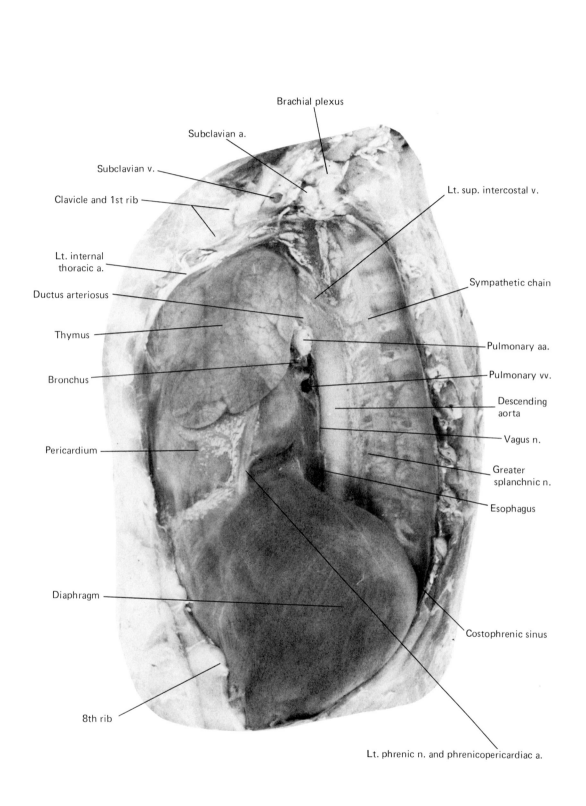

Brachial plexus

Subclavian a.

Subclavian v.

Lt. sup. intercostal v.

Clavicle and 1st rib

Lt. internal
thoracic a.

Sympathetic chain

Ductus arteriosus

Thymus

Pulmonary aa.

Bronchus

Pulmonary vv.

Descending
aorta

Pericardium

Vagus n.

Greater
splanchnic n.

Esophagus

Diaphragm

Costophrenic sinus

8th rib

Lt. phrenic n. and phrenicopericardiac a.

DISSECTION
OF THE
MEDIASTINUM I

The thymus has been removed to expose the upper part of the pericardium and the great vessels, and the strap muscles of the neck have been divided and retracted to show the structures entering or leaving the superior mediastinum.

The intact *pericardial sac* shown here consists of two layers — an outer supportive fibrous tunic and an inner serous layer, the *parietal pericardium.* Inferiorly, the fibrous layer is firmly attached to the central tendon of the *diaphragm,* and superiorly it blends with the connective tissue around the great vessels in the superior mediastinum. The parietal serous layer is reflected around the roots of the great vessels and is turned back over the surface of the heart as the visceral serous layer, the *epicardium.* The lateral walls of the fibrous pericardium are covered externally with pleura and are therefore sandwiched between two serous laminae.

In the fetus the combined layers of the pericardium are still quite transparent, and the major features of the heart and vessels may be visualized through them.

The most anterior great vessels are the *superior vena cava* and the *right* and *left brachiocephalic veins.* Both brachiocephalics are formed by the junctures of the subclavian and jugular vessels and drain into the superior vena cava. Because the left vein is longer and crosses the mediastinum, it receives the tributaries from the thymus and pericardium.

As valves are first encountered in the proximal sections of the subclavian, jugular and iliac veins, the valveless caval system has been filled from the umbilical vein by a retrograde injection of blue Neoprene. It should be noticed that very little of the injection medium penetrated distal to the brachiocephalic veins.

The right and left *phrenic nerves* can be seen traveling down each side of the mediastinum to reach the diaphragm. They pass anterior to the roots of the lungs and should never be confused with vagal branches that run posterior to these structures.

Plate 60

Mediastinum: Dissection I   129

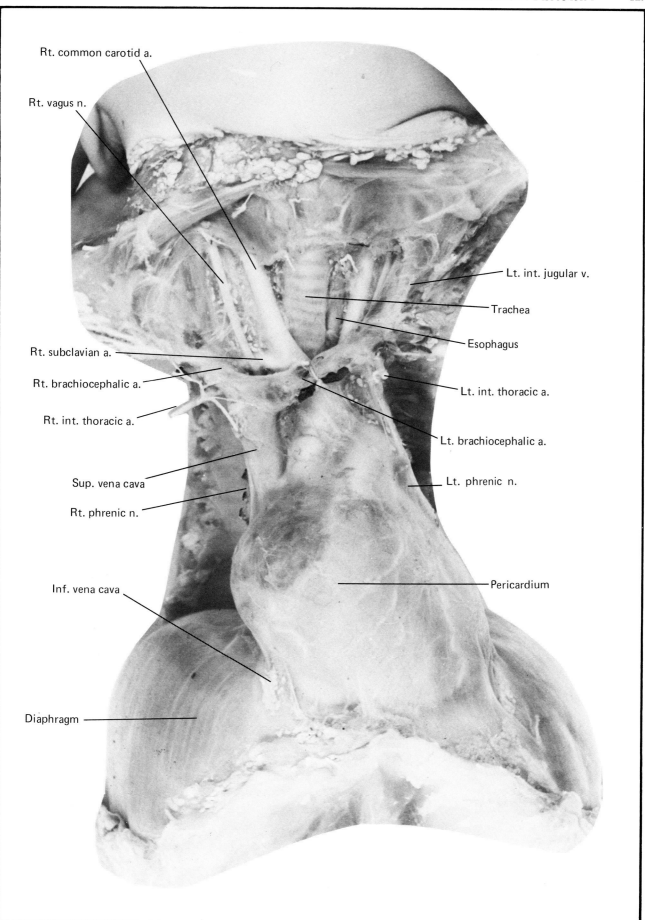

Rt. common carotid a.

Rt. vagus n.

Lt. int. jugular v.

Trachea

Esophagus

Rt. subclavian a.

Rt. brachiocephalic a.

Lt. int. thoracic a.

Rt. int. thoracic a.

Lt. brachiocephalic a.

Sup. vena cava

Lt. phrenic n.

Rt. phrenic n.

Inf. vena cava

Pericardium

Diaphragm

DISSECTION OF THE MEDIASTINUM II

This is a sequential dissection of the same specimen shown in the previous plate. The brachiocephalic veins and the anterior wall of the pericardium have been removed. The extent of the pericardial cavity, which is topographically equivalent to the middle mediastinum, is easily comprehended.

The base of the heart is fixed in position by the afferent and efferent great vessels, but the ventricular part is free to slide anteriorly and inferiorly during its rhythmic excursions.

The *right auricle* is readily defined by the contrasting dark blue Neoprene forced into it from the caval system. Because of the patent interatrial foramen (foramen ovale) the blue medium also filled the *left atrium*, whose *auricle* is visible to the right of the *pulmonary trunk*. The injected *venous vasa vasorum* of the aorta and pulmonary trunk form fine plexuses on the surfaces of these vessels. These drain into pericardial veins superiorly, and directly into the right atrium inferiorly.

On the aorta and pulmonary trunk, the line of *pericardial reflections* shows the upper limits of the pericardial cavity and indicates that the intrapericardial segments of these vessels are sheathed by epicardium. Above the reflections, which are approximately at the level of the fourth intervertebral disc, the *arch of the aorta* lies in the superior mediastinum. Here it can be seen giving off the *brachiocephalic artery* that is the source of the *right common carotid* and *subclavian arteries*. The *left common carotid* arises from the highest part of the arch. It forms an inverted triangle with its right counterpart that frames the *trachea* and *esophagus* as they descend into the mediastinum. The *left subclavian*, being more posterior, is not visible, but its position is revealed by its branch, the *left internal thoracic artery*.

The carotid sheath, which has been dissected open here, is the common investment of the *vagus nerve, carotid artery* and *jugular vein*. Because the vein lay superficial to the other two structures it was removed.

The *right vagus* nerve descends along the carotid to the level of the right subclavian, where its major component abruptly takes a deeper course to pass posterior to the root of the lung. A recurrent branch loops 180 degrees around the subclavian and ascends between the trachea and esophagus to supply these structures and the larynx as the right inferior laryngeal nerve. The *left vagus*, however, must descend to the level of the ductus arteriosus and bend under this structure to pass deep to the root of the left lung. It also sends a branch upward to the trachea, esophagus and larynx as the left inferior laryngeal nerve.

Like all dissections prepared for this atlas, this specimen was photographed while immersed in water to eliminate highlights. At the upper right, the dissector's thumb provides comparative reference for size, and the water level is indicated by the white highlights around the thumbnail.

Plate 61   Mediastinum: Dissection II   131

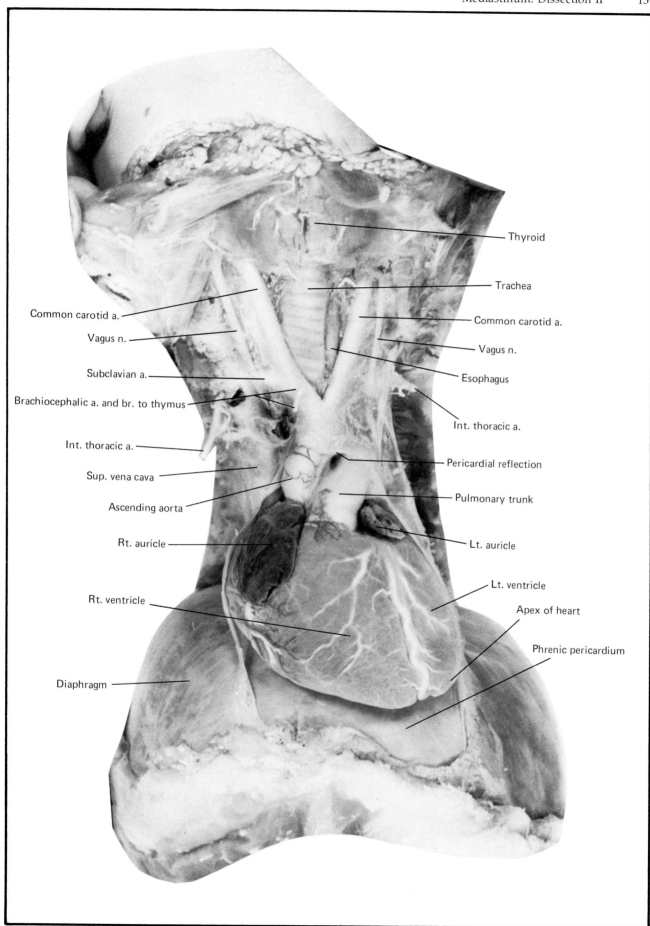

Thyroid

Trachea

Common carotid a.

Common carotid a.

Vagus n.

Vagus n.

Subclavian a.

Esophagus

Brachiocephalic a. and br. to thymus

Int. thoracic a.

Int. thoracic a.

Pericardial reflection

Sup. vena cava

Pulmonary trunk

Ascending aorta

Rt. auricle

Lt. auricle

Rt. ventricle

Lt. ventricle

Apex of heart

Phrenic pericardium

Diaphragm

DISSECTION OF THE MEDIASTINUM III

The heart has been removed and the intrapericardial segments of the great vessels have been sectioned close to or at the level where the parietal pericardium was reflected onto the vessels.

The relations between the pericardium and the vessels can be understood more easily if their development is briefly recalled. The early embryonic heart was a sinuous muscular tube that received all venous structures at one end and discharged into a single arterial conus at the other. A thin sleeve of parietal pericardium ensheathed this tube and was turned upon its surface as a single reflection of primitive epicardium at each end. In subsequent development, the heart tube was folded upon itself so that the arterial and venous ends were brought into close approximation of each other at what would become the base of the heart, and the bulge of the fold would become the ventricular region.

Despite the series of subdivisions that occur to form the definitive heart chambers, all of the venous structures remain bound together in a single complex fold of pericardial reflection that may be traced around the pericardial entrance of both the *superior* and *inferior venae cavae* and both sets of *right* and *left pulmonary veins*. With an intact heart still attached to its vessels, a blunt probe or finger may be passed beneath and posterior to the ventricles until it is stopped by this pericardial reflection. The space thus probed (indicated by the two arrows) is the *oblique sinus* of the pericardium.

The conal (arterial) end of the heart becomes subdivided into the *pulmonary trunk* and *ascending aorta*, but these also remain with a common reflection of the pericardium. The interval that persistently separated this arterial reflection from the venous reflection is called the *transverse sinus* (indicated here by the long, double headed arrow).

Plate 62   Mediastinum: Dissection III   133

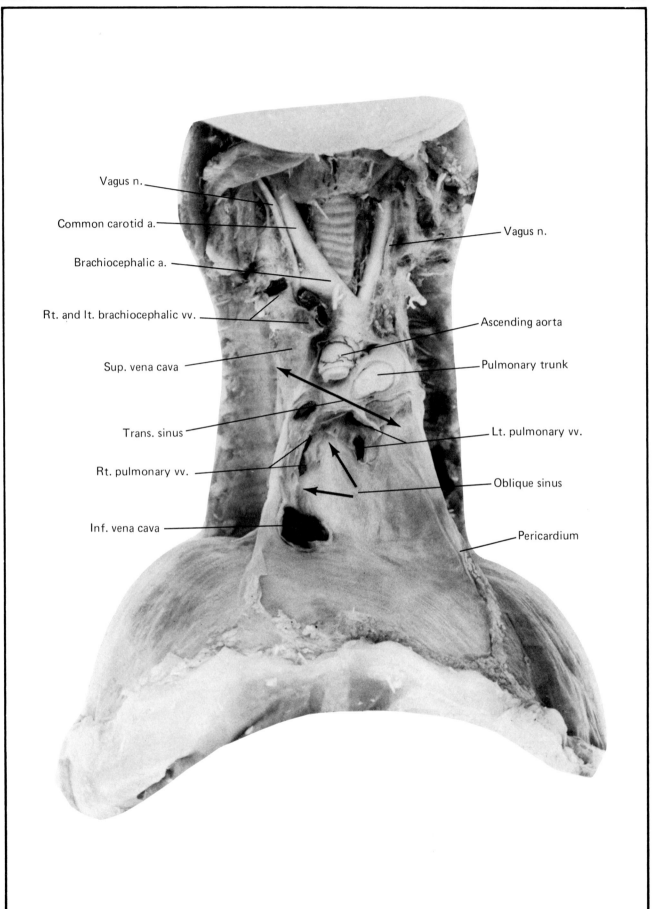

Vagus n.

Common carotid a.

Brachiocephalic a.

Rt. and lt. brachiocephalic vv.

Sup. vena cava

Trans. sinus

Rt. pulmonary vv.

Inf. vena cava

Vagus n.

Ascending aorta

Pulmonary trunk

Lt. pulmonary vv.

Oblique sinus

Pericardium

DISSECTION OF THE MEDIASTINUM IV

As a continued dissection of the specimen shown in Plate 60, this view shows the deepest structures of the posterior mediastinum. The posterior pericardium and the immediately subjacent esophagus have been removed to expose the *azygos vein* as it ascends from the lumbar region below the *diaphragm*. It collects the right intercostal veins from the posterior thoracic wall before it arches anteriorly over the root of the right lung to join the superior vena cava. The left lower intercostals are drained by the *hemiazygos vein* shown in the next figure.

The formation of the right *greater splanchnic nerve* is well shown as it descends through the diaphragm to join the celiac and superior mesenteric ganglia.

The anterior edge of the diaphragm has been slightly retracted downward to display the high domes formed by the right and left hemidiaphragms. The right dome is higher than the left to accommodate the greater mass of the liver that lies inferior to this part. The domes are covered by phrenic pleura and the central tendon is covered by the *phrenic pericardium*. The large *caval hiatus* that is filled with blue Neoprene also serves to pass the *right phrenicopericardial artery* and the *right phrenic nerve*, whereas the *left phrenic nerve* and corresponding vessels pierce the diaphragm independently.

Posteriorly, between the domes, the *esophageal hiatus* lies anterior to the thoracic aorta and marks the position of the cardiac region of the stomach situated immediately below the diaphragm.

Plate 63   Mediastinum: Dissection IV   135

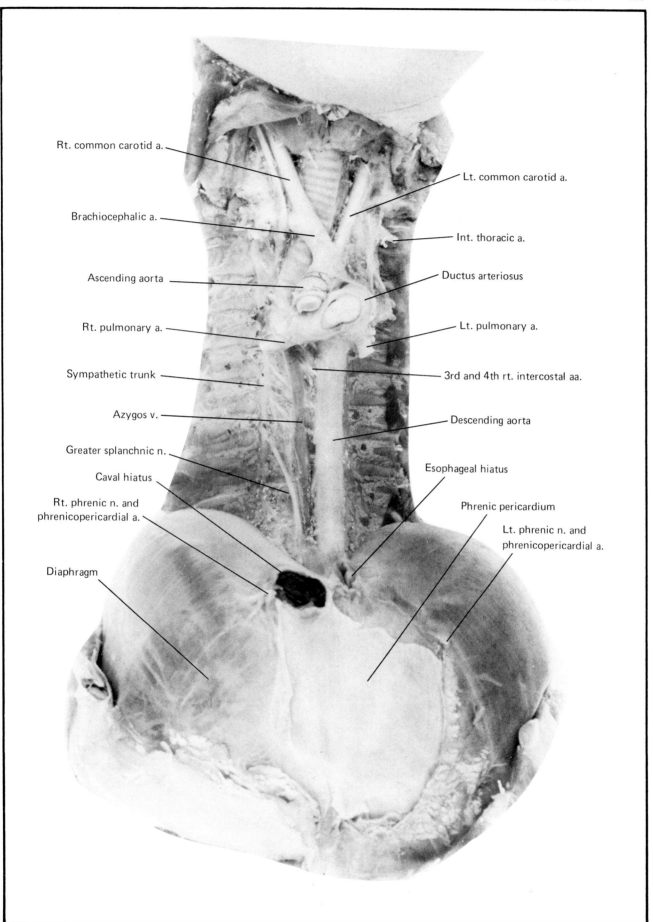

Rt. common carotid a.

Brachiocephalic a.

Ascending aorta

Rt. pulmonary a.

Sympathetic trunk

Azygos v.

Greater splanchnic n.

Caval hiatus

Rt. phrenic n. and
phrenicopericardial a.

Diaphragm

Lt. common carotid a.

Int. thoracic a.

Ductus arteriosus

Lt. pulmonary a.

3rd and 4th rt. intercostal aa.

Descending aorta

Esophageal hiatus

Phrenic pericardium

Lt. phrenic n. and
phrenicopericardial a.

DISSECTION OF THE MEDIASTINUM V

This lateral view of the previous dissection shows the sequential derivation of the large branches of the aortic arch and the arrangement of the vessels and nerves that pass over the first rib.

Note that a short segment of the *subclavian vein* lies anterior to the *left subclavian artery*. Before dissection these vessels were separated by the anterior scalene insertion on the first rib. Directly posterior and superior to the left subclavian artery lie the trunks of the *brachial plexus*.

The manner in which both vagi loop beneath arterial structures can be better appreciated in terms of their developmental history. The series of early aortic arches formed ventral to the pharyngeal region when the vagal branches became associated with the post-branchial mesenchyme that formed the laryngeal musculature. As the definitive remnants of the right fourth arch (right subclavian) and left sixth arch *(ductus arteriosus)* engaged the vagal laryngeal branches in their descent, they drew these nerves into recurrent loops. The marked asymmetry of the two vagal loops is caused by the persistence of a sixth arch on the left side only.

In this illustration the *right vagus* can be traced to its abrupt posterior turn under the *right subclavian artery*, while the *left vagus* descends between the *left common carotid* and the *left subclavian* to bend under the ductus arteriosus.

The *left sympathetic trunk* descends from the neck and shows an enlargement at the level of the subclavian artery that results from the fusion of the lower cervical and first thoracic ganglia to form the large *stellate ganglion*. The thoracic sympathetic trunk passes anterior to the heads of the ribs and gives off sympathetic rami at each intercostal space; it also contributes to the *greater splanchnic nerve* in the lower thorax.

A rather inconspicuous *hemiazygos vein* ascends immediately posterior to the *aorta;* it receives the left intercostals before it crosses the fifth vertebral body to join the azygos on the left side.

Plate 64   Mediastinum: Dissection V   137

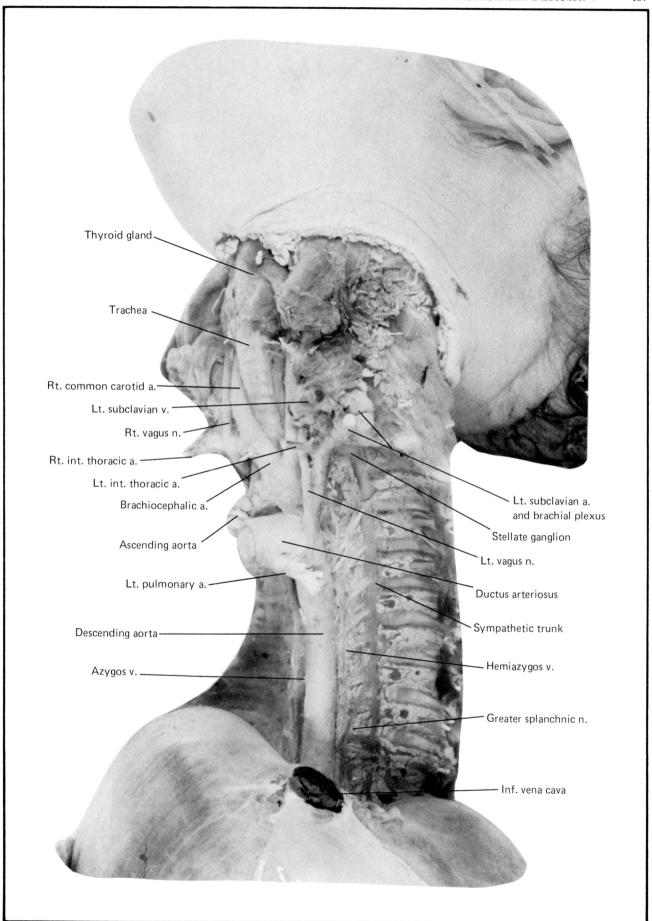

Thyroid gland

Trachea

Rt. common carotid a.

Lt. subclavian v.

Rt. vagus n.

Rt. int. thoracic a.

Lt. int. thoracic a.

Brachiocephalic a.

Ascending aorta

Lt. pulmonary a.

Descending aorta

Azygos v.

Lt. subclavian a.
and brachial plexus

Stellate ganglion

Lt. vagus n.

Ductus arteriosus

Sympathetic trunk

Hemiazygos v.

Greater splanchnic n.

Inf. vena cava

DISSECTION OF THE MEDIASTINUM VI

The previous plates showed progressive dissections of the same specimen. In this posterior view of the mediastinum, a differently prepared specimen is presented. The lungs have been injected intratracheally with Neoprene to render them firm so that their retraction shows accurate impressions formed by contiguous mediastinal structures. Because of some retained fluid, the intraalveolar filling of the lung was not complete, but the mosaic appearance accurately demonstrates the secondary pulmonary lobulations.

The entire thoracic viscera has been dissected from the posterior thoracic wall, and the midthoracic section of the *aorta* has been removed to expose the posterior relations of the *vagus nerves*.

In the superior mediastinum, the aorta has been sectioned at the confluence of the *aortic arch* and the *ductus arteriosus.* Descending anterior to the *left subclavian artery,* the *left vagus* passes lateral to the ductus and gives off its *recurrent inferior laryngeal nerve* that loops under the ductus and ascends between the trachea and *esophagus.* The main part of the vagus then continues posterior to the *pulmonary arteries* and *veins* where it provides numerous fibers to the pulmonary and cardiac plexuses. The former nerves enter the lung with the hilar structures, and the latter become involved with the cardiac autonomic plexuses found in association with the aortic arch.

In the midregion of the posterior mediastinum, both vagi break up into a plexus that enmeshes the esophagus. Because of the leftward rotation of the stomach and lower esophagus, the derivatives of the left vagus tend to enter the abdomen or the anterior surface of the esophagus, and those of the right vagus run on its posterior surface.

Just posterior to the left pulmonary veins, a small sectioned ventral branch of the removed segment of the aorta gives rise to *bronchial* and *esophageal arteries.* At the level where the aorta has been sectioned inferiorly, another ventral branch, the *esophagopericardial artery,* may be seen.

Note that the left atrium is located in the midline of the mediastinum and the right and left pulmonary veins are therefore equal in length. This view clearly shows that the esophagus lies immediately posterior to the posterior wall of the *pericardium.*

Plate 65   Mediastinum: Dissection VI   139

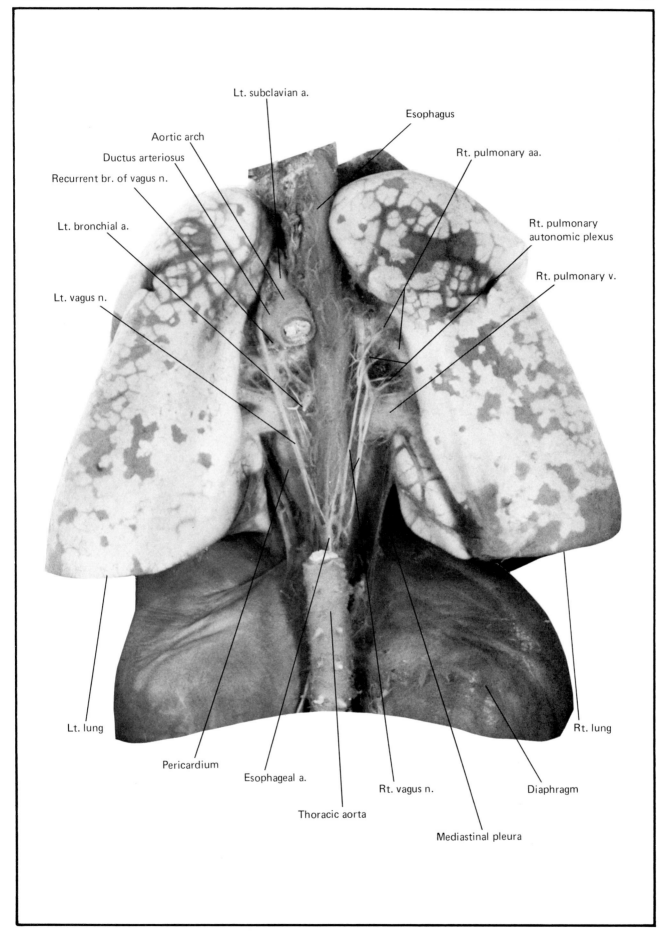

Lt. subclavian a.

Esophagus

Aortic arch

Rt. pulmonary aa.

Ductus arteriosus

Recurrent br. of vagus n.

Rt. pulmonary
autonomic plexus

Lt. bronchial a.

Rt. pulmonary v.

Lt. vagus n.

Lt. lung

Rt. lung

Pericardium

Esophageal a.

Rt. vagus n.

Diaphragm

Thoracic aorta

Mediastinal pleura

CROSS SECTION THROUGH THE UPPER THORAX

This section of the thorax shows the mediastinum at the level of the fourth thoracic vertebra and the structures in the base of the neck that are related to the apices of the pleural cavities. The plane of section has passed between the arch of the aorta and the ductus arteriosus so that only the *aortic arch* has been included in the specimen. As the ascending aorta has been cut just below the level of the pericardial reflection, the most superior recess of the *pericardial cavity* may be seen anterior to this structure. The posterior part of the aortic arch shows the characteristic narrowing that occurs just before it joins the ductus arteriosus (refer to Plate 77).

To the right of the ascending aorta the *superior vena cava* is shown containing a mixture of Neoprene and clotted blood. This venous injection is the result of a failure of the pulmonary valve that allowed the Neoprene to enter the venous system from the right chambers of the heart.

The proximal sections of the *right* and *left main bronchi* indicate that the plane of this view lies just below the tracheal bifurcation. Dorsal to the bronchi and to the right of the descending aorta, the *esophagus* runs along the anterior surface of the vertebral bodies.

The apical lobes of the lungs extend above the first ribs and are separated from the vessels and nerves in the base of the neck only by a layer of pleura and the supporting scalene fascia. It is obvious that neoplastic or septic processes in the lung apex could affect the vascular and nervous structures that are seen lying directly against the apical pleura.

On the right side, the *subclavian artery* crosses from the mediastinum to the medial border of the first rib. Anteriorly, it gives off the *internal thoracic artery* that can be seen providing the anterior intercostal arteries to the first two intercostal spaces. Posteriorly, the *subclavian* sends out the *costocervical trunk* that supplies the posterior region of the neck and the first two posterior intercostal arteries by a descending branch. Just medial to the origin of both of these arteries, the *sympathetic trunk* may be seen looping the subclavian to form the *stellate ganglion*. Lung or mediastinal lesions that affect this structure cause the loss of sympathetic innervation to the same side of the neck and face (Horner's syndrome).

On the left side, the *left subclavian vein* is apparent because some of the white Neoprene entered this vessel. Usually, as on the right side, venous valves prevent the filling of the subclavians. Also injected is the *left vertebral vein* that here runs an atypical course inferior, rather than superior, to the left subclavian artery. The *anterior scalene muscle* separates the subclavian veins from the arteries by its insertion on the upper border of the first rib.

Plate 66   Cross Section through Upper Thorax   141

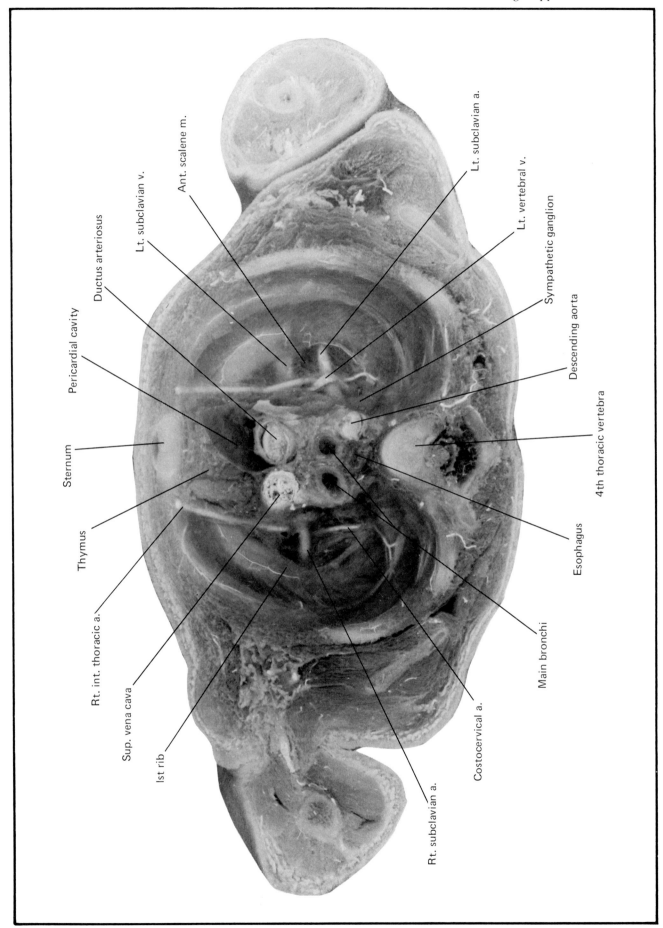

Ant. scalene m.

Lt. subclavian v.

Ductus arteriosus

Pericardial cavity

Sternum

Thymus

Rt. int. thoracic a.

Sup. vena cava

1st rib

Lt. subclavian a.

Lt. vertebral v.

Sympathetic ganglion

Descending aorta

4th thoracic vertebra

Esophagus

Main bronchi

Costocervical a.

Rt. subclavian a.

SUPERFICIAL ANATOMY OF THE HEART: STERNOCOSTAL ASPECT

In the anterior view of the heart in its normal anatomic position, the right chambers form the greatest part of its sternocostal surface. The *right border* of the heart is entirely formed by the proximal venae cavae and the less distensible part (sinus venarum) of the *right atrium*. The *right auricle* is the dark, ear-shaped (hence its name) contractile anterior appendage of the right atrium that is separated from the right ventricle by a deep groove, the *atrioventricular sulcus*. Carrying the major coronary arteries and cardiac veins, this sulcus encircles the heart except in the anterior region of the *conus arteriosus*.

The left lateral extent of the *right ventricle*, which forms most of the *inferior margin* of the heart, is marked by the *anterior interventricular sulcus* that bears the left *anterior descending artery* and corresponding branch of the *great cardiac vein*. The position of this sulcus indicates the internal anterior attachment of the interventricular septum that separates the right and left ventricular chambers.

The *left border* of the heart is formed by the *apex* and left wall of the *left ventricle* plus the lobe of the *left auricle* that extends forward under the root of the *pulmonary trunk*.

The *conus arteriosus*, which leads up to the root of the *pulmonary trunk*, is the most superior part of the right ventricle. It was derived from the proximal portion of the single channeled primitive conus that eventually was subdivided into the pulmonary trunk and ascending aorta and their immediately attached parts of the right and left ventricles.

Although the proximal right and left coronary arteries lie deep in the atrioventricular sulcus under the auricles and cannot be seen in a superficial inspection, the anterior descending branch of the left coronary is the most prominent consistent feature of the coronary system observable on the anterior heart surface. The *marginal artery*, a branch of the right coronary that follows the inferior margin of the right ventricle, is also visible. In this specimen, the blue injection mass has filled the *anterior cardiac veins* that drain the anterior wall of the right ventricle. Unlike the rest of the cardiac veins which are confluent upon the coronary sinus, the anterior cardiacs drain directly and individually into the right atrium.

Plate 67   Sternocostal Aspect of Heart   143

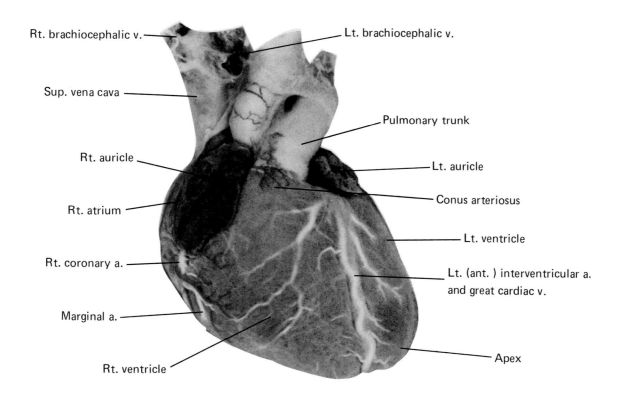

Rt. brachiocephalic v.

Lt. brachiocephalic v.

Sup. vena cava

Pulmonary trunk

Rt. auricle

Lt. auricle

Conus arteriosus

Rt. atrium

Lt. ventricle

Rt. coronary a.

Lt. (ant.) interventricular a.
and great cardiac v.

Marginal a.

Apex

Rt. ventricle

SUPERFICIAL ANATOMY OF THE HEART: INFEROPOSTERIOR (PHRENIC) ASPECT

For this illustration the entire thoracic viscera were excised and photographed in an inverted position to indicate the relations of the heart to the diaphragm and to the other thoracic organs. During dissection of the diaphragm, the adherent inferior mediastinal pleura and phrenic pericardium were also removed.

This specimen shows the "double injection" phenomenon that was very common in the preparation of fetal cadavers. When sufficient pressure was applied to the arterial injection of Neoprene, failure of either the aortic or pulmonary valves permitted the Neoprene to enter the right side of the heart and the venous system. In this case, it filled the right atrium, the coronary sinus and the cardiac veins. Although both arteries and veins are injected, the latter are easily distinguished from the coronary arteries by their wider lumina and more irregular outline.

The left ventricle, right atrium and a lesser contribution by the right ventricle form the phrenic surface of the heart. As on the anterior surface, the delineation between the two ventricles is revealed by the position of the *descending artery*, and the deep *atrioventricular sulcus* separates the ventricular and atrial regions. Here the *right atrium* shows its full relative size, as it is impacted with clotted blood and Neoprene. Anterior and to the left of the sectioned *inferior vena cava* a cylindrical bulge in the inferior atrial wall reveals the position of the *coronary sinus* that empties into the right atrium. This remnant of the embryonic duct of Cuvier functions as a venous manifold that receives all of the cardiac veins except the several small anterior cardiacs of the right ventricle. The confluence of the *small* and *middle cardiac veins* drains into the coronary sinus near its ostium, and the *great cardiac vein* that receives the venous drainage from the anterior and lateral areas of the left ventricle can be seen joining the left end of the sinus.

Note that although the lungs embrace two thirds of the heart, they have not reached the full adult relationship in which their anterior margins nearly meet at the sternum.

Part of the *pericardium* is still adherent to the posterior atrial wall at its reflections around the veins and forms the only separation between the *esophagus* and the *atrium*.

Plate 68   Inferoposterior Aspect of Heart   145

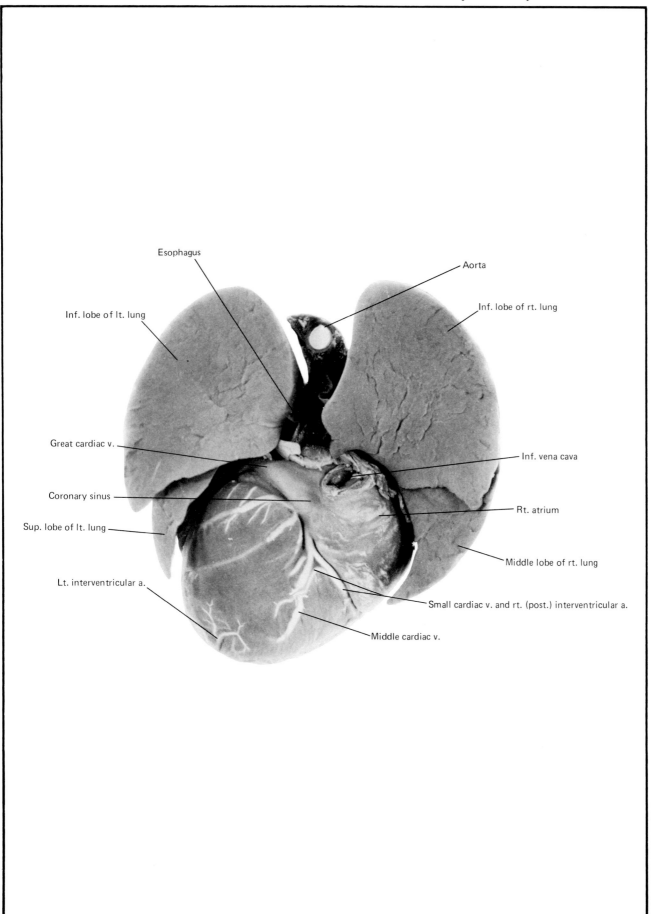

Esophagus

Aorta

Inf. lobe of lt. lung

Inf. lobe of rt. lung

Great cardiac v.

Inf. vena cava

Coronary sinus

Rt. atrium

Sup. lobe of lt. lung

Middle lobe of rt. lung

Lt. interventricular a.

Small cardiac v. and rt. (post.) interventricular a.

Middle cardiac v.

ANTEROPOSTERIOR ARTERIOGRAM OF THE CORONARY ARTERIES

The right and left coronary arteries encircle the heart in the atrioventricular sulcus and form a vascular crown (hence the name coronary) that sends off numerous ventricular branches. These vessels tend to converge toward the apex and supply the myocardium with many smaller penetrating arteries. The total arterial pattern shows considerable variation from one specimen to the next, and only a small number of the larger ventricular branches are sufficiently constant in their location to be given specific names. Even the ventricular areas supplied by either the right or left coronary artery are quite variable, and the complete lack of one or the other of these vessels in a normally functioning heart is not so infrequent as to be surprising. However, one certain statement that may be made about the coronary circulation is that every region of the myocardium in a normally functioning heart must receive ample vascularization from some branch of coronary system, and the sudden interruption of this blood supply produces disastrous consequences to the area involved.

Because of a mutual reciprocity in the territories covered by the right or left coronary arteries, the pattern formed in any single individual may be called a "right predominant" system if the right coronary artery provides an obviously greater share of the myocardial circulation, or a "left predominant" system if the reverse is true.

The subject of this arteriogram shows a "balanced" or nearly typical coronary distribution. Although the *left coronary* arises a little higher than usual from above the left aortic sinus, its conventional course takes it behind the *pulmonary sinuses*, where it divides into a larger *anterior descending branch* and a *circumflex branch*. The first of these follows the anterior ventricular walls down to the right of the apex and around the inferior margin to the inferoposterior ventricular walls. The entire length of this artery superficially marks the location of the interventricular septum into which it sends numerous perpendicular branches.

The circumflex branch of the left coronary artery follows the atrioventricular sulcus. It gives off a variable series of descending branches to the wall of the left ventricle and some small ascending branches to the left atrium and proximal pulmonary veins. As in this specimen, the circumflex branch usually anastomoses with the right coronary in the atrioventricular sulcus posterior to the left chambers, but in a left predominant situation it would provide the posterior descending branch and anastomose in the sulcus of the right chambers.

The *right coronary artery* can be seen arising in the conventional manner from the right sinus and coursing in the atrioventricular sulcus between the right chambers. In the region of the inferior margin of the heart it provides the fairly constant and conspicuous *marginal artery* to the wall of the right ventricle. The right coronary continues along the posterior atrioventricular sulcus where, inferior to the coronary sinus, it sends off the *posterior descending branch* before it anastomoses with the terminals of the circumflex artery.

The major *arteries of the atria* are beautifully illustrated in this arteriogram. Most frequently the larger superior branch is derived just distal to the ostium of the right coronary, but here it arises from the left coronary behind the aorta. It runs over the top of the atria supplying branches to both right and left chambers and the interatrial septum. Its major continuation toward the right atrium supplies the root of the superior vena cava and the *sinoatrial node*. A second atrial branch of the right coronary provides vascularity to the auricle and inferior part of the sinus venarum.

The atrial branches to the great veins and the vasa vasorum of the great arteries form coronary-mediastinal anastomoses through pericardial connections.

Plate 70   Arteriogram of Proximal Ventricular Section   149

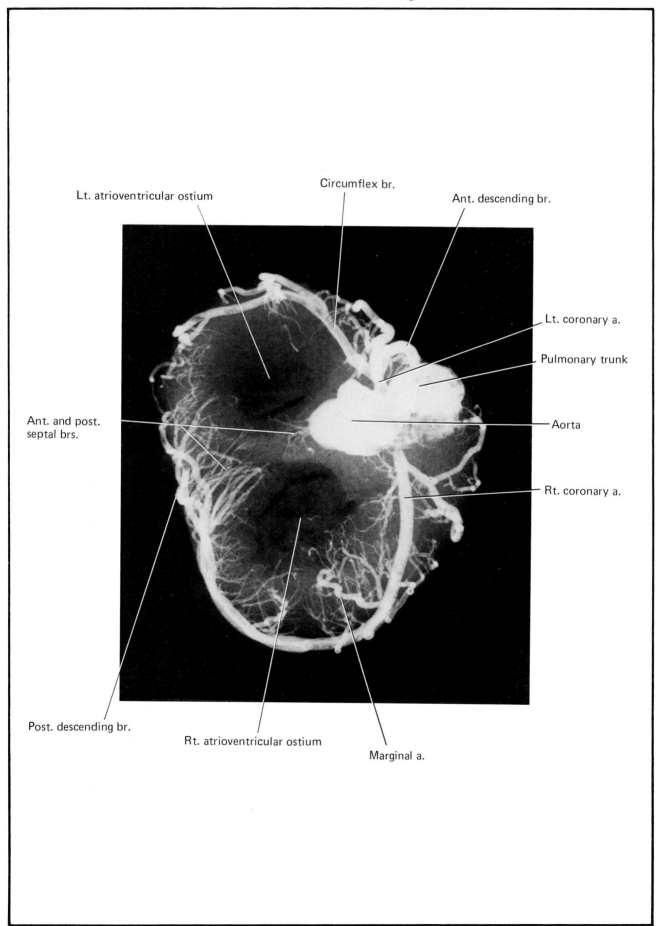

Circumflex br.

Lt. atrioventricular ostium

Ant. descending br.

Lt. coronary a.

Pulmonary trunk

Ant. and post.
septal brs.

Aorta

Rt. coronary a.

Post. descending br.

Rt. atrioventricular ostium

Marginal a.

DISSECTION OF THE HEART: RIGHT ATRIUM

The right atrium of the heart has been opened by an incision parallel to the atrioventricular sulcus, and its anterior wall has been folded back at the *crista terminalis*.

The blood enters the heart through the venae cavae. The *inferior vena cava* opens into the lower part of the *sinus venarum*, a less distensible part of the right atrium that is formed by the confluence of the caval veins and is delineated from the auricular part of the atrium by the crista terminalis. The *valve of the inferior vena cava* is a fold of tissue that directs the fetal blood from the inferior vena cava toward the *foramen ovale,* through which it enters the left atrium and the systemic circulation. This valve is usually resorbed or very much attenuated in the adult.

Anterior to the foramen ovale lies the *ostium of the coronary sinus* that discharges the greatest part of the venous return of the cardiac veins into the right atrium. It is often guarded by an incomplete valvular cusp.

The *right auricle* has been sectioned, leaving the lobular extension of its chamber lying as a flap over the right ventricle. However, the reflected part shows the characteristic structures of its internal wall. As in all contractile chambers of the heart, the innermost part of the myocardium is arranged in prominent bundles of muscle that are coated with endocardial epithelium and separated from each other by deep furrows. These muscular projections are generically called *trabeculae carneae* (girders of flesh), but specific terms may be applied to topographically or morphologically distinct types.

In the right auricle the muscular bundles generally are arranged to radiate toward the free edge of the auricle like the parallel teeth of a comb. Hence, collectively they are called the *musculi pectinati*.

The left anterior boundary of the right atrium is formed by the atrioventricular ring that supports the *tricuspid valve*. Through the ostium of this valve the auricular contraction sends the blood into the right ventricle.

Plate 71   Right Atrium   151

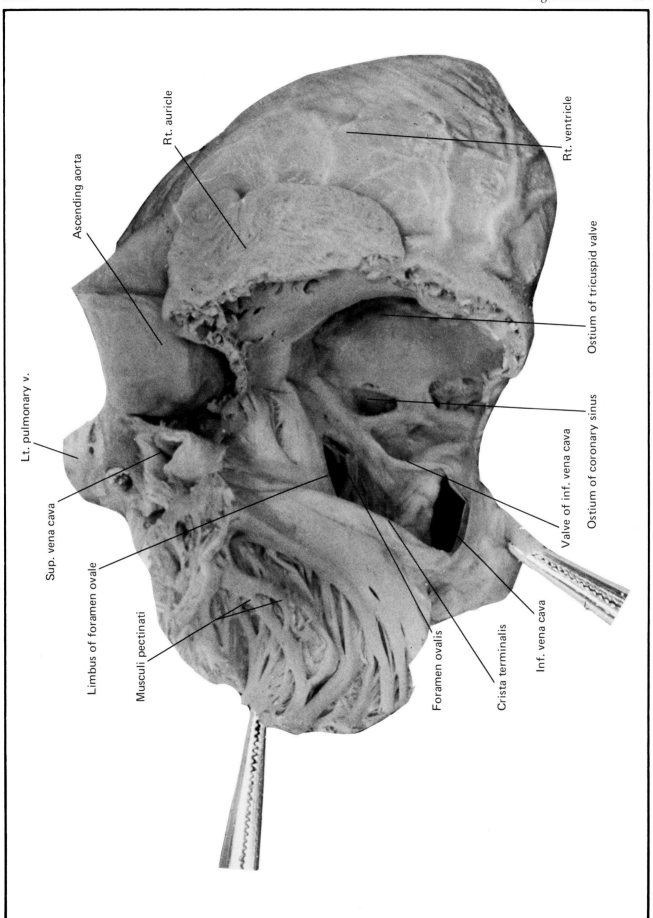

Rt. auricle

Ascending aorta

Rt. ventricle

Ostium of tricuspid valve

Lt. pulmonary v.

Ostium of coronary sinus

Valve of inf. vena cava

Sup. vena cava

Limbus of foramen ovale

Musculi pectinati

Foramen ovalis

Crista terminalis

Inf. vena cava

DISSECTION OF THE HEART: RIGHT VENTRICLE

A spiraling incision has been made through the anterior walls of the *right ventricle, conus arteriosus* and the *pulmonary trunk* to reveal their internal morphology.

The anterior aspect of the *tricuspid valve* and its associated structures is prominently displayed. Inversion of the valve is prevented by three sets of *chordae tendineae* that are tensed by *papillary muscles* during myocardial contractions.

Although the position, size and subdivision of the papillary muscles tend to be quite variable, usually three distinct groups can be identified. The *anterior papillary muscle* arises from the anterior ventricular wall next to the incision, and a set of *posterior papillary muscles* may be seen arising from the inferoposterior wall. The third set of the short *septal papillary muscles* originate on the surface of the septum.

The chordae tendineae from each group of papillary muscles are distributed over approximately one half of the ventricular surface of two adjacent valve cusps, so that the position of the papillary muscles is more directly related to the *commissures* between the valves than to the cusps themselves. Nevertheless, the valve cusps are also designated as *anterior, posterior* and *septal* in their positions.

Toward the apical end of the right ventricular chamber, the size and number of the *trabeculae carneae* increase, and one modified version of these structures, the *septomarginal band,* bridges the interval between the septum and the base of the anterior papillary muscle. A white strip of modified myocardial tissue can be seen beneath the endocardium as it descends the septum and crosses on the septomarginal band. This is part of the right ventricular arm of the impulse-conducting *bundle of His* that initiates contraction in the anterior ventricular wall and the attached papillary muscle.

The part of the chamber that extends into the *conus arteriosus* is called the *infundibulum* because it funnels the blood into the pulmonary trunk. Its walls are relatively smooth, particularly near the superior region where the right, left and anterior cusps of the *pulmonary valve* are found.

Within the opened pulmonary trunk, the orifices of the two *pulmonary arteries* and the *ductus arteriosus* are displayed.

Plate 72   Right Ventricle   153

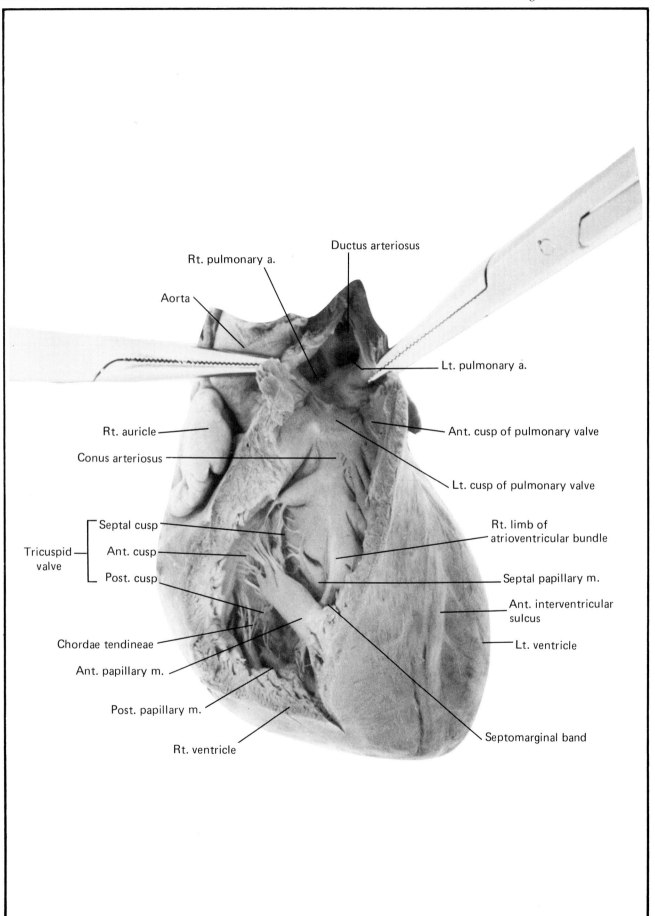

Rt. pulmonary a.

Ductus arteriosus

Aorta

Lt. pulmonary a.

Rt. auricle

Ant. cusp of pulmonary valve

Conus arteriosus

Lt. cusp of pulmonary valve

Septal cusp

Rt. limb of
atrioventricular bundle

Tricuspid
valve

Ant. cusp

Post. cusp

Septal papillary m.

Ant. interventricular
sulcus

Chordae tendineae

Lt. ventricle

Ant. papillary m.

Post. papillary m.

Septomarginal band

Rt. ventricle

DISSECTION OF THE HEART: LEFT ATRIUM

The left atrium shows less internal complexity than the right. It is located on the posterior aspect of the heart in the midline of the mediastinum and therefore receives *right* and *left pulmonary veins* of equal length. Here the ostia of these veins have been reflected upward or split when the posterior atrial wall was opened and retracted. During fetal life the major quantity of blood enters the left atrium through the *foramen ovale* of the *interatrial septum.* The dual nature of the septum is indicated by the heavier anterior *septum secundum* and the thinner posterior *septum primum.* The structure of these septa should be such that the altered hemodynamics of parturition brings them into apposition to seal the interatrial opening. In this specimen, however, the obvious deficiency in the septum primum produced a persistent interatrial defect and probably contributed to its neonatal death.

The contractile sac of the *left auricle* extends over the border of the left ventricle, and the trabeculations of its *musculi pectinati* are revealed.

The atrioventricular ring supports the two cusped *mitral valves,* whose ostium passes the blood into the left ventricle.

Plate 73   Left Atrium   155

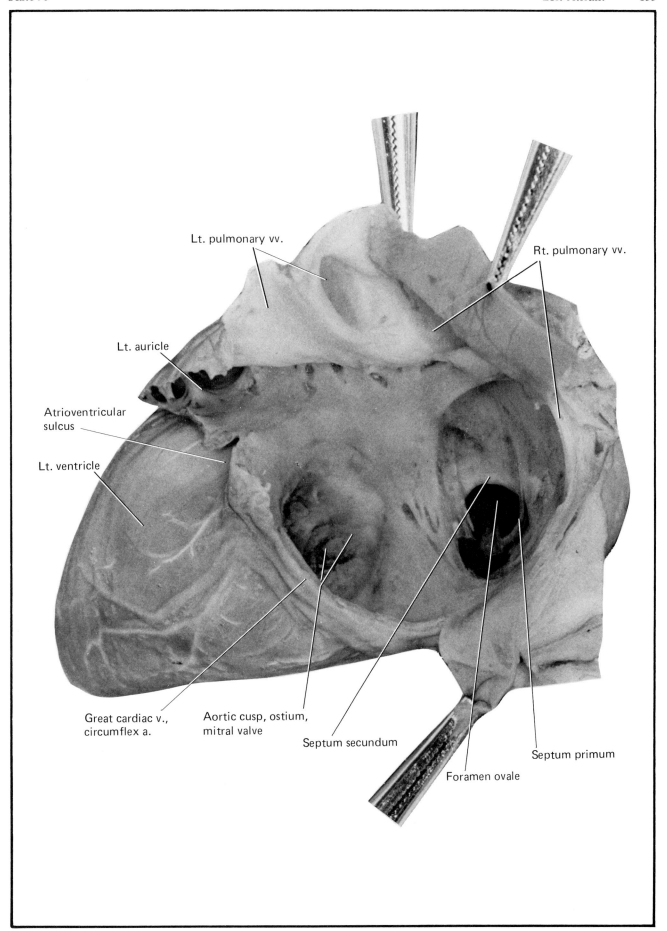

Lt. pulmonary vv.

Rt. pulmonary vv.

Lt. auricle

Atrioventricular
sulcus

Lt. ventricle

Great cardiac v.,
circumflex a.

Aortic cusp, ostium,
mitral valve

Septum secundum

Foramen ovale

Septum primum

DISSECTION OF THE HEART: LEFT VENTRICLE

An incision parallel to the anterior attachment of the interventricular septum has permitted the retraction of the anterolateral wall of the left ventricle. The superior continuation of this incision has also opened the ascending aorta to expose its sinuses and their valves.

In the posterior region of the left ventricle two sets of stout *anterior* and *posterior papillary muscles* are attached to the two cusps of the *mitral valve*. The anterior or aortic cusp is the larger of the two and separates the mitral ostium from the aortic orifice. Unlike the other atrioventricular cusps, it has a relatively smooth ventricular surface. Only the free edge of the posterior cusp is visible here, but it is obvious that each set of papillary muscles sends *chordae tendineae* to both cusps.

Near the apical part of the ventricular chamber the *trabeculae carneae* are quite numerous, and many are of the type that is attached at both ends but free in the middle.

The ventricular entrance to the aortic orifice is called the *vestibule*. It is devoid of trabeculae and its upper walls are fibrous rather than muscular. The orifice is guarded by three semilunar valve cusps whose upper surfaces face their respective *aortic sinuses*. The right and left aortic sinuses each contain the ostium of their corresponding *coronary artery*. In this specimen the *posterior aortic sinus* bears the small ostium of *the artery of the conus* that supplies a part of the upper anterior interventricular septum in 40 percent of the cases.

In the perinatal cadaver, the thickness of the myocardium is approximately equal in both ventricles, but the wall of the left ventricle eventually becomes three times thicker than that of the right. This situation roughly reflects the disparity between the blood pressures of the pulmonary and systemic systems.

Plate 74   Left Ventricle   157

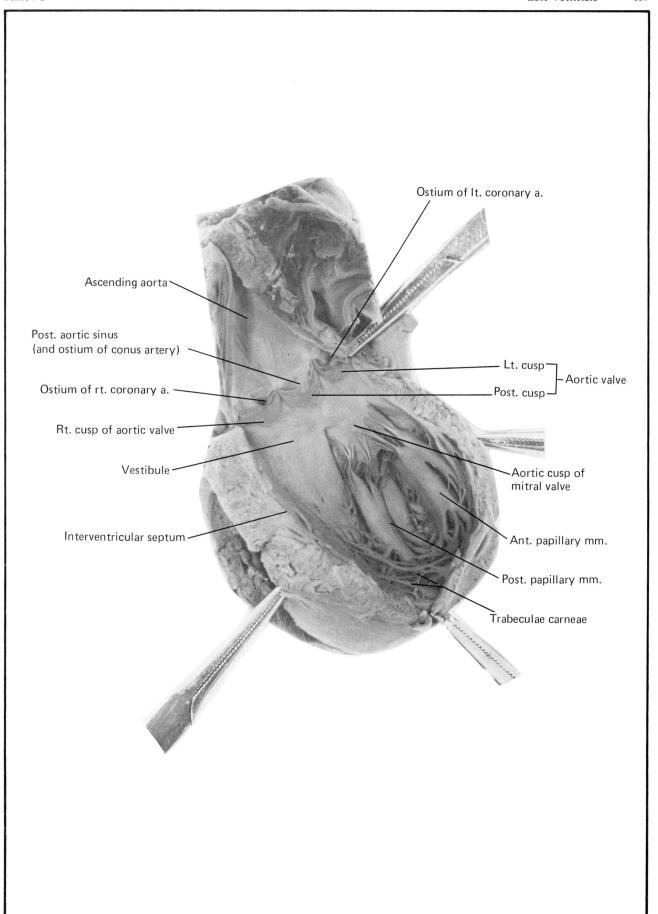

Ostium of lt. coronary a.

Ascending aorta

Post. aortic sinus
(and ostium of conus artery)

Lt. cusp ⌐
                    ⌐ Aortic valve
Post. cusp ⌐

Ostium of rt. coronary a.

Rt. cusp of aortic valve

Aortic cusp of
mitral valve

Vestibule

Ant. papillary mm.

Interventricular septum

Post. papillary mm.

Trabeculae carneae

CROSS SECTION OF THE THORAX THROUGH THE SIXTH THORACIC VERTEBRA

This view is particularly instructive of the topographic relations of the individual heart chambers to the anterior thoracic wall, lungs and posterior mediastinum. The plane of section has passed through all four heart chambers and the ostia of the atrioventricular valves. The attachment of the *chordae tendineae* to the ventricular surfaces and edges of the *tricuspid valve* is easily discernible.

Note the rich vascularity indicated by the Neoprene injection of the myocardium and the position of the *coronary arteries* in the *atrioventricular sulcus*.

In this specimen failure of the pulmonary valve permitted the Neoprene injection mass to enter the *right ventricle* and the *right* and *left atria*. For clarity the mass has been removed from the heart chambers, but its continued presence in the pulmonary veins marks the topographic and functional relations of these structures to the left atrium.

The posterior mediastinum here shows relative positions of the *esophagus* and *descending aorta* to the *left atrium* and its veins.

A very important structure of the posterior mediastinum, the *thoracic duct*, runs along the anterior surface of the vertebral bodies, but its small size and very thin walls preclude its labeling with any certainty in this section.

Plate 75   Cross Section through 6th Thoracic Vertebra   159

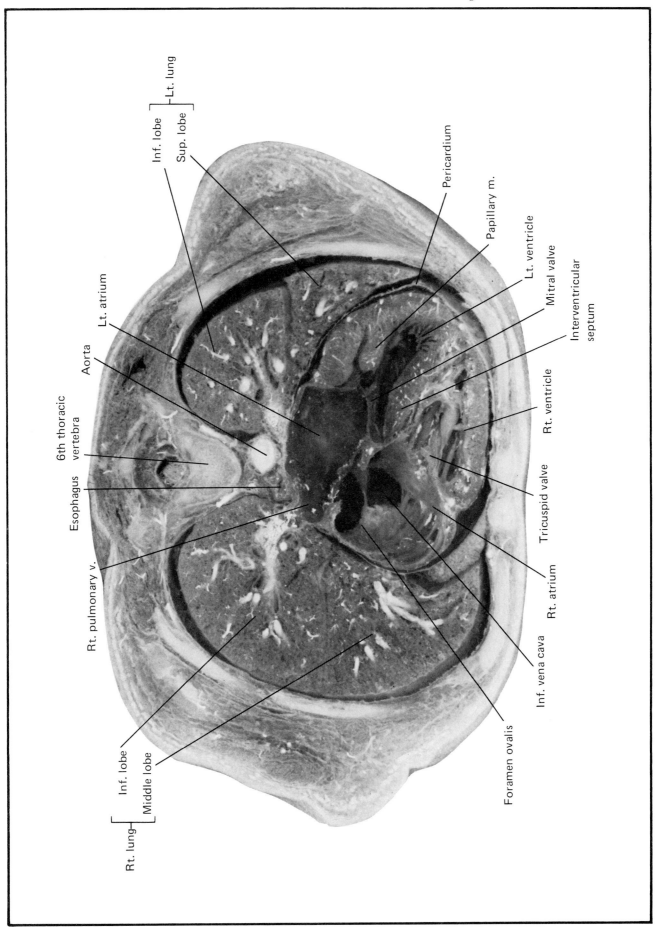

Inf. lobe ⎤ Lt. lung
Sup. lobe ⎦

Pericardium

Papillary m.

Lt. ventricle

Mitral valve

Interventricular septum

Rt. ventricle

Tricuspid valve

Rt. atrium

Inf. vena cava

Foramen ovalis

Lt. atrium

Aorta

6th thoracic vertebra

Esophagus

Rt. pulmonary v.

Inf. lobe ⎤ Rt. lung
Middle lobe ⎦

CORROSION CAST OF THE GREAT ARTERIES: ANTERIOR ASPECT

Because of the difficulty in appreciating the spatial relationships of the large arteries of the fetal thorax, a Neoprene cast of the lumina of these vessels is presented.

The bulges of the *pulmonary* and *aortic sinuses* show some irregular pitting because of air bubbles trapped in these structures during the injection, but their essential form and the origins of the *right* and *left coronary arteries* are well illustrated.

The short *pulmonary trunk* empties directly into the large *ductus arteriosus*, and the more inferior and laterally directed *pulmonary arteries* receive but a fraction of blood discharged by the fetal right ventricle.

The sequential origins of the large arteries from the aortic arch show a minor variation in which the *left common carotid* arises from the same root as the *brachiocephalic artery*.

Plate 76   Anterior Aspect of Great Arteries   161

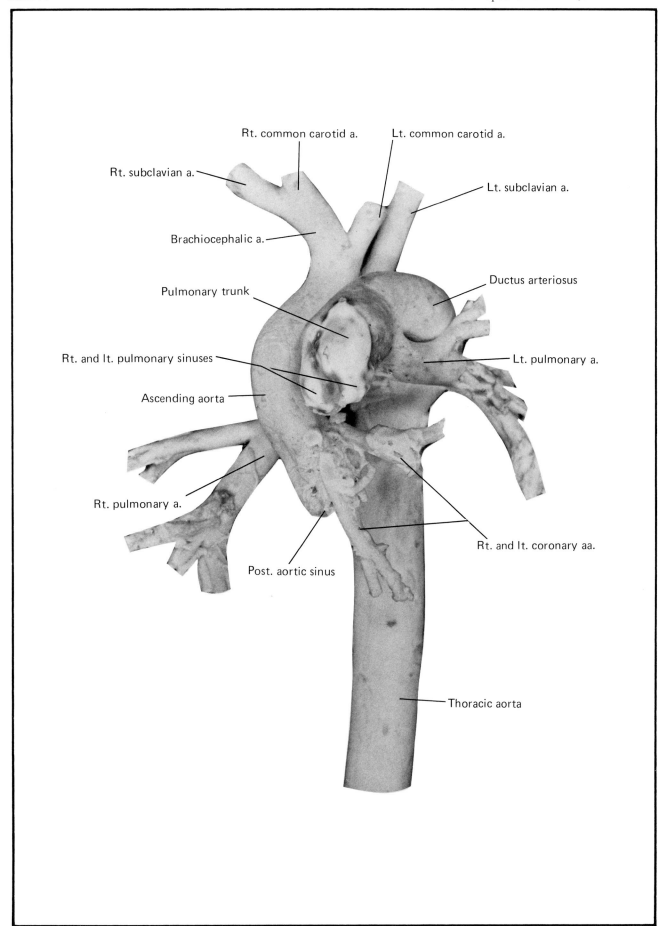

Rt. common carotid a.

Lt. common carotid a.

Rt. subclavian a.

Lt. subclavian a.

Brachiocephalic a.

Ductus arteriosus

Pulmonary trunk

Rt. and lt. pulmonary sinuses

Lt. pulmonary a.

Ascending aorta

Rt. pulmonary a.

Rt. and lt. coronary aa.

Post. aortic sinus

Thoracic aorta

CORROSION CAST OF THE GREAT ARTERIES: POSTERIOR ASPECT

This view is more informative than the preceding one. The relative sizes of the posterior part of the *aortic arch* and the *ductus arteriosus* at their junction is indicative of the dual distribution of the returned placental blood to the body regions of the fetus.

The placental blood is recycled to the fetus via the umbilical vein and inferior vena cava. On entering the right atrium it passes in either of two directions. The stream that is directed through the fossa ovalis into the left atrium and left ventricle is the only one that supplies the head and upper extremities. It is discharged into the carotids and subclavians from the aortic arch, and only a lesser fraction of it is destined for the lower body through the narrow descending part of the posterior arch.

The stream of caval blood that enters the right atrioventricular ostium to the right ventricle is discharged to the lungs via the pulmonary trunk and to the lower torso and lower extremities by the ductus arteriosus.

Analysis of this figure should indicate the extent of morphologic modification that these vessels must rapidly undergo at parturition. The massive ductus arteriosus must become rapidly stenosed, and the narrow posterior aortic arch must enlarge to permit the left ventricle to supply the entire systemic circulation.

Plate 77   Posterior Aspect of Great Arteries   163

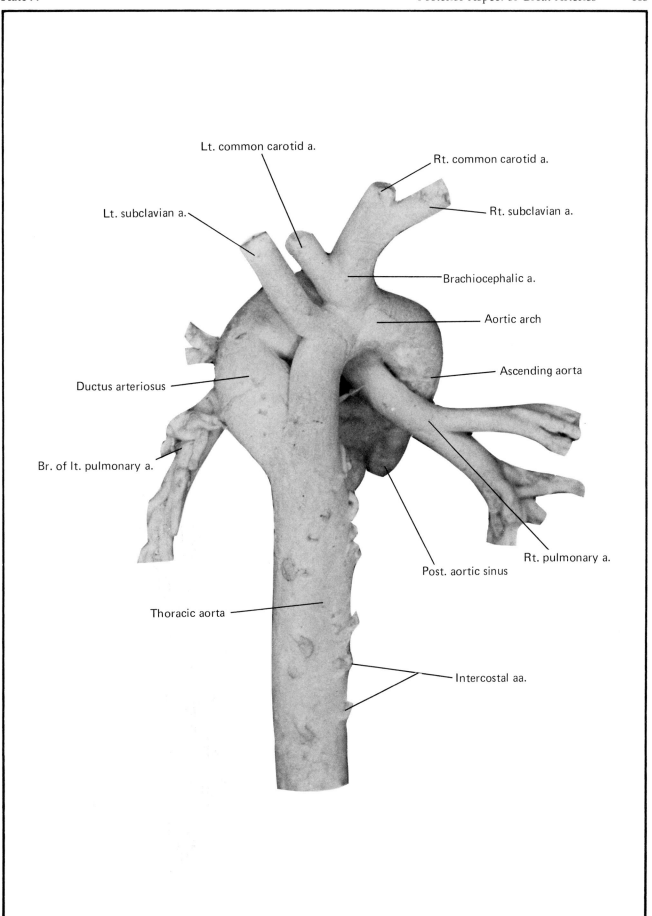

Lt. common carotid a.

Rt. common carotid a.

Lt. subclavian a.

Rt. subclavian a.

Brachiocephalic a.

Aortic arch

Ascending aorta

Ductus arteriosus

Br. of lt. pulmonary a.

Rt. pulmonary a.

Post. aortic sinus

Thoracic aorta

Intercostal aa.

SUPERFICIAL ANATOMY OF THE LUNG: ANTERIOR ASPECT

The lungs are the largest organs in the thoracic cavity. Their parenchyma consists of a great number of small chambers (alveoli) in which aspirated air is brought into physiologic proximity with the blood. They therefore contain a system of air ducts (the *tracheobronchial tree*), a vascular system that circulates the blood for respiratory processing (the *pulmonary arteries* and *veins*) and a separate systemic arterial supply for their own nutrition (the *bronchial arteries*).

The lungs prove to be quite plastic in their development. Although the major pattern of the bronchial branching and the general lobation are determined genetically, the final shape of the lung is virtually a cast of the thoracic space that accurately reflects, in projections and depressions, its intimate relations with other structures.

In this anterior view of the excised lungs, a negative mold of the mediastinal organs is seen formed by their medial surfaces. These examples were taken from a stillborn fetus of 28 weeks' gestation and are therefore fixed in the prenatal uninflated condition.

The perinatal lung has not reached its full development; it is relatively smaller and lacking the full elaboration of the adult bronchial system. The bronchi may have up to 17 orders of subdivision at birth, but continued postnatal development eventually produces up to 24 orders of branches.

The right lung is shorter, wider and more voluminous than the left. The asymmetry is mainly attributable to the increased height of the right hemidiaphragm that shortens the right lung and the leftward displacement of the heart that markedly encroaches on the volume of the left lung.

For convenience, the form of each lung may be conceptualized as a half of a cone that has been split from its apex to its base with the mediastinal surface being on the plane of section. It then presents an apex; an anterior, a posterior and an inferior border; and a medial (mediastinal), a lateral (costal) and a basal (diaphragmatic) surface.

Plate 78   Anterior Aspect of Lung   165

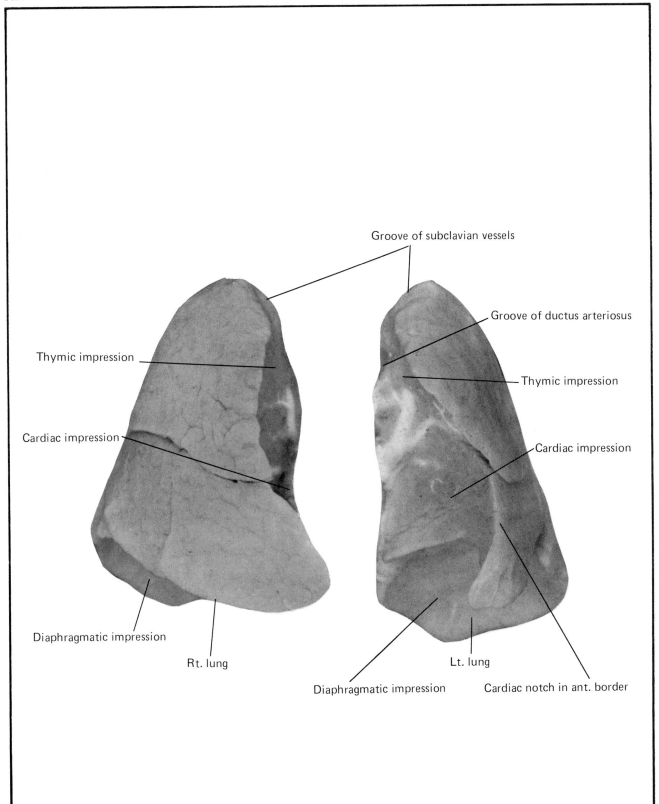

Groove of subclavian vessels

Groove of ductus arteriosus

Thymic impression

Thymic impression

Cardiac impression

Cardiac impression

Diaphragmatic impression

Rt. lung

Lt. lung

Diaphragmatic impression

Cardiac notch in ant. border

SUPERFICIAL ANATOMY OF THE LUNG: LATERAL ASPECT

The right lung is divided into three lobes by two inter-lobar fissures. The *oblique fissure* virtually bisects the organ on a plane of about 45 degrees from the perpendicular and separates the *inferior lobe* from the *middle* and *superior lobes*. The *horizontal fissure* separates the superior and middle lobes.

Because the lung is fixed at the hilum and the greatest volumetric changes occur near the diaphragm, the vectors of lung expansion are not equal in all directions. The slippage between the parietal and visceral pleurae permits differential movement between the thoracic wall and the lung, but the functional significance of the interlobar fissures is to relieve intrapulmonary differential stresses by the slipping of the opposing interlobar surfaces.

Because the bend of the fetal ribs around the thoracic wall is more horizontal than in the adult, the relations between specific intercostal spaces and the underlying lung lobations change with postnatal growth. In addition, the fetal lungs have a much greater relative anteroposterior depth and a shorter apical-basal length than the adult, so that the interlobar fissures are generally 1.5 intercostal spaces higher in the fetus.

Plate 79   Lateral Aspect of Lung   167

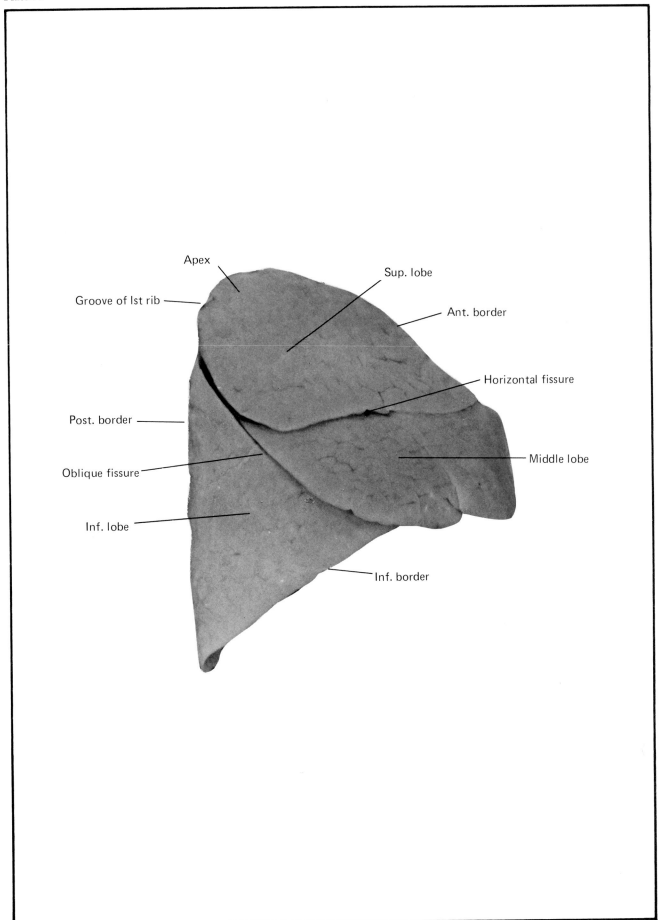

Apex

Groove of lst rib

Sup. lobe

Ant. border

Horizontal fissure

Post. border

Oblique fissure

Middle lobe

Inf. lobe

Inf. border

SUPERFICIAL ANATOMY OF THE LUNG: MEDIAL ASPECT

The medial (mediastinal) view of the right lung shows the large concavities formed by the right side of the heart and right hemidiaphragm. In the apical and posterior regions the individual grooves and depressions formed by large mediastinal vessels can be determined. Although the hilar anatomy will be discussed in subsequent plates, the root of the lung is used as a reference point for other mediastinal structures.

Between the apex and the groove for the dorsal part of the first rib, the *right subclavian artery* has left its impression as it passed from the mediastinum to the axillary region. Below this area, a hook-shaped groove that arches over the root of the lung marks the course of the *azygos vein* where it leaves the posterior mediastinum to reach the superior vena cava. Medial to the posterior border of the inferior lobe, a shallow depression indicates the relationship of the *esophagus* to the lung in the posterior mediastinum. Note that the oblique fissure commences at the dorsum of the lung root and, after girdling the lung, ends at the inferior ventral surface of the root.

Plate 80   Medial Aspect of Lung   169

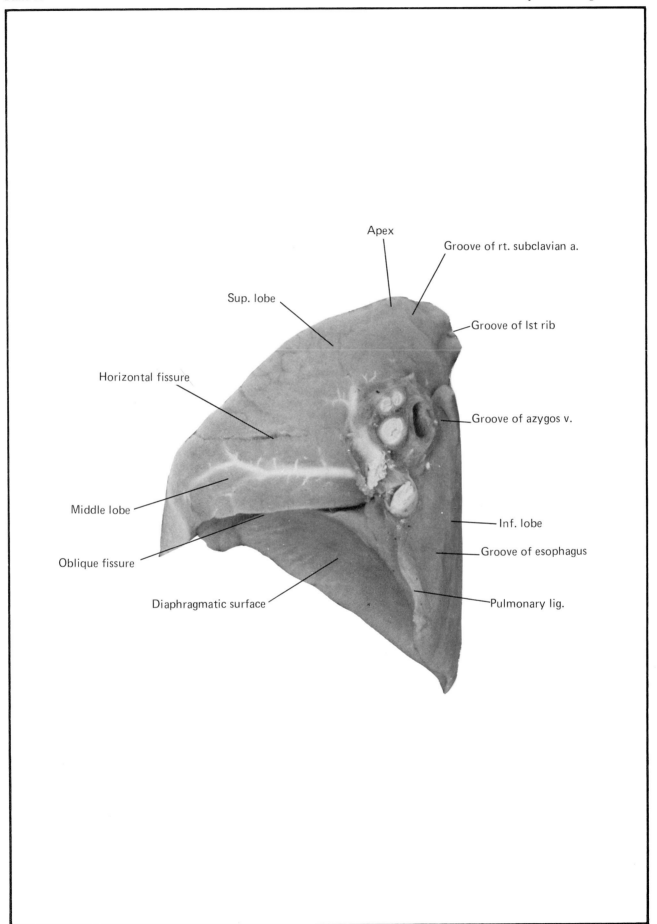

Apex

Groove of rt. subclavian a.

Sup. lobe

Groove of lst rib

Horizontal fissure

Groove of azygos v.

Middle lobe

Inf. lobe

Groove of esophagus

Oblique fissure

Diaphragmatic surface

Pulmonary lig.

BRONCHOPULMONARY SEGMENTS OF THE RIGHT LUNG: LATERAL ASPECT

Each tertiary bronchus bears a resectable broncho-vascular unit, the *bronchopulmonary segment*. The bronchus with its corresponding branch of the *pulmonary artery* and its entwining *bronchial artery* forms an anatomic triad that is the central element of the segment. Adjoining segments are separated by a cleavage plane that is readily divided by blunt dissection to reveal the radicles of the *pulmonary vein*. These veins are therefore intersegmental and can drain blood from two or more segments that share a common boundary.

This morphologic arrangement is best understood through the developmental history of the bronchopulmonary segment. At an intermediate stage of lung morphogenesis, the segments are represented as individual mesenchymal bulbs overlying the buds of the growing tertiary bronchi, so that in aggregate they give the early lung the appearance of a bunch of tightly packed grapes. The branches of the pulmonary and bronchial arteries develop within the mesenchyme along the tubes of bronchial epithelium, whereas the pulmonary veins form on the ventral surface of the lung with their radicles lying in the groove between the segmental bulges. With further elaboration of the lung, the surfaces of these segmental lobules are brought into apposition to form the intersegmental planes and thus enfold the tributaries of the pulmonary veins.

The delineation of the individual bronchopulmonary segments in the postnatal specimen is best accomplished by selectively inflating the individual tertiary bronchi, but in the material shown here, the injected pulmonary veins were followed from the hilum by blunt separation of their intersegmental planes.

The lungs have a total of 18 bronchopulmonary segments, 10 in the right lung and 8 in the left. This lateral view of the right lung shows that all segments except the medial and posterior basals are projected against the lateral costal surface. The individual segments have been labeled to indicate their location with respect to the major lung lobes.

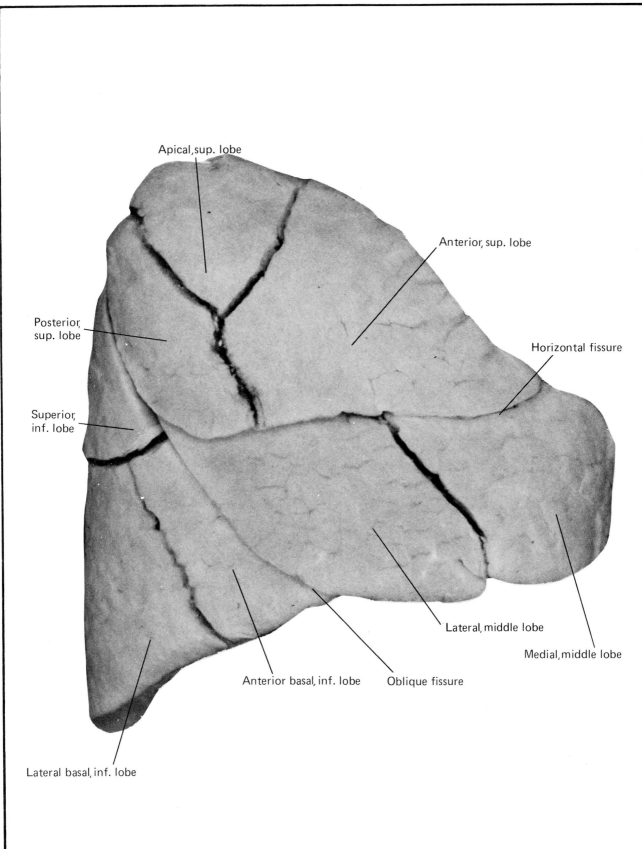

Apical, sup. lobe

Anterior, sup. lobe

Posterior, sup. lobe

Horizontal fissure

Superior, inf. lobe

Lateral, middle lobe

Medial, middle lobe

Anterior basal, inf. lobe

Oblique fissure

Lateral basal, inf. lobe

THE HILUM AND BRONCHOPULMONARY SEGMENTS OF THE RIGHT LUNG: MEDIAL ASPECT

The hilum of the lung is the potential concavity through which the structures in the root of the lung enter or leave its substance.

The *right pulmonary artery* commences to branch within the lung root; but because its major branch must pass under the first lateral bronchus (eparterial bronchus), it lies anterior to the main bronchus in the hilum. However, within the lung the pulmonary branches typically run in a dorsolateral relation to their respective bronchi.

Dorsal and inferior to the sectioned stump of the bronchus, *bronchial arteries* may be seen coursing in the peribronchial tissue. These fine systemic arteries are direct branches of the aorta on the left side and derivatives of an upper intercostal artery on the right. Because the pulmonary arteries carry only blood of low oxygenation, it is the bronchial arteries that provide the vascular nutrition to the nonalveolar lung tissues and the pleura.

The *pulmonary veins* are found ventral and inferior to the bronchus in the hilum. They are formed by the confluence of the intersegmental veins that tend to lie equidistant between two adjacent segmental bronchi. A large superficial pulmonary vein courses along the medial surface of the medial lobe to empty into the right inferior vein. This variant is found quite frequently and serves to illustrate the original superficial and ventral relationship of the pulmonary veins to the developing lung tissue.

In this medial view, all bronchopulmonary segments of the right lung are shown except the lateral segment of the middle lobe. The intersegmental plane that separates the posterior basal from the medial basal segment is one that is most constant in position and easily located as it lies along the attachment of the pulmonary ligament.

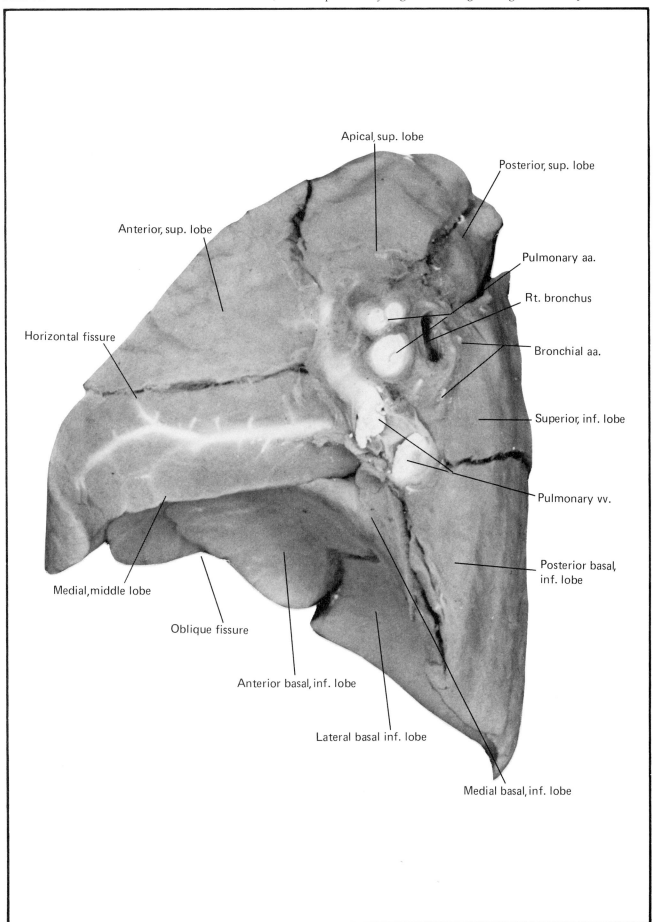

Apical, sup. lobe

Posterior, sup. lobe

Anterior, sup. lobe

Pulmonary aa.

Rt. bronchus

Horizontal fissure

Bronchial aa.

Superior, inf. lobe

Pulmonary vv.

Medial, middle lobe

Posterior basal, inf. lobe

Oblique fissure

Anterior basal, inf. lobe

Lateral basal inf. lobe

Medial basal, inf. lobe

SUPERFICIAL ANATOMY OF THE LEFT LUNG: LATERAL ASPECT

The left lung has only two lobes separated by a single interlobar *oblique fissure*. The large, irregular *superior lobe* is the morphologic equivalent of the combined middle and superior lobes of the right lung. In this lateral view it shows its two most salient characteristics: a *lingula* that projects beneath the heart apex and a marked *cardiac notch* in its *anterior border*. Both of these features are the result of the sinistral disposition of the ventricles which encroach on the left pleural cavity.

The presence here of an incomplete atypical fissure that partially separates the inferior or lingular division from the rest of the left superior lobe is a fairly frequent occurrence. Supernumerary sublobar fissures frequently are found in any lobe of both lungs and are indicative of one or more of the intersegmental planes between the bronchopulmonary segments.

Plate 83   Lateral Aspect of Left Lung   175

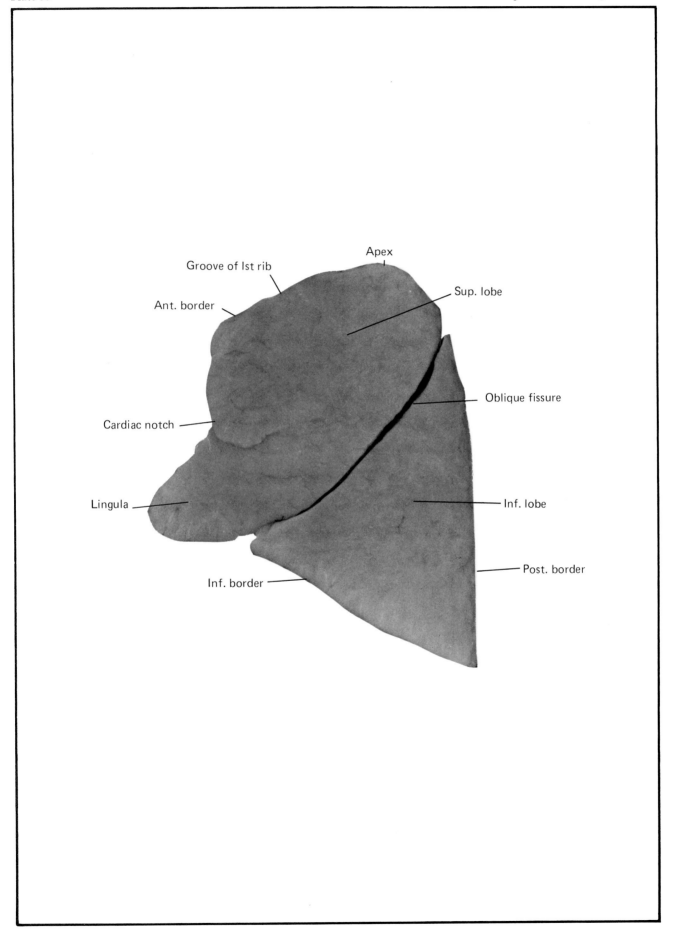

Groove of Ist rib

Apex

Ant. border

Sup. lobe

Oblique fissure

Cardiac notch

Lingula

Inf. lobe

Inf. border

Post. border

SUPERFICIAL ANATOMY OF THE LEFT LUNG: MEDIAL ASPECT

The subpleural structures of the left side of the mediastinum leave deeper impressions on the medial surface of the left lung than those of the right side. The concavity caused by the ventricular projection of the heart considerably attenuates the thickness of the anterior regions of the left superior lobe. The groove of the *aortic arch* is also quite pronounced where it loops over the root of the lung and descends in the posterior mediastinum.

The more posterior origin of the *left subclavian artery* can be determined by following its groove over the apex of the lung.

The *ductus arteriosus* lies inferior to the *aortic arch* and is in direct contact with the superior surface of the lung root. Its presence forces the aortic arch to make a wider arc, and it also serves to deepen the aortic impression.

Plate 84   Medial Aspect of Left Lung   177

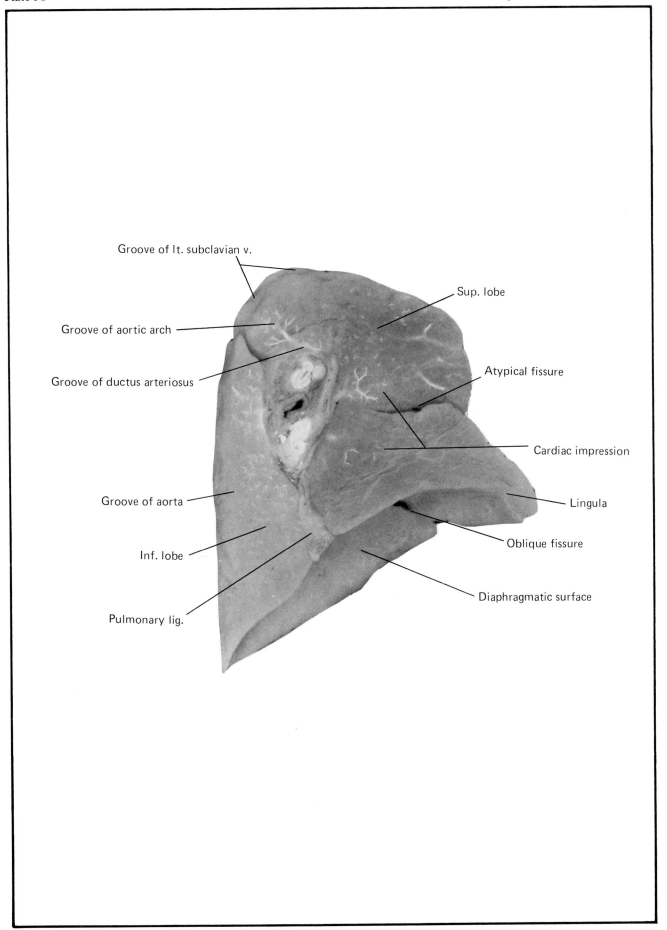

Groove of lt. subclavian v.

Groove of aortic arch

Groove of ductus arteriosus

Groove of aorta

Inf. lobe

Pulmonary lig.

Sup. lobe

Atypical fissure

Cardiac impression

Lingula

Oblique fissure

Diaphragmatic surface

BRONCHOPULMONARY SEGMENTS OF THE LEFT LUNG: LATERAL ASPECT

The left lung contains eight bronchopulmonary segments, giving it two less than the right lung. Although the left lung has less volume than the right, this structural asymmetry is mostly an artificial imposition to maintain the consistency of the definition of the bronchopulmonary segment (i.e., the single segment must arise from a tertiary bronchus). The discrepancy in the segment number is caused by the combining of the areas of the apical and posterior segments of the superior lobe and the anterior and medial basal segments of the inferior lobe. The rationale for this lies in the fact that what were segmental tertiary bronchi on the right side arise as quarternary branches of very short common tertiary roots on the left.

The *superior lobe* of the left lung is divided into *superior* and *inferior divisions.* The superior division consists of the *anterior* and *apical-posterior segments,* and the *inferior division,* which corresponds to the right middle lobe, contains the *superior and inferior lingular segments.* These latter segments are dependent on long, slender bronchial derivatives of the upper lobe and are frequently the subjects of surgical resection.

In the inferior lobe the *superior, anterior-medial* and *lateral basal segments* are projected onto the costal surface of the pleura.

Plate 85   Bronchopulmonary Segments of Right Lung: Lateral Aspect   179

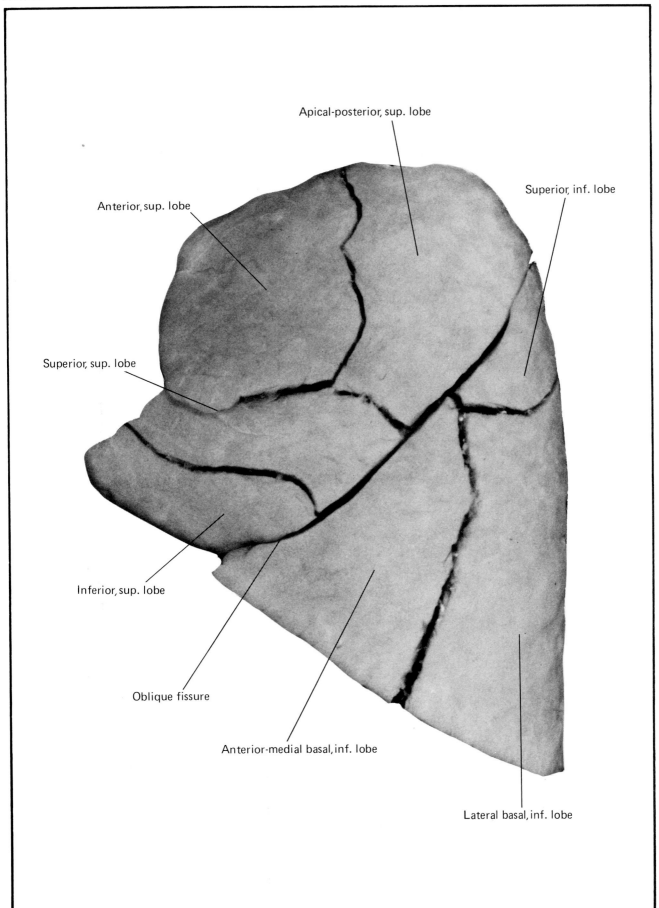

Apical-posterior, sup. lobe

Superior, inf. lobe

Anterior, sup. lobe

Superior, sup. lobe

Inferior, sup. lobe

Oblique fissure

Anterior-medial basal, inf. lobe

Lateral basal, inf. lobe

THE HILUM AND BRONCHOPULMONARY SEGMENTS OF THE LEFT LUNG: MEDIAL ASPECT

The hilar anatomy of the left lung differs from that of the right in that the *pulmonary artery* does not pass inferior to the first lateral bronchus, but instead passes directly over and dorsal to the *main bronchus*.

The *bronchial arteries* are seen ventral and inferior to the stump of the bronchus, and the combined *superior* and *inferior pulmonary veins* have been sectioned at the point where they enter the left atrium.

This view is particularly instructive in that the branches forming the superior pulmonary vein may be observed emerging from the *intersegmental planes* of both the *superior* and *inferior divisions* of the *superior lobe*.

All of the injected finer subpleural vessels of the mediastinal surface are small venous radicles. Note that they are more prominent where the lung has been impressed by mediastinal structures.

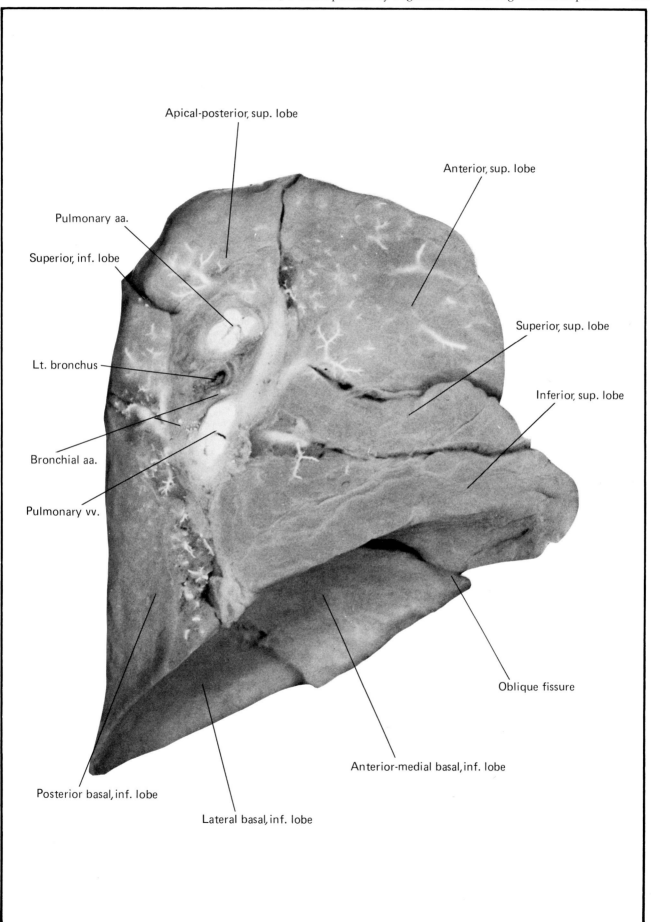

Apical-posterior, sup. lobe

Anterior, sup. lobe

Pulmonary aa.

Superior, inf. lobe

Lt. bronchus

Superior, sup. lobe

Inferior, sup. lobe

Bronchial aa.

Pulmonary vv.

Oblique fissure

Posterior basal, inf. lobe

Anterior-medial basal, inf. lobe

Lateral basal, inf. lobe

ANTEROPOSTERIOR ARTERIOGRAM OF THE RIGHT PULMONARY ARTERY

Within the lung the pulmonary arteries faithfully follow the bronchial ramifications and can, therefore, be labeled according to their segmental distributions. Fortunately, there is sufficient density in the peripheral parenchyma to visualize the contours and fissures of the three lobes. The three dimensional relations of the arteries of the superior lobe can be understood more easily when compared with the lateral view, but the long course of middle lobar branches here is well displayed. It can be seen why the root of the middle lobe is more liable to compression that leads to the "middle lobe syndrome." The four descending segmental branches of the inferior lobe can be seen spreading to the four basal segments.

Plate 87   Anteroposterior Arteriogram of Right Pulmonary Artery   183

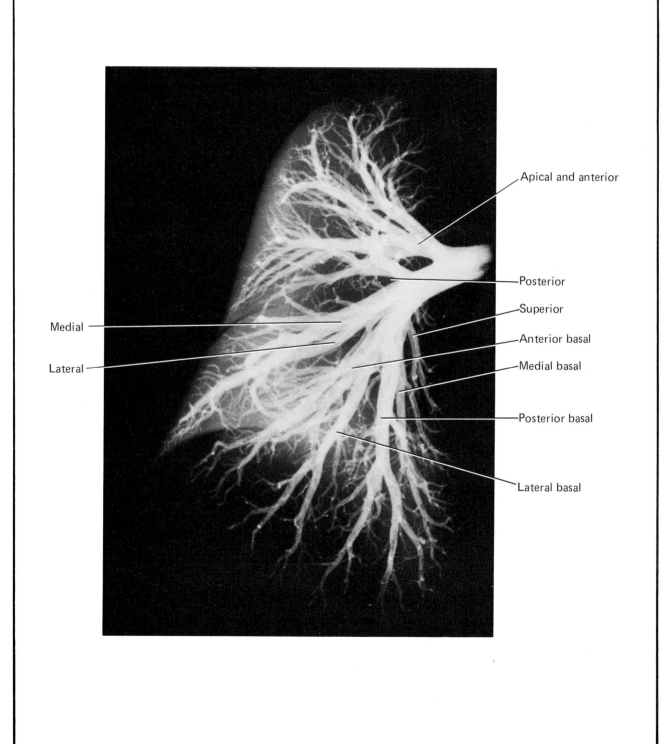

LATERAL ARTERIOGRAM OF THE RIGHT PULMONARY ARTERY

Because the fetal lungs have a greater anteroposterior depth and are relatively thinner than the adult lung in width, the distribution of the segmental arteries is better revealed in the lateral view.

The location and comparative sizes of the three bronchopulmonary segments of the upper lobe can be readily determined, as can the lateral and medial segmental arteries of the middle lobe.

In the inferior lobe, the dorsally directed *superior segmental branch* reveals why its segmental bronchus and that of the *posterior segment* of the *superior lobe* have postural drainage problems when the body is kept too long in the supine position. The large posterior and lateral basal branches show why these segments would tend to be the greater recipients of foreign material aspirated into the stem bronchus.

Plate 88   Lateral Arteriogram of Right Pulmonary Artery   185

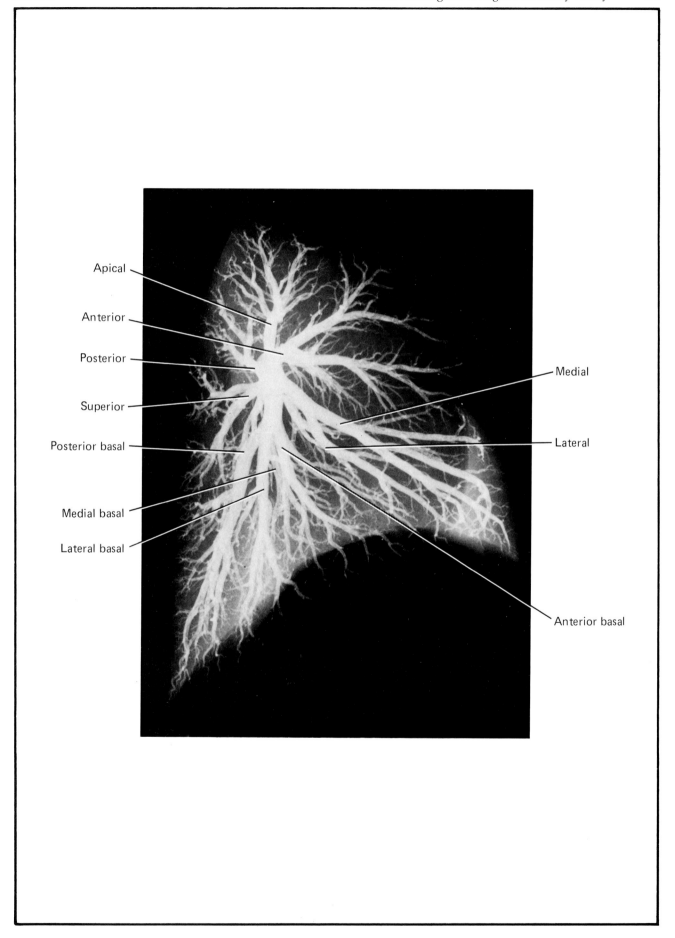

Apical

Anterior

Posterior

Superior

Posterior basal

Medial basal

Lateral basal

Medial

Lateral

Anterior basal

ANTEROPOSTERIOR ARTERIOGRAM OF THE LEFT PULMONARY ARTERY

The left pulmonary artery is a large, short vessel that subdivides almost immediately after arising from the left inferior surface of the junction point between the *pulmonary trunk* and *ductus arteriosus.* The artery, like the bronchus, usually divides into major *superior* and *inferior divisions* that supply their respective lobes, but variations to this rule most frequently involve the segmental arteries to the lingular divisions and the branch to the superior segment of the inferior lobe.

Because the cardiac impression forces both lobar and segmental branches to the left, the superior segmental branch of the inferior lobe is visualized without obstruction in this view. Also, the branches to the anteromedial basal segment arise from a common root off the inferior lobar artery and thus mimic the bronchial pattern that causes these areas to be classified as a single segment.

Plate 89   Anteroposterior Arteriogram of Left Pulmonary Artery   187

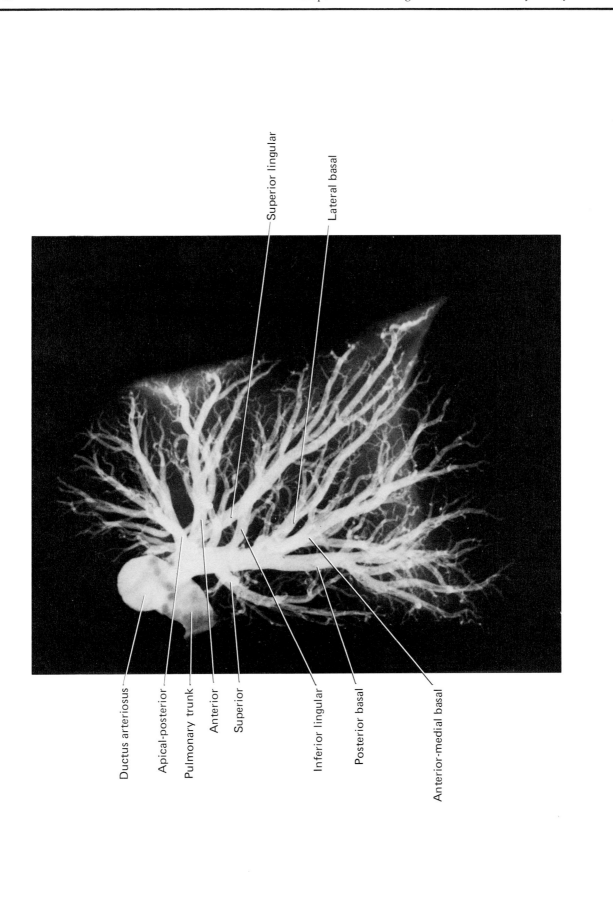

Superior lingular

Lateral basal

Ductus arteriosus

Apical-posterior

Pulmonary trunk

Anterior

Superior

Inferior lingular

Posterior basal

Anterior-medial basal

LATERAL ARTERIOGRAM OF THE LEFT PULMONARY ARTERY

In this lateral view the pulmonary trunk and ductus arteriosus have been removed because they overshadowed the proximal upper segmental branches.

Despite the common origin of the apical-posterior subsegmental bronchi, their arterial equivalents show separate derivations from the lobar artery.

The only pronounced variation in the arterial distribution shown here occurs in the inferior division of the left superior lobe. Typically, the two bronchopulmonary segments of the lingula have a superior-inferior relationship, but in this case a medial-lateral arrangement prevails. A single artery, derived in common with the branch of the anterior segment of the superior lobe, supplies the lateral aspect of the inferior division and all of the lingular projection, whereas a medial branch from the inferior lobar artery supplies an atypical medial segment of the superior lobe's inferior division.

The distribution of the segmental branches of the left inferior lobe is typical and the individual segmental branches may be identified.

Plate 90   Lateral Arteriogram of Left Pulmonary Artery   189

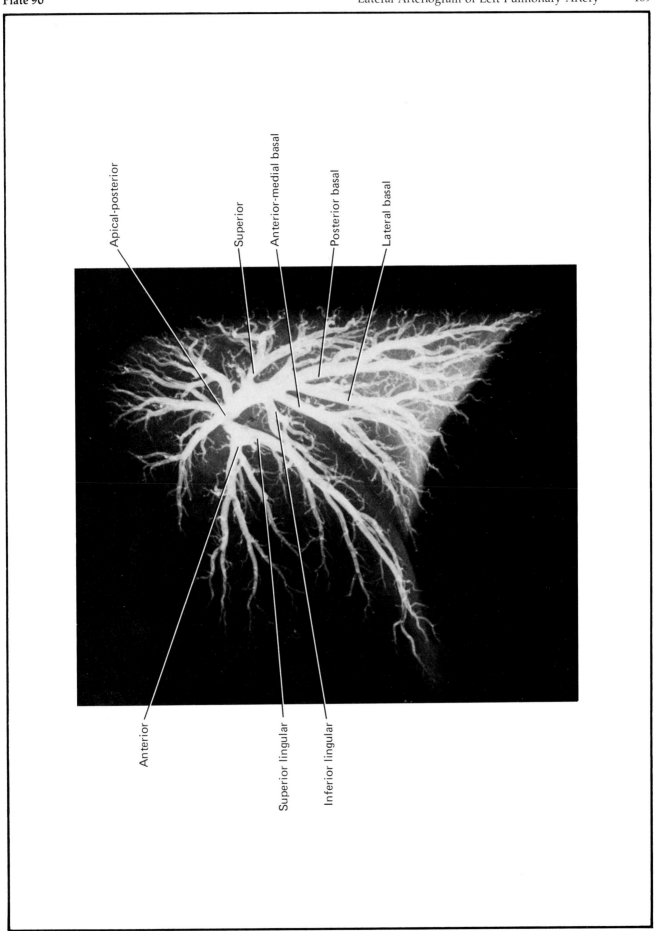

Apical-posterior

Superior

Anterior-medial basal

Posterior basal

Lateral basal

Anterior

Superior lingular

Inferior lingular

ANGIOGRAM
OF THE
PULMONARY VEINS

This specimen was prepared by injecting barium sulfate directly into the left atrium. The portal system was also injected separately for the illustration of that region. This accounts for the radiopaque mass in the liver and spleen.

The central position of the *left atrium* and its saccular *auricle* are well shown, and the major veins can be identified according to their lobar affiliations.

Compare this illustration with the pulmonary arteriograms, and it will become apparent that there are about one half the number of pulmonary veins as arteries at the segmental level. The reason for this numerical discrepancy becomes clear when it is realized that a single intersegmental vein may drain two or more contiguous segments that are supplied by individual segmental arteries.

Note that some of the injection medium had gained access to the superior vena cava via the hepatic veins and faintly outlines the right and left *brachiocephalic veins* and the valves that guard the jugulars and subclavians.

Plate 91   Angiogram of Pulmonary Veins   191

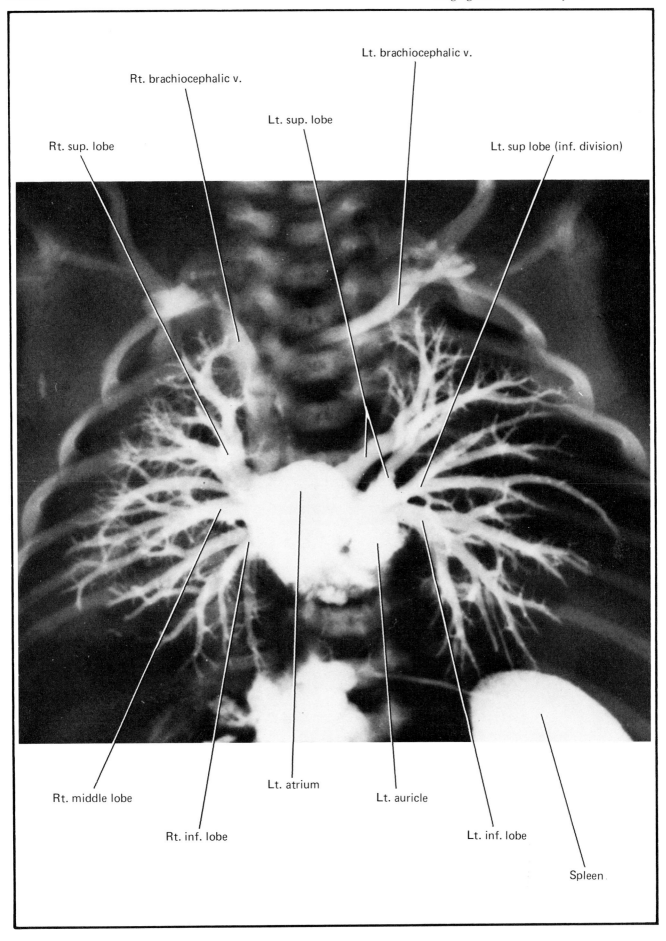

Rt. brachiocephalic v.

Lt. brachiocephalic v.

Lt. sup. lobe

Rt. sup. lobe

Lt. sup lobe (inf. division)

Rt. middle lobe

Lt. atrium

Lt. auricle

Rt. inf. lobe

Lt. inf. lobe

Spleen

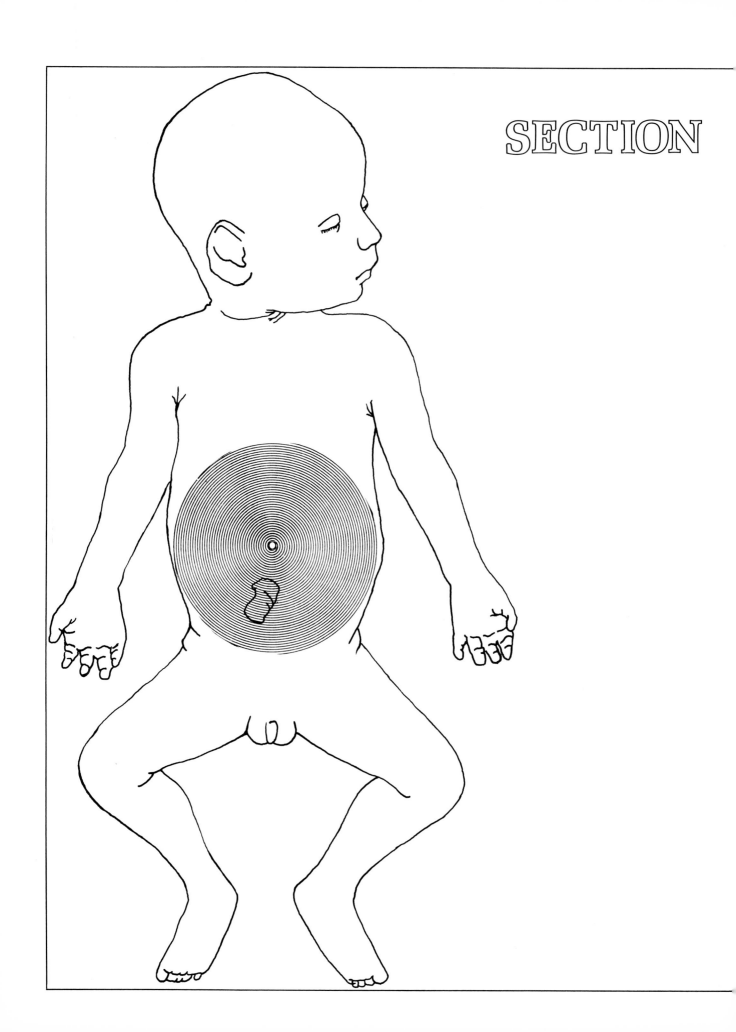

SECTION

FIVE

ABDOMEN AND POSTERIOR ABDOMINAL WALL

THE ANTERIOR ABDOMINAL WALL

This superficial dissection of the abdominal wall has exposed the abdominal musculature, the superficial inguinal region and the femoral triangle. The abdominal peritoneum is supported anteriorly by three musculoaponeurotic layers and a ventral pair of straplike muscles. The most external layer consists of the *external oblique,* whose muscular fibers arise from the thoracolumbar fascia of the back, the inferior ribs and the crest of the ilium. The fibers are directed antero-inferiorly, but midway between the lateral body wall and the umbilicus they blend into an aponeurotic sheet that extends ventrally superficial to the *rectus abdominis* and forms part of the sheath that encases this muscle. The rectus muscle is attached to the ribs and sternum superiorly and to the pubic symphysis inferiorly. It is irregularly divided by *tendinous inscriptions* that indicate its segmental origin. The *internal oblique* lies immediately beneath the external layer, and its muscle fibers may be seen where the external aponeurosis has been dissected away just above the *inguinal ligament.* The fibers generally run in an anterosuperior direction and, in the midabdominal region, its aponeurosis splits to completely ensheath the rectus muscle before inserting on the *linea alba.* The deepest muscular layer is formed by the horizontal fibers of the *transversus abdominis,* whose internal layer of investing fascia (tranversalis fascia) supports the serous peritoneum.

In the inguinal region, the inguinal ligament spans the interval between the anterior superior iliac spine and the pubic crest. It is formed from the rolled-under part of the external oblique aponeurosis and serves as an inferior attachment for the abdominal muscles. It thus provides a space between it and the underlying pubic ramus that permits muscles, vessels and nerves to pass from the posterior abdominal wall into the thigh.

The inguinal region is further complicated, especially in the male, by the passage of genital structures through the abdominal wall. Before the testes descend, the peritoneum protrudes to line the scrotal sac and takes with it contributions from all three layers of the abdominal wall to form the corresponding layers of the spermatic cord. The extensions of the external oblique and transversus abdominis remain thin and fibrous, but a relatively thick layer of looping muscle fibers extends from the internal oblique to form the *cremaster muscle* that elevates the cord.

The *external inguinal ring,* an opening between the fibers of the external oblique, is reinforced by the *superior* and *inferior crura* of the medial attachment of the inguinal ligament. Its relation to the internal inguinal ring is illustrated in the section on the pelvis.

The *iliohypogastric* and *ilioinguinal nerves* are readily exposed by superficial dissection. The first may be seen coursing on the exposed surface of the internal oblique as it supplies the lower abdominal musculature and skin. The ilioinguinal also innervates the lower abdominal wall and sends a branch along the spermatic cord to supply nerve endings to the skin of the scrotum.

In combination, all of the abdominal muscles flex the trunk and compress the abdominal cavity. This latter action assists in expelling the contents of the gastrointestinal and urogenital systems as well as raising the diaphragm in forced expiration.

This illustration provides a good cross section of the *umbilical cord* where the single superior *umbilical vein* and inferior pair of thick walled *umbilical arteries* respectively enter and leave the abdomen. This relationship is found only where the cord is sectioned very close to the wall, since the vessels are much entwined in the more distal regions of the cord.

Plate 92   Anterior Abdominal Wall   195

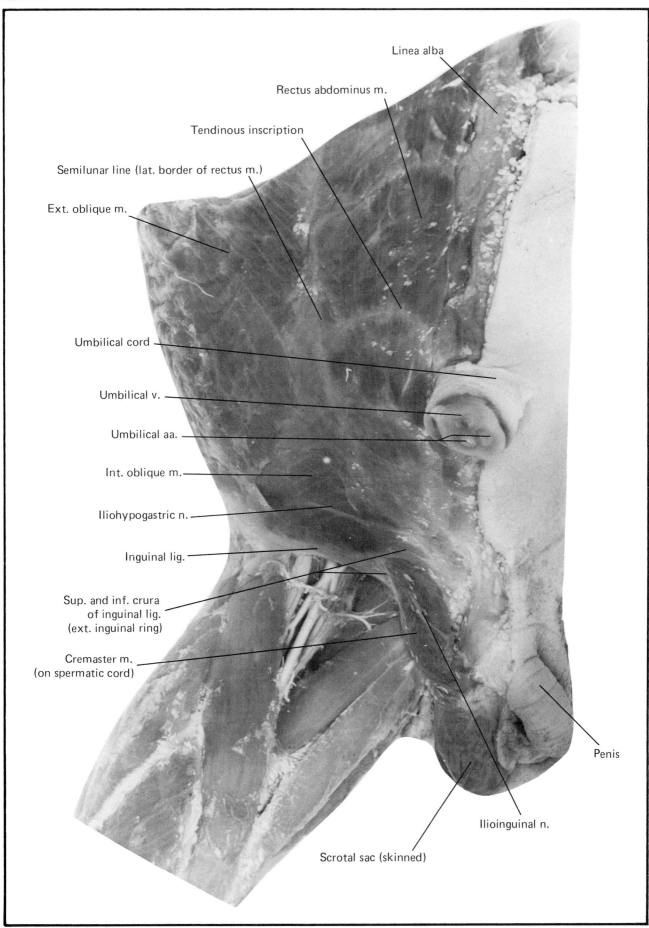

Linea alba

Rectus abdominus m.

Tendinous inscription

Semilunar line (lat. border of rectus m.)

Ext. oblique m.

Umbilical cord

Umbilical v.

Umbilical aa.

Int. oblique m.

Iliohypogastric n.

Inguinal lig.

Sup. and inf. crura
of inguinal lig.
(ext. inguinal ring)

Cremaster m.
(on spermatic cord)

Penis

Ilioinguinal n.

Scrotal sac (skinned)

ARTERIOGRAM OF THE ANTERIOR BODY WALL

The anterior thoracic wall is supplied primarily by the intercostal arteries. The *posterior intercostal arteries* are derived from the aorta, and the *anterior intercostal arteries* are derivatives of the *internal thoracic arteries*. Both sets of intercostals usually subdivide into superior and inferior intercostal branches within each intercostal space with their anteroposterior anastomoses usually occurring lateral to a vertical line intersecting the nipple. Branches of the thoracoacromial and *lateral thoracic artery* share numerous anastomoses with the intercostals.

At the junction of the sixth rib and the sternum, the musculophrenic artery leaves the internal thoracic and follows the subchondral margin of the rib cage. It supplies anterior intercostal branches to the lower five intercostal spaces and sends many branches to the marginal regions of the diaphragm.

The anterior abdominal wall receives its major arterial vascularization from the *superior* and *inferior epigastric arteries,* with lateral contributions from the *subcostal* and *lumbar arteries.* The superior epigastric is an inferior continuation of the internal thoracic vessels. It descends in the rectus sheath and gives off arborizations between the layers of the abdominal muscles. The *inferior epigastric* arteries arise from the external iliac vessels just as they pass under the inguinal ligaments. The inferior epigastrics ascend the internal surface of the abdominal wall posterior to the rectus abdominis muscle and eventually form anastomotic connections with the superior epigastrics lateral to the umbilicus. The deep circumflex arteries also arise from the external iliacs and laterally follow the inguinal ligament and iliac crest to anastomose with lumbar branches and supply the lower lateral abdominal wall.

In this arteriogram the two umbilical arteries can be seen ascending to the umbilicus lateral to the urachal extension of the bladder. In postnatal life the umbilical arteries and the bladder extension are obliterated and become cords of connective tissue (the urachus and medial umbilical ligaments).

Plate 93

Arteriogram of Anterior Body Wall   197

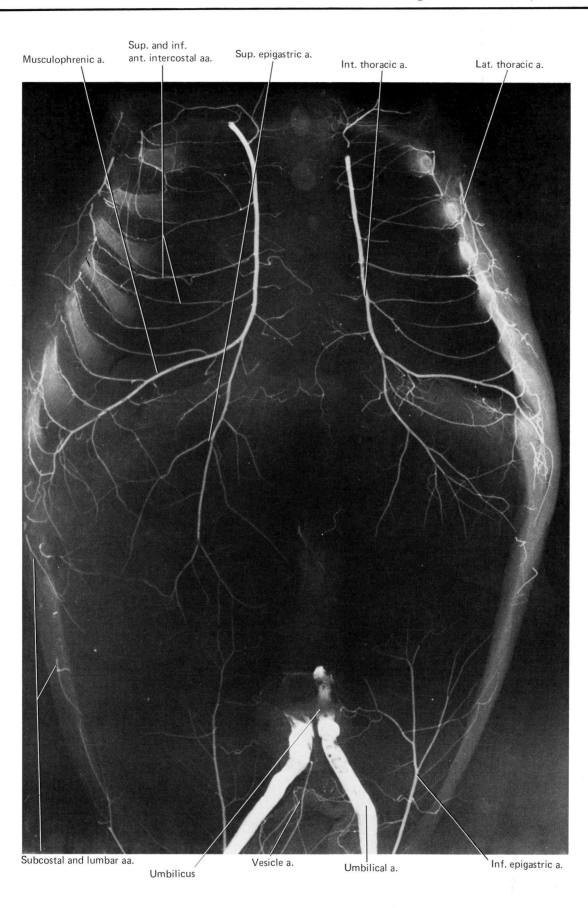

Musculophrenic a.

Sup. and inf.
ant. intercostal aa.

Sup. epigastric a.

Int. thoracic a.

Lat. thoracic a.

Subcostal and lumbar aa.

Umbilicus

Vesicle a.

Umbilical a.

Inf. epigastric a.

SUPERFICIAL ASPECT OF THE SUPRACOLIC REGION

Using the *transverse colon* as a landmark, the abdominal cavity is conveniently divided into an upper supracolic region and a lower infracolic region. The liver, gall bladder, bile ducts, stomach, duodenum, pancreas and spleen comprise the supracolic organs which, for the most part, are supplied by branches of the celiac artery.

Here the liver has been retracted upward to expose the subhepatic viscera. The specific anatomy of each organ is treated in subsequent plates so that only an overview is presented now. The stomach lies under the left lobe of the liver and presents its anterior surface (developmentally its left side). This organ may be traced from its junction with the esophagus at the *cardiac antrum* to where it enters into the *duodenal bulb* through the *pylorus*. The lesser curvature is rimmed by the *right* and *left gastric arteries* and marks the gastric attachment of the *lesser omentum*, a ventral mesentery comprised of the thin hepatogastric and the thicker hepatoduodenal ligaments. The latter part contains branches of the *hepatic artery*, the *common bile duct* and, deep to these two, the *portal vein*. The free edge (right border) of the lesser omentum transmits the bile duct, and a probe inserted behind this structure from right to left will enter the *omental bursa*.

The first part of the duodenum, the *duodenal bulb,* is supplied by the *supraduodenal artery*. Here its muscular layer has been dissected away to show the intricate submucosal plexus of arteries. The second part, the *descending duodenum,* shows the branches of the *anterior superior pancreatoduodenal artery;* these, in conjunction with their posterior counterparts, supply the duodenum and the head of the pancreas. The superior pancreatoduodenal arteries join the inferior pancreatoduodenal arteries to form anastomotic arcades between the celiac and superior mesenteric systems.

The greater curvature of the stomach is well delineated by the *right gastroepiploic artery,* which also indicates the attachment of the *greater omentum*. This redundant fold of the early dorsal mesogaster was thrown to the left and downward when the dorsum of the stomach turned to the left during the developmental rotation of the gut. In combination with the lesser omentum and the stomach, this large mesenteric fold seals off the retrogastric part of the abdominal cavity to form the omental bursa, whose communication with the remainder of the cavity exists only through the epiploic foramen. In this photograph, the *caudate lobe* of the liver can be seen extending downward into the bursa.

The greater omentum retains its original attachment to the posterior body wall in the region of the celiac artery so that the posterior layers of the fold come in contact with and, postnatally, will eventually adhere to the surface of the transverse mesocolon and the colon itself. The resulting gastrocolic ligament represents the fusion of four membranes, a fact not so unusual when it is recalled that all mesenteries originally consist of a double layer of peritoneum. The inferior extension of the greater omental fold falls freely over the transverse colon to form a protective apron anterior to the infracolic viscera. In the adult, the omentum becomes opaque through the accumulation of much fat, but in the fetus it is quite transparent and readily exhibits the omental branches of the epiploic arteries.

Plate 94   Superficial Aspect of Supracolic Region   199

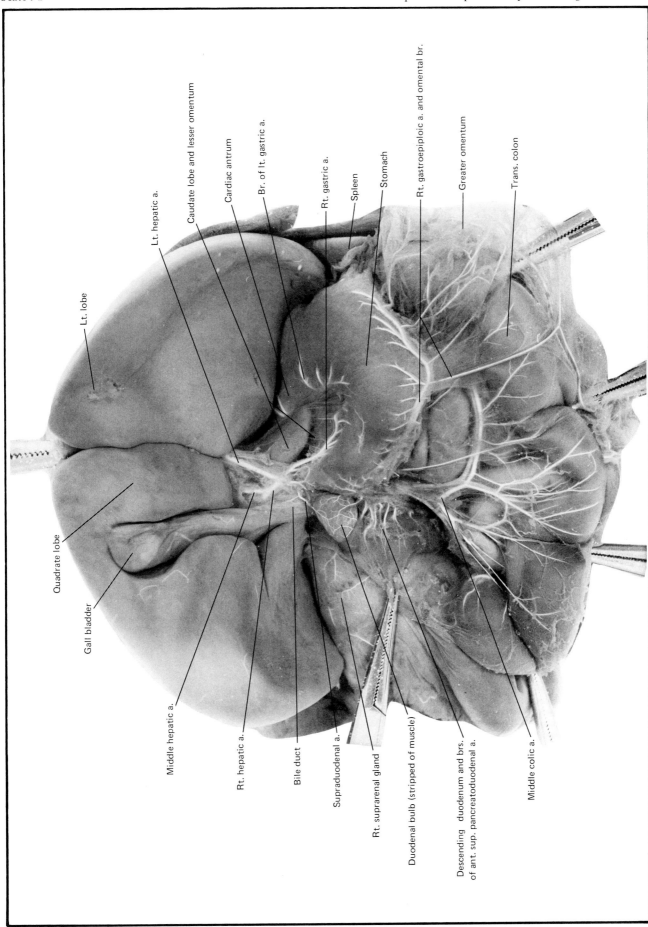

Lt. lobe

Lt. hepatic a.

Caudate lobe and lesser omentum

Cardiac antrum

Br. of lt. gastric a.

Rt. gastric a.

Spleen

Stomach

Rt. gastroepiploic a. and omental br.

Greater omentum

Trans. colon

Quadrate lobe

Gall bladder

Middle hepatic a.

Rt. hepatic a.

Bile duct

Supraduodenal a.

Rt. suprarenal gland

Duodenal bulb (stripped of muscle)

Descending duodenum and brs.
of ant. sup. pancreatoduodenal a.

Middle colic a.

RETROGASTRIC STRUCTURES OF THE SUPRACOLIC REGION

This is a continued dissection of the preceding specimen. Most of the stomach, superior duodenum, hepatogastric and gastrocolic ligaments have been removed to expose the retrogastric supracolic organs. The stomach was cut through the superior part of its body, leaving its sectioned edge and fundus visible under the left lobe of the liver.

It is obvious here that the major arteries to the supracolic organs have a common origin from the celiac trunk of the aorta. In their tripartite arrangement the *hepatic artery* will be considered the first major celiac branch. It courses anteriorly to the left to divide into the proper hepatic artery of the liver and the *gastroduodenal artery* that provides the *pancreatoduodenal* and right *gastroepiploic* arteries. A long, thin unlabeled vessel that descends from the bifurcation of the proper hepatic artery represents the right gastric artery. The *left gastric artery*, the next large branch of the celiac trunk, ascends toward the cardiac antrum of the stomach to contribute to the arterial loop that runs along the lesser curvature. This artery also has anastomotic connections with the esophageal vessels. The third large branch of the celiac trunk is the *splenic artery*, which travels along the superior border of the pancreas and terminates in several branches that enter the spleen. The *left gastroepiploic* branch of the splenic artery ascends in the gastrosplenic ligament (part of the original dorsal mesogaster) to supply the fundus

and contribute to the arterial loop of the greater curvature.

The initial part of the *superior mesenteric artery* can be seen passing inferior to the neck of the pancreas and anterior to the third (horizontal) part of the duodenum. Its first branch, the *middle colic artery*, sends contributions right and left to the marginal artery of the transverse colon.

The duodenum, the spleen, the body and the tail of the pancreas develop between the layers of a freely suspended area of the primitive dorsal mesentery and remain in this condition throughout the life of most mammals. However, the upright posture of man required additional support for some abdominal viscera, so that the second and third parts of the duodenum, the pancreas and the ascending and descending parts of the colon became secondarily retroperitoneal and adhered to the posterior abdominal wall. Also, since the gut loop that formed the small and large intestine rotated counterclockwise around the axis formed by the superior mesenteric artery, the transverse colon was thrown across the duodenum and pancreas. This necessitated that the transverse mesocolon should become adherent to the anterior surface of the second part of the duodenum and the pancreas.

Thus in this illustration, the dorsal attachment of the thin, transparent mesocolon may be traced across the suprarenal gland, the second part of the duodenum and the inferior border of the pancreas in a horizontal line that intersects the superior mesenteric artery where it emerges between the pancreas and duodenum. Deep to the transverse mesocolon the fourth (ascending) part of the duodenum can be seen where it becomes continuous with the superior coils of the jejunum.

Plate 95

Retrogastric Structures of Supracolic Region   201

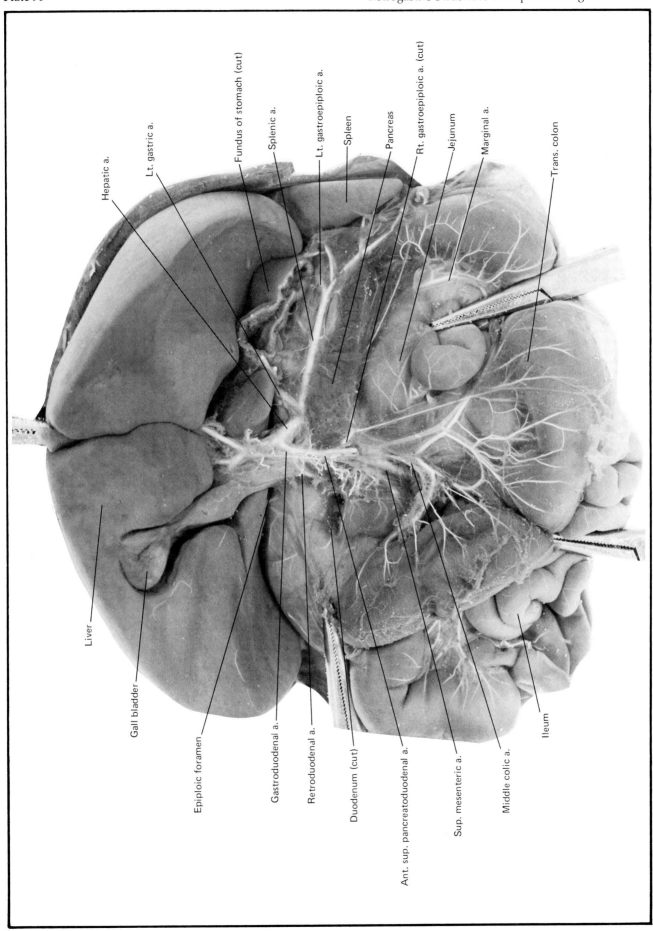

Hepatic a.

Lt. gastric a.

Fundus of stomach (cut)

Splenic a.

Lt. gastroepiploic a.

Spleen

Pancreas

Rt. gastroepiploic a. (cut)

Jejunum

Marginal a.

Trans. colon

Liver

Gall bladder

Epiploic foramen

Gastroduodenal a.

Retroduodenal a.

Duodenum (cut)

Ant. sup. pancreatoduodenal a.

Sup. mesenteric a.

Middle colic a.

Ileum

202 Abdomen and Abdominal Wall

ANTERIOR ASPECT OF THE LIVER

The liver is the largest gland in the body, and its total range of functions is yet to be appreciated. The adult liver normally is confined within the concavity of the diaphragm and is not readily palpated below the inferior margins of the rib cage. In the fetus, however, the liver is relatively twice as massive with the *right lobe* extending below the umbilicus. Furthermore, the prenatal liver is more symmetrical; the left lobe is approximately four fifths the size of the right. During postnatal growth, the left lobe becomes progressively more attenuated until it achieves but less than one third the volume of its bilateral equivalent. Since the liver is primarily an accessory gland of the digestive tract, its size in the fetus may seem paradoxical because very little substance is absorbed by the fetal intestine. Nevertheless, it is already the major organ of biosynthesis and the detoxification of noxious metabolites. In addition, the liver is the primary hematopoietic center until the postnatal intramedullary blood cell-forming areas develop within the bones.

The liver develops from an outgrowth at the juncture of the primitive foregut and midgut regions. This hepatic diverticulum invades the inferior layers of the transverse septum that forms the greater part of the central diaphragm. Therefore, the organ is eventually suspended from the inferior surface of the diaphragm by the reflections of its peritoneal sac. Collectively, these reflections comprise the triangular *coronary ligament*.

In this anterior view, only a small section of the attachment of the coronary ligament is visible where it converges to be continuous with the *falciform ligament*. This latter structure is an anterior fold of ventral mesentery that is reflected from the internal surface of the upper abdominal wall. In the inferior free edge of the falciform ligament, the *umbilical vein* passes from the umbilicus to the porta of the liver. Postnatally, the lumen of this vessel becomes obliterated, leaving a fibrous remnant, the ligamentum teres.

Note that the fundus of the gall bladder is hidden by the anteroinferior margin of the right lobe. With differential growth and the relative diminution of the postnatal liver, the gall bladder usually becomes visible from the anterior aspect.

Plate 96   Anterior Aspect of Liver   203

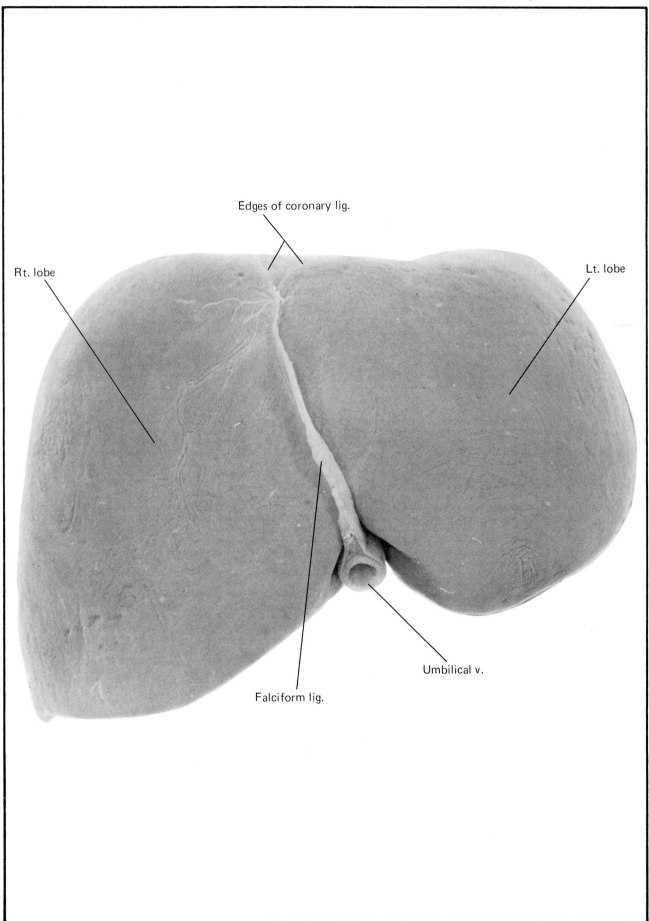

Edges of coronary lig.

Rt. lobe

Lt. lobe

Falciform lig.

Umbilical v.

INFEROPOSTERIOR ASPECT OF THE LIVER

The major anatomic subdivisions of the liver are clearly indicated in this view. The organ is approximately bisected into right and left halves by the *fossa of the umbilical vein* and its dorsal continuation, the *fossa of the ductus venosus*. The latter lies between the *left lobe* and the *caudate lobe* and receives the attachment of the *hepatogastric ligament*.

In the depths of both fossae lies the large developmental venous channel that shunts the major part of the returning placental blood directly through the liver and into the inferior vena cava. The umbilical vein and ductus venosus are represented postnatally as the ligamentum teres and the ligamentum venosum, respectively.

A laterally directed groove intersects the umbilical fossa and receives the *hepatoduodenal ligament* and its contained *hepatic artery*, *portal vein* and *bile ducts*. The large opening in the medial part of this fissure has been called the hepatic porta (entranceway), which gives the portal vein its name.

The *gall bladder* lies in a depression, the fossa of the gall bladder, that subdivides the anteroinferior surface of the right half of the liver and separates the *quadrate lobe* from the *right lobe*. Posterior to this, the groove of the *inferior vena cava* isolates the caudate lobe, except for a narrow isthmus, the caudate process. The *papillary process* of the caudate lobe is much enlarged in the fetus and retracts in subsequent development. The subdivisions of the gall bladder are not sharply defined in the fetal liver, but the rounded terminal part, the fundus, and its more proximal portion, the body, can be seen leading to a constriction forming the narrower neck of the gall bladder that eventually leads into the cystic duct. On the surface of the duct, fine ramifications of the cystic artery may be discerned.

Plate 97   Inferoposterior Aspect of Liver   205

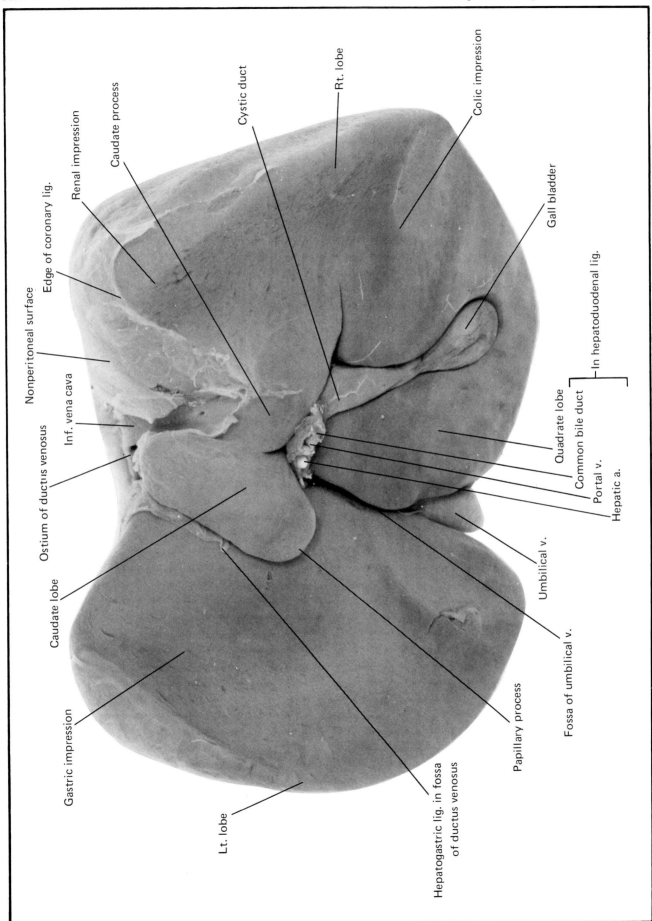

Caudate process

Cystic duct

Rt. lobe

Colic impression

Renal impression

Edge of coronary lig.

Nonperitoneal surface

Gall bladder

Inf. vena cava

In hepatoduodenal lig.

Ostium of ductus venosus

Quadrate lobe

Common bile duct

Portal v.

Hepatic a.

Caudate lobe

Umbilical v.

Fossa of umbilical v.

Gastric impression

Papillary process

Lt. lobe

Hepatogastric lig. in fossa
of ductus venosus

POSTERIOR ASPECT OF THE LIVER

The attachment of the *coronary ligament* and the relations of the great veins are best appreciated in a posterior view of the liver. The wide discrepancies between the edges of the ligament indicate that the organ is not suspended by a simple mesenteric fold, but has a peritoneal relationship to the diaphragm that roughly suggests the shape of a colonial tricornered hat. The anterior triangle of the coronary ligament converges to join the falciform ligament while its right and left extremities form the right and left *triangular ligaments*. It is obvious, then, that the large part of the posterior and superior surfaces of the organ that lies between the margins of the peritoneal reflections is without a serosal covering and is referred to as the "bare area" of the liver. Since the coronary ligament is also reflected around the inferior vena cava as it penetrates the diaphragm, the groove that passes this vessel along the posterior hepatic surface can be observed in the bare area. Deep in this groove, a number of ostia indicate where hepatic veins drain into the inferior vena cava. The large caval connection to the ductus venosus becomes much reduced after parturition.

The oblique view of the inferior hepatic surface shows the impressions of related viscera that were preserved when the organ was hardened by fixation.

Plate 98   Posterior Aspect of Liver   207

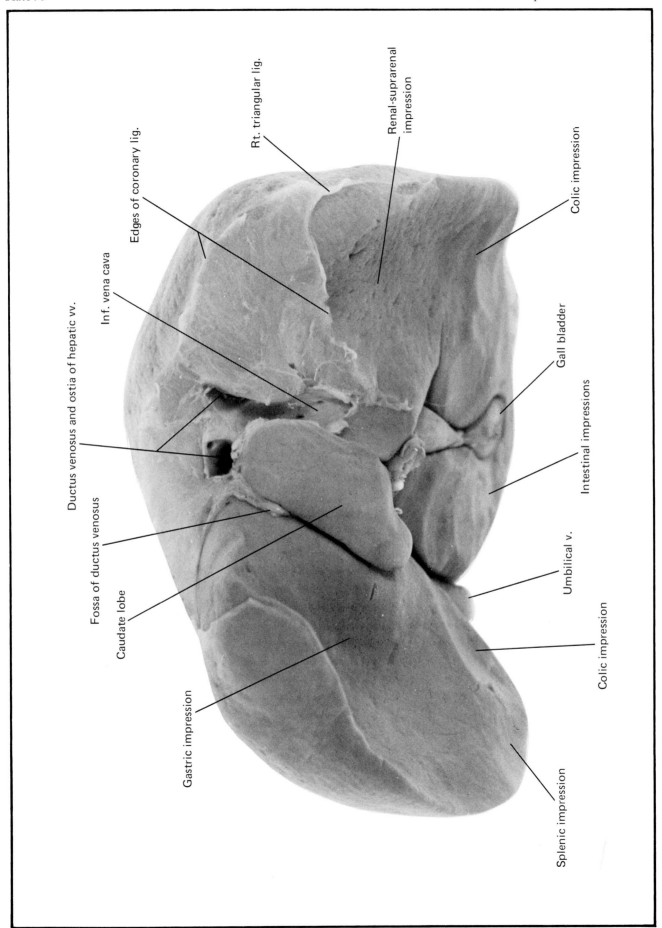

Rt. triangular lig.

Renal-suprarenal impression

Colic impression

Edges of coronary lig.

Inf. vena cava

Ductus venosus and ostia of hepatic vv.

Gall bladder

Intestinal impressions

Fossa of ductus venosus

Caudate lobe

Umbilical v.

Colic impression

Gastric impression

Splenic impression

ANGIOGRAM OF INTRAHEPATIC ARTERIAL CIRCULATION

During development the endodermal hepatic diverticulation subdivides within its surrounding mesenchymal mass to form the liver. The resulting system of tubules remains as the intrahepatic biliary tract. Because each duct is accompanied by a branch of the hepatic artery, the relative positions of the larger intrahepatic ducts can be conceptualized in this arteriogram. The liver is subdivided into eight segments that are supplied by their corresponding area arteries. The area arteries are subdivisions of their regional segmental branches that, in turn, are derived from their respective right or left hepatic arteries.

It should be noted that the classic anatomic division of the liver into right and left major lobes by the falciform and hepatogastric ligaments does not coincide with the distribution of the biliary and arterial systems. The quadrate lobe, which is "anatomically" associated with the right side of the liver, is actually served by the medial inferior area artery of the left hepatic branch, and the caudate lobe is supplied by branches of both the right and left hepatics.

The cystic artery has a variable origin, but is usually derived from the right hepatic, and its terminals on the hepatic side of the gall bladder contribute to the vascularization of the liver.

Plate 99   Angiogram of Intrahepatic Arterial Circulation   209

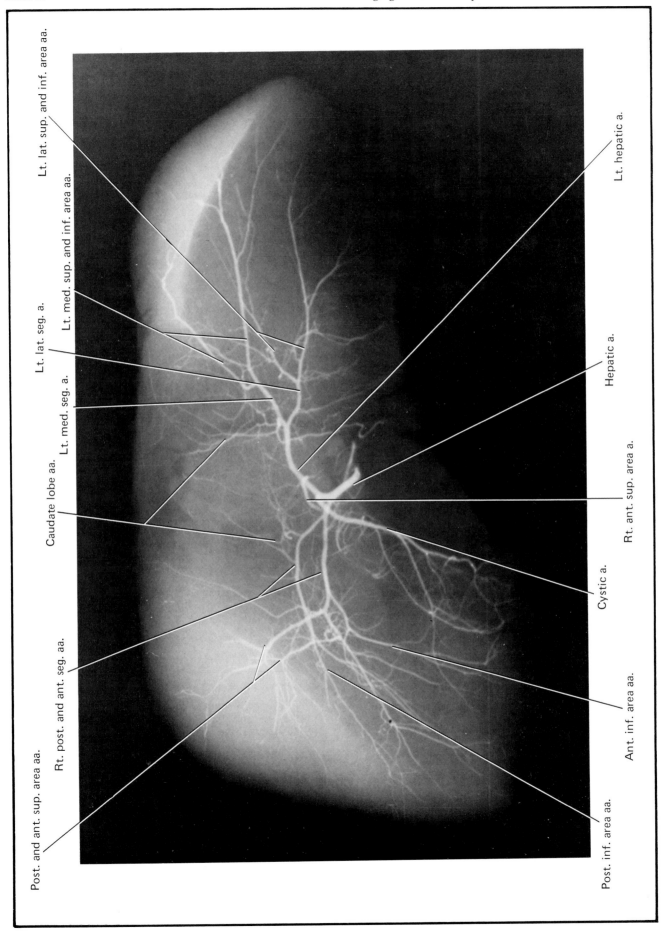

Lt. lat. sup. and inf. area aa.

Lt. med. sup. and inf. area aa.

Lt. lat. seg. a.

Lt. med. seg. a.

Caudate lobe aa.

Post. and ant. sup. area aa.

Rt. post. and ant. seg. aa.

Lt. hepatic a.

Hepatic a.

Rt. ant. sup. area a.

Cystic a.

Ant. inf. area aa.

Post. inf. area aa.

VINYLITE LATEX CAST OF A FETAL LIVER

Depicted here is a corrosion cast of a doubly injected fetal liver. Clear vinyl acetate had been injected into the umbilical vein and has filled the branches of both the portal vein and the hepatic veins from their connections with the ductus venosus and the inferior vena cava. A subsequent injection of black colored latex into the umbilical artery had also filled the ramifications of the hepatic artery. The tissues of the liver were then corroded away in a solution of potassium hydroxide. In this view of the inferior surface of the resulting specimen, the proximal sections of the *umbilical vein, portal vein* and *inferior vena cava* are labeled. It can also be noted that the arterial injection, for some unknown reason, did not penetrate the caudate lobe.

If one equates the intrahepatic portal veins and hepatic veins with the pulmonary arteries and veins, the hepatic arteries with the bronchial arteries and the bile ducts with the bronchi, it becomes apparent that the liver and lung share many features in common. The similarities in the structural organization of the two organs are attributable to their essential functions involving the processing of large volumes of blood that pass through the tissues by way of large afferent and efferent vessels. However, the blood in these systems is insufficiently oxygenated or, as in the case of the pulmonary veins, has insufficient pressure to support the organ's own tissues. Therefore, the fine, high pressure systemic arteries such as the hepatics and bronchials form a "private" blood that must include even the vasa vasorum of the greater vessels.

Plate 100   Vinylite Latex Cast of Liver   211

Portal v.   Inf. vena cava   Caudate lobe

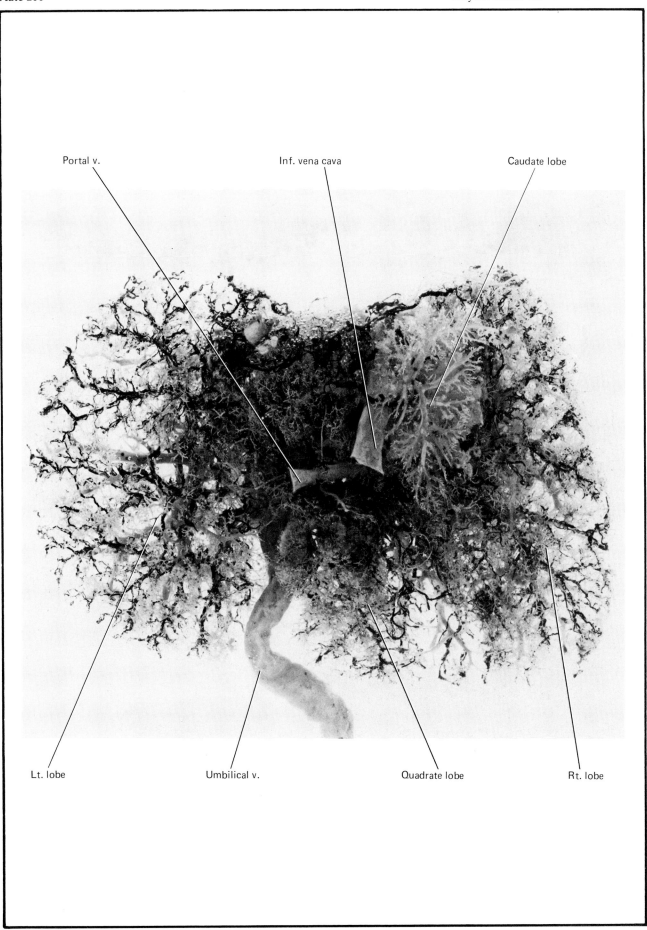

Lt. lobe   Umbilical v.   Quadrate lobe   Rt. lobe

VASCULAR DETAIL IN THE LIVER CAST

In this finer detail of the previously illustrated specimen, the organizational similarities between the liver and the lung may be further appreciated. The bile ducts, hepatic arteries and portal veins, the three structures observed at the porta of the liver, form an inseparable triad throughout their intrahepatic ramifications and thus resemble the close association of the bronchus, bronchial artery and pulmonary artery. In addition, the vascular relations at the subsegmental level are identical to the patterns found in the bronchopulmonary segment. Note here that each ramification of the *portal vein* (white) is entwined by the black latex of the *hepatic artery*, which also would have been shown to entwine a bile duct had it been injected. This combination runs through the center of the subsegment, but the regional *hepatic vein* (clear white) is intersegmental and drains two or more adjacent subsegments.

Plate 101   Vascular Detail of Liver   213

Portal v. (white)   Hepatic a. (black)

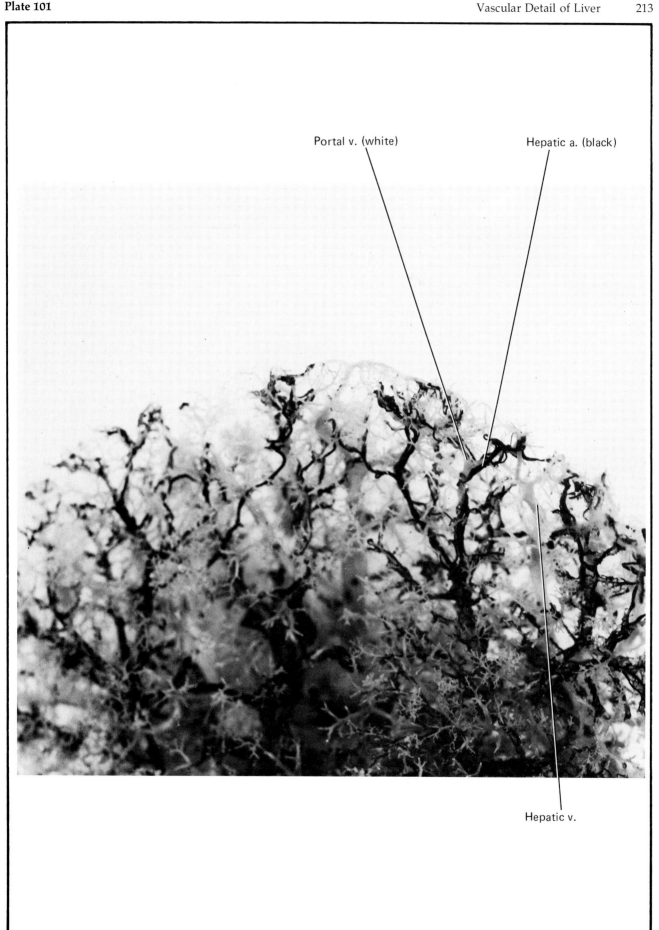

Hepatic v.

THE STOMACH

The stomach is a dilated part of the digestive tract that serves as the immediate receptacle for ingested food and initiates some of the digestive processes. It conventionally appears in cadavers as a J-shaped organ occupying the left supracolic region.

The part inferior to the esophageal hiatus of the diaphragm is called the *cardiac antrum*, presumably because of its close relation to the posteroinferior aspect of the heart. The antrum leads into the much expanded *body* and is delineated from the domelike *fundus* by the *cardiac notch*. Inferiorly, the body turns to the right and becomes constricted as the *pyloric antrum*. A thick muscular sphincter, the *pylorus*, controls the passage of the gastric contents into the first part of the duodenum.

The stomach and the superior duodenum developed with both dorsal and ventral mesenteries. The ventral mesentery attaches to the lesser curvature as the hepatogastric and hepatoduodenal ligaments, and the dorsal mesentery, which attaches to the entire length of the *greater curvature*, forms the greater omentum and subdivisions of the gastrocolic and gastrosplenic ligaments. This double mesenteric support also permits the stomach to receive vascularization from two arterial arcades. The *left* and *right gastric arteries* form an anastomotic connection along the lesser curvature, and the *right* and *left gastroepiploic arteries* form another marginal arterial loop along the greater curvature. Because of a slight obliquity in the view presented here, the left gastroepiploic arteries lie behind the fundus.

This specimen includes part of the diaphragm to indicate how the muscle fasciculae surrounding the esophageal hiatus may have a sphincteric action on the lower esophagus. Because the dorsum of the stomach rotates to the left during development, what is presented here as the anterior gastric surface was formerly its left side.

Plate 102   Stomach   215

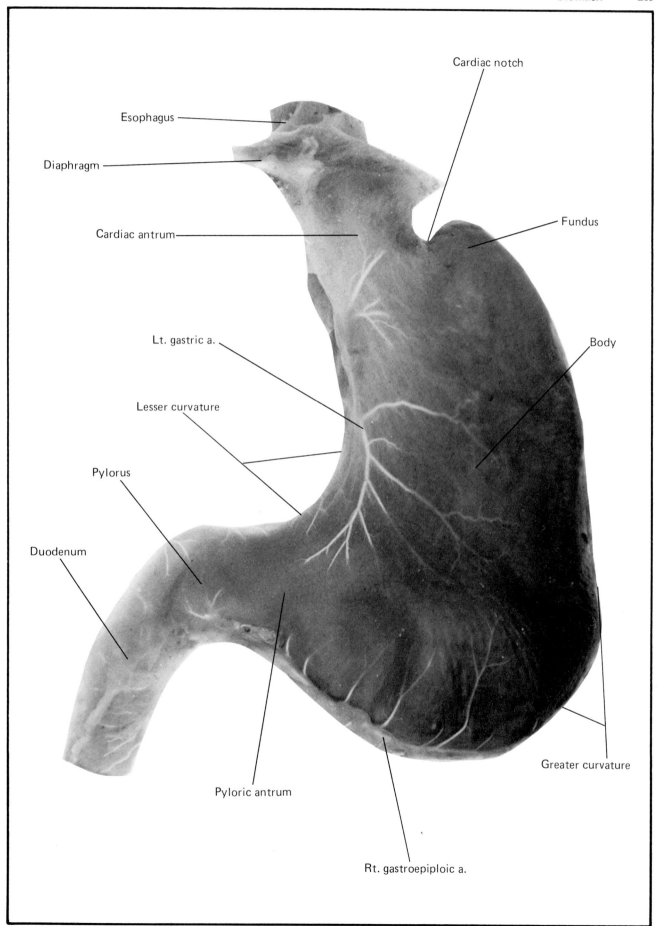

Cardiac notch

Esophagus

Diaphragm

Cardiac antrum

Fundus

Lt. gastric a.

Body

Lesser curvature

Pylorus

Duodenum

Greater curvature

Pyloric antrum

Rt. gastroepiploic a.

THE DUODENUM, PANCREAS AND SPLEEN

Removal of the stomach and the transverse meso-colon reveals the deeper supracolic organs, the duodenum, pancreas and spleen. Most of the duodenum and pancreas are secondarily re-troperitoneal. They developed in the free suspension of the early mesenteries, but the gut rotation forced them against the posterior abdominal wall where the right side of their peritoneal surfaces adhered to form a fusion fascia. Characteristically, this plane of fusion may be readily separated again without fear of disrupting any consequential vessels.

The duodenum is the first part of the small intestine. Having been formed between the developing foregut and midgut regions, it derives its blood supply from anastomotic loops between the foregut (celiac) artery and the midgut (superior mesenteric) artery. The duodenum receives the biliary and pancreatic ducts through a common orifice, the ampulla, located in the concavity of its loop. The common bile duct and pancreatic duct are united and controlled by a single sphincter just before entering the intestinal lumen.

In this illustration the four parts of the duodenum may be observed. The *superior part* lies to the right of the pylorus and is suspended from the *hepato-(pancreato-) duodenal ligament*. It blends into the *descending part* that arcs around the head of the pancreas. The *horizontal part* passes posteroinferior to the *superior mesenteric artery* and *vein*, and the *ascending part* joins the *jejunum* behind the body of the pancreas. The juncture of the duodenum and jejunum forms an acute flexure that is supported by a strong fibrous attachment to the crura of the diaphragm, the suspensory ligament (of Treitz).

The pancreas is a combined exocrine-endocrine organ that, like the liver, developed from endodermal outgrowths from the transitional area between the primitive foregut and midgut regions. Originally there were two pancreatic primordia. An evagination of the hepatic diverticulum expanded into the ventral mesentery and formed the ventral pancreas, and a dorsal pancreas grew from an independent gut diverticulum in the dorsal mesentery. Through subsequent gut rotation the two pancreatic masses fused. The ventral pancreas was incorporated into the head of the definitive organ, and its main duct was joined by that of the dorsal pancreas. In early vertebrate evolution, it was the dorsal pancreas that contained the islet cells, so that it is not surprising that most of the endocrine function is still confined to the pancreatic *body* and *tail*.

The *head of the pancreas*, like the duodenum, is supplied by branches from both the celiac and superior mesenteric arteries. The superior mesenteric vessels pass between the horizontal duodenum and the pancreas, producing a notch in the latter that forms the constricted neck of the pancreas. As the vessels leave the pancreas, they are ensheathed in the root of the mesentery that carries their branches and supports the small intestines. Here the mesentery is thick and contains many nerve filaments, accounting for the indistinct appearance of the vessels at this point.

The large *splenic artery* passes along the dorso-superior edge of the pancreas and supplies numerous branches to its body and tail before dividing into several terminals that enter the spleen.

The *spleen* is an organ of the cardiovascular system with immunologic functions. Because it developed within the dorsal mesogaster, it is attached to the greater curvature of the stomach by the *gastrosplenic ligament* that conveys the *short gastric* and *left gastroepiploic* branches of the *splenic artery*. It is also attached to the posterior abdominal wall by the lienorenal ligament. The spleen has a crescentic configuration, and its surfaces are named according to their relation to other structures. The hilus of the spleen receives the vessels and is located in a concavity called the *gastric impression*. Its convex *external phrenic surface* lies in contact with the diaphragm, and its upper posterior surface is situated against the kidney to form the renal impression.

The spleen is protected by the ribs overlying the left hemidiaphragm, but certain blood dyscrasias will cause its enlargement and inferior extension where it becomes more exposed to injury.

Plate 103   Duodenum, Pancreas and Spleen   217

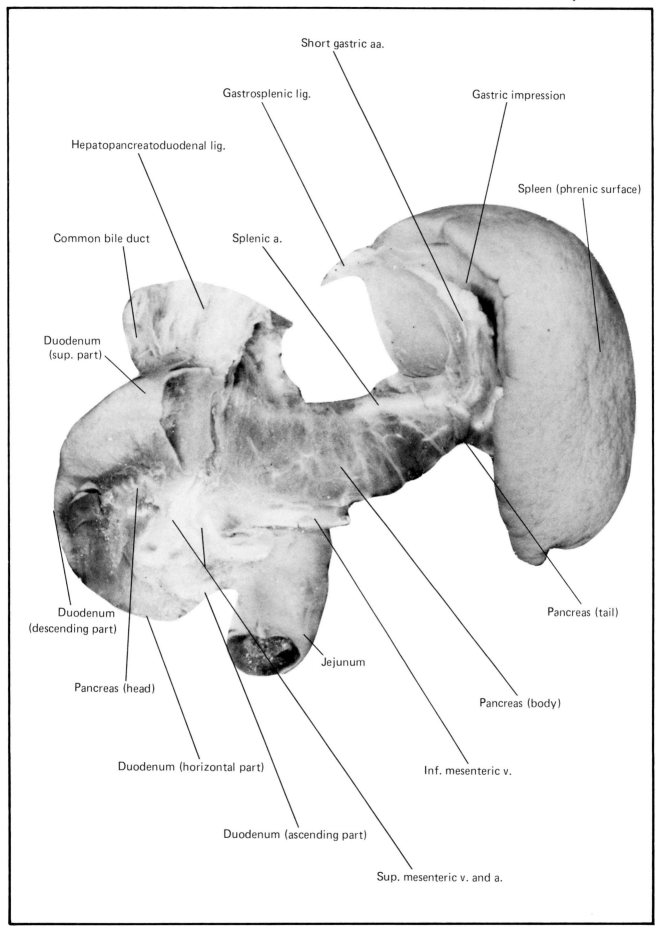

Short gastric aa.

Gastrosplenic lig.

Gastric impression

Hepatopancreatoduodenal lig.

Spleen (phrenic surface)

Common bile duct

Splenic a.

Duodenum
(sup. part)

Duodenum
(descending part)

Pancreas (head)

Pancreas (tail)

Jejunum

Duodenum (horizontal part)

Pancreas (body)

Inf. mesenteric v.

Duodenum (ascending part)

Sup. mesenteric v. and a.

ARTERIOGRAM OF THE SUPRACOLIC ORGANS

As this angiogram shows, the blood supply of the supracolic organs is essentially a study of the branches of the celiac artery. This vessel is the first visceral branch of the abdominal aorta and arises between the crura of the diaphragm. Because it is short and stout and its length may often be less than its diameter, it is frequently referred to as the *celiac axis* or *trunk*. The vessel divides simultaneously into the *common hepatic artery* on the right, the *splenic artery* on the left and the *left gastric artery* superiorly.

The common hepatic artery divides into the roughly equal "proper" *hepatic artery* to the liver and gall bladder, and the *gastroduodenal artery,* which provides the superior pancreatoduodenal and *left gastroepiploic vessels.* The *right gastric artery* is seen as a small branch descending from the midportion of the hepatic artery to the antrum of the stomach. The left gastric courses anterosuperiorly toward the cardia of the stomach, where it supplies an arcade along the lesser curvature. The splenic artery, the largest of the celiac triad, travels left toward the spleen. Its first major branch, the *inferior pancreatic artery,* supplies the major part of the pancreatic body and tail. In addition to branches to the substance of the spleen, the terminals of the splenic artery include *short gastric arteries* to the gastric fundus, and *left gastroepiploic* to the greater curvature and omentum.

The inferior phrenic arteries are often derived from the celiac axis, but are not usually classified with its visceral branches.

Plate 104   Arteriogram of Supracolic Organs   219

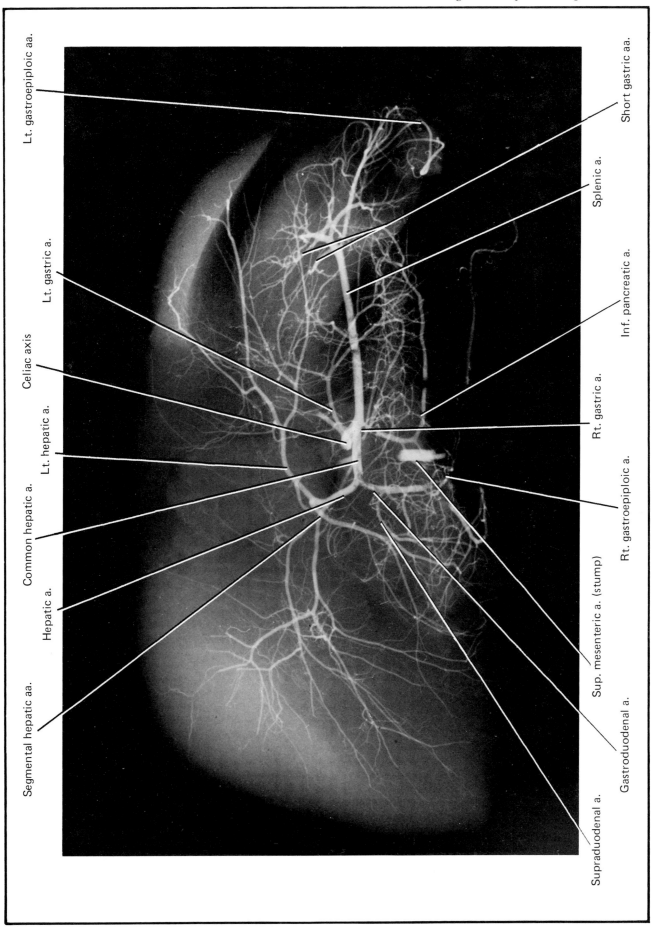

Lt. gastroepiploic aa.

Short gastric aa.

Splenic a.

Lt. gastric a.

Inf. pancreatic a.

Celiac axis

Lt. hepatic a.

Rt. gastric a.

Common hepatic a.

Rt. gastroepiploic a.

Hepatic a.

Sup. mesenteric a. (stump)

Segmental hepatic aa.

Gastroduodenal a.

Supraduodenal a.

INFRACOLIC VISCERA: SUPERFICIAL ASPECT

Elevation of the *transverse colon* exposes the extent of the transparent mesocolon and the distribution of the *middle colic artery*. This vessel is usually the first branch of the superior mesenteric artery and tends to favor the left side of the transverse colon. On approaching the large bowel, the artery forms part of a large arterial arcade that travels along the mesenteric side of the entire colon. This marginal artery supplies the gut with numerous vasa recta and provides ample collateral circulation that permits the ligation of a major colic branch. Just inferior to the origin of the middle colic artery, the root of the mesentery fans out to support the small intestines. It contains the superior *mesenteric arteries* and *veins*. The root is quite thick here because a great number of lymph nodes and nerves surround the major vessels, and the fat that will become quite thick in postnatal life is beginning to be deposited. Some individual lymph nodes are apparent around the origin of the middle colic artery.

In the center of the infracolic region the *jejunum* may be seen emerging from behind the root of the mesentery. It forms roughly two fifths of the small bowel and is supplied by the more proximal branches of the superior mesenteric artery. Retracted to the right, the *ileum* comprises the remaining three fifths of the small intestines and is supplied by the more distal superior mesenteric branches.

Posterior to the ileum, the ascending colon may be seen rising to the hepatic flexure, where it makes an abrupt turn anteriorly and becomes the freely suspended transverse colon. Most of the ascending colon is supplied by the right colic branch of the superior mesenteric artery.

Plate 105

Superficial Aspect of Infracolic Viscera

221

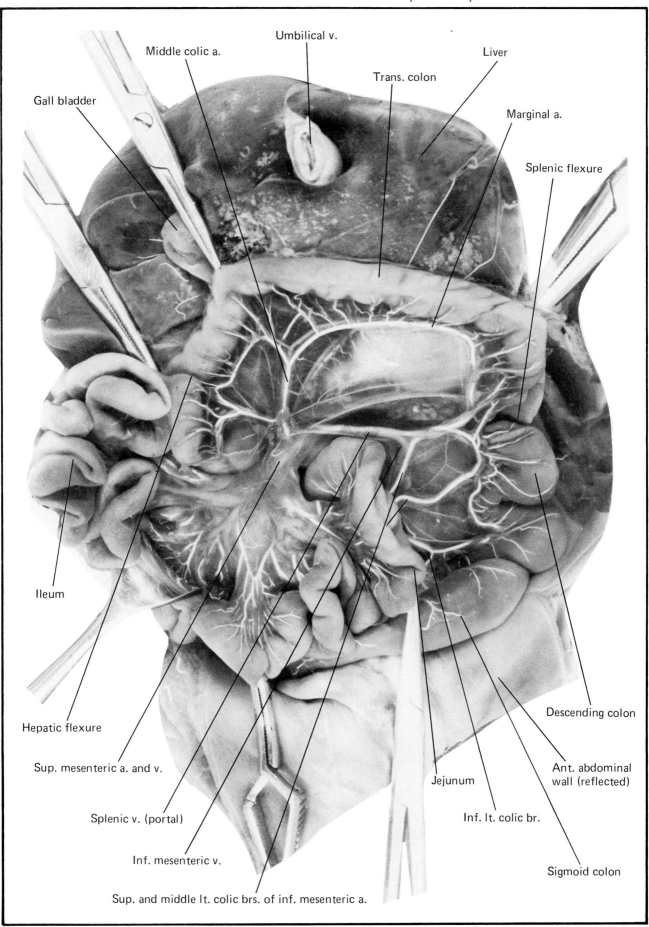

Middle colic a.

Umbilical v.

Liver

Trans. colon

Marginal a.

Gall bladder

Splenic flexure

Ileum

Hepatic flexure

Sup. mesenteric a. and v.

Descending colon

Jejunum

Ant. abdominal
wall (reflected)

Splenic v. (portal)

Inf. lt. colic br.

Inf. mesenteric v.

Sup. and middle lt. colic brs. of inf. mesenteric a.

Sigmoid colon

INFRACOLIC VISCERA: DEEPER ASPECT

This is a deeper exposure of the specimen in the preceding illustration. The entire small intestine has been retracted to the right to expose the vascular relations of the lower abdominal aorta and the inferior surface of the root of the mesentery. Note that the course of the proximal part of the *superior mesenteric artery* is more obvious in this exposure, and the origin of the *middle colic artery* is clearly defined.

In the center of the specimen, the inferior section of the abdominal aorta shows the origin of the *inferior mesenteric artery* just above the bifurcation that forms the two *common iliac arteries*. The inferior mesenteric artery is the definitive expression of the embryonic hindgut artery. Therefore, its vascular domain includes the left third of the *transverse colon,* the *splenic flexure,* the *descending colon,* the *sigmoid colon* and the *rectum* (refer to labels on previous illustration). The inferior mesenteric artery shortly branches into the *superior* and *middle left colic arteries* to the transverse colon, hepatic flexure and descending colon. The inferior left colic arteries supply the lower descending colon and proximal sigmoid, and the most inferior branch continues inferiorly as the *superior rectal artery.* The number of colonic branches of the inferior mesenteric is quite variable, but all of them contribute to the marginal artery. However, the marginal anastomotic loop is often deficient between the lower colic and superior rectal vessels (Sudeck's critical point).

In the right lower quadrant of this exposure, the *ureter* may be seen crossing the external iliac branch of the *right common iliac artery.* Lateral to these structures, the *right testicular artery* marks the path of descent of the *right testicle,* which here lies above the internal inguinal ring just prior to its descent into the scrotum. Posterior to the testicular artery, the cecum may be seen lying on the pelvic brim.

Plate 106   Deeper Aspect of Infracolic Viscera   223

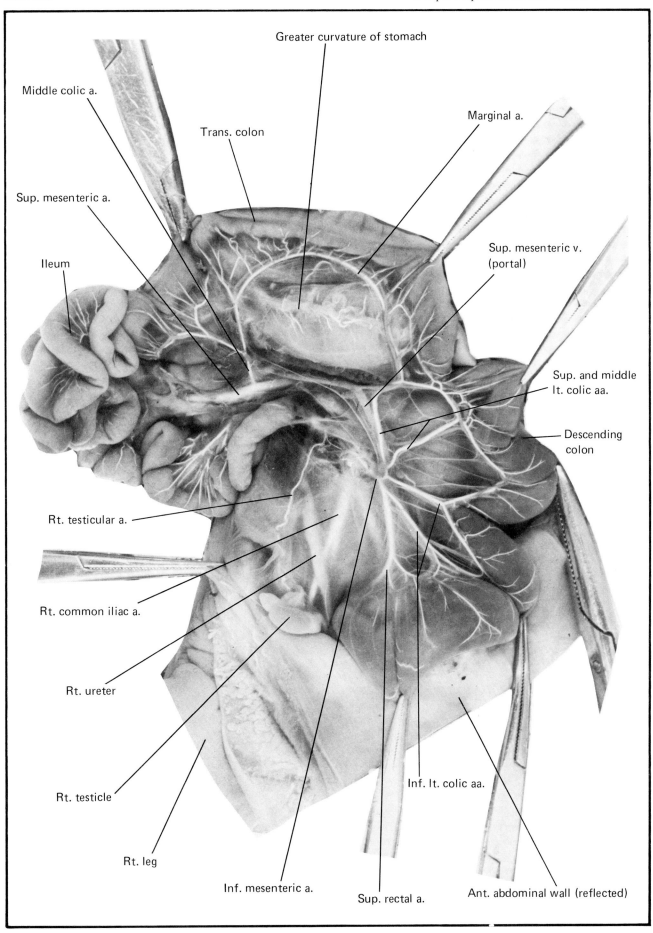

Greater curvature of stomach

Middle colic a.

Trans. colon

Marginal a.

Sup. mesenteric a.

Sup. mesenteric v. (portal)

Ileum

Sup. and middle lt. colic aa.

Descending colon

Rt. testicular a.

Rt. common iliac a.

Rt. ureter

Rt. testicle

Inf. lt. colic aa.

Rt. leg

Inf. mesenteric a.

Sup. rectal a.

Ant. abdominal wall (reflected)

THE JEJUNUM AND ILEUM: DIFFERENCES IN VASCULARITY

Although characteristic sections of the jejunum and ileum may be differentiated by the greater abundance of semilunar plicae and wider lumen of the former, these are internal characteristics. Externally, however, these two regions of the small intestine may be distinguished by their vascularity. The *jejunal branches* of the superior mesenteric artery are the longest of the intestinal series of branches, and upon approaching the gut, they break up into a row of wide vascular loops before providing rather long vasa recta to the intestine (Plate 107). The *ileal branches,* on the other hand, are shorter and more numerous for a given length of the gut. They divide into a more complex arrangement of vascular loops, often three or four tiers deep, and supply the intestinal wall with very many closely arranged vasa recta (Plate 108).

The fat deposition in the mesentery of the fetus is usually sparse and equal in both sections of the intestine, but postnatally the mesentery of the ileum builds up a very thick fat layer that obscures much of the vascularity. On the other hand, the jejunal mesentery remains relatively fat-free, and transparent mesenteric areas may be seen between its readily observable vascular loops.

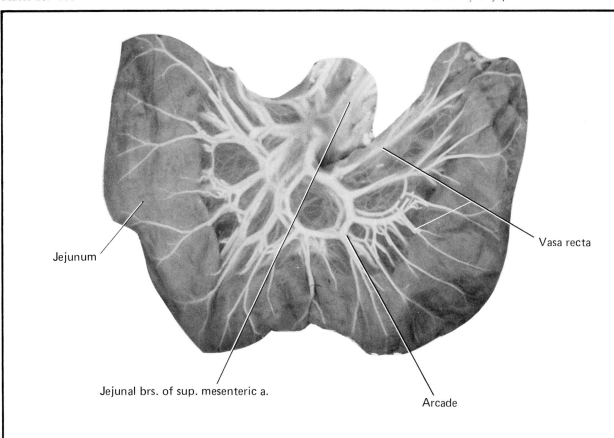

Jejunum

Vasa recta

Jejunal brs. of sup. mesenteric a.

Arcade

Ilial br. of sup. mesenteric a.

Secondary arcades

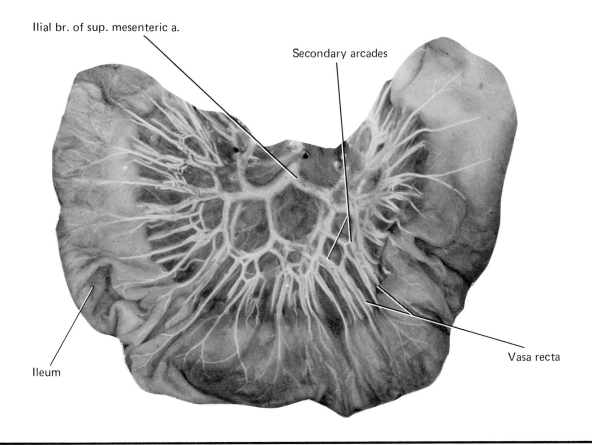

Ileum

Vasa recta

THE ILEOCECAL REGION AND THE APPENDIX

The ileum does not simply expand into the colon but forms a complex valved union with the large intestine called the ileocecal junction. In diverse forms of other mammals, the large bowel possesses a long, coiled diverticulum called the cecum. The cecum served as an accessory digestive chamber where substances (particularly cellulose) unaffected by the secreted digestive enzymes were subjected to bacterial decomposition so that their simpler fractions could be absorbed. In the omnivorous human, the cecum is represented by a blind pouch inferior to the ileocecal junction that bears a condensed remnant of the original cecal extension called the *appendix*. This structure has no obvious digestive function but seems to be retained as an accessory immunologic organ.

The blood supply to the cecum, appendix and inferior part of the ascending colon is provided by the *ileocecal artery*. This vessels runs in the mesentery in approximation to the terminal part of the ileum, which it supplies with vasa recta, and terminates in an *ascending branch* that is the initial part of the marginal artery of the ascending colon. Because of the complexities of the ileocecal union, the suspending mesentery forms a series of folds and fossae. Anterior to the ileocecal union, a branch of the ileocecal artery runs in the free edge of a mesenteric duplication called the *superior ileocecal fold*. This structure creates a blind pouch, the ileocecal fossa, that is here marked by an inserted paper wedge. Along the inferior aspect of the terminal ileum, another vessel raises the *inferior ileocecal fold* that guards the inferior ileocecal fossa.

Posterior to the ileum, the ileocecal artery provides the *appendicular artery* that descends along the appendix in the mesoappendix.

Plate 109   Ileocecal Region and Appendix   227

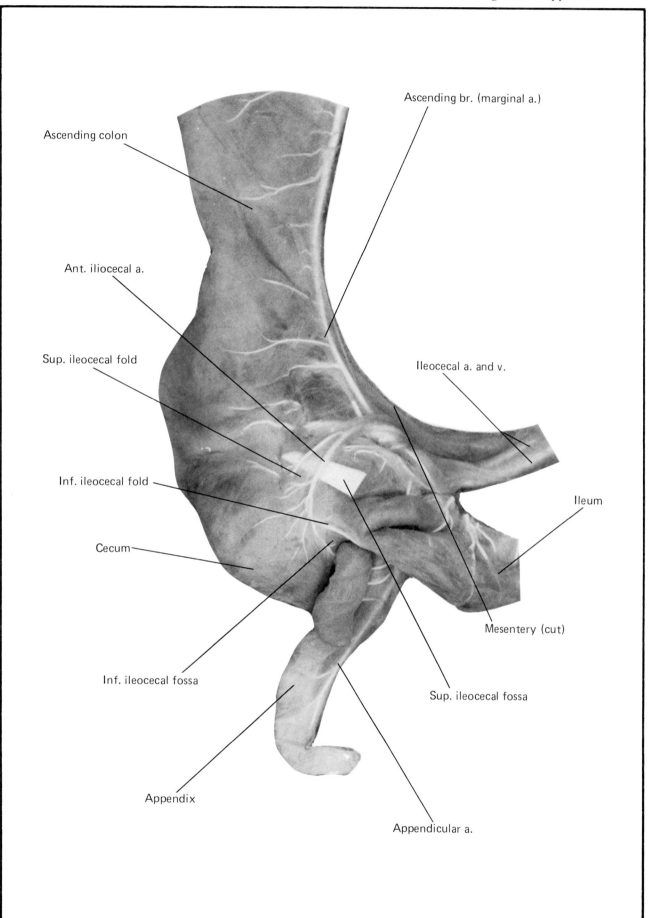

Ascending colon

Ascending br. (marginal a.)

Ant. iliocecal a.

Sup. ileocecal fold

Ileocecal a. and v.

Inf. ileocecal fold

Cecum

Ileum

Inf. ileocecal fossa

Mesentery (cut)

Sup. ileocecal fossa

Appendix

Appendicular a.

ANGIOGRAM OF THE SUPERIOR MESENTERIC ARTERY

In this illustration, the parts of the digestive tract that are dependent upon the superior mesenteric artery were dissected out of the body and radiographed separately. The contrast medium shows the major artery severed at its origin on the abdominal aorta. The first branch, the *middle colic artery*, here runs a short distance to the right and reaches the transverse colon just medial to the hepatic flexure. As mentioned previously, the so-called "middle" colic artery most frequently is associated with the left side of the transverse colon. The extent of the marginal artery and its anastomoses with the *superior left colic branches* of the inferior mesenteric artery can be appreciated.

The *jejunal branches* comprise the first four left lateral derivatives of the superior mesenteric. They are typically longer and have fewer vasa recta and terminal anastomotic loops than the *ileal branches*. The main shaft of the superior mesenteric artery seems to terminate in a loop proximal to the ileocecal junction. The loop that is completed by the *ileocolic artery* bears the appendicular artery to the appendix. The marginal artery commences with the right loop of the ileocolic and is reinforced by contributions from the right colic branch of the superior mesenteric.

Plate 110   Angiogram of Superior Mesenteric Artery   229

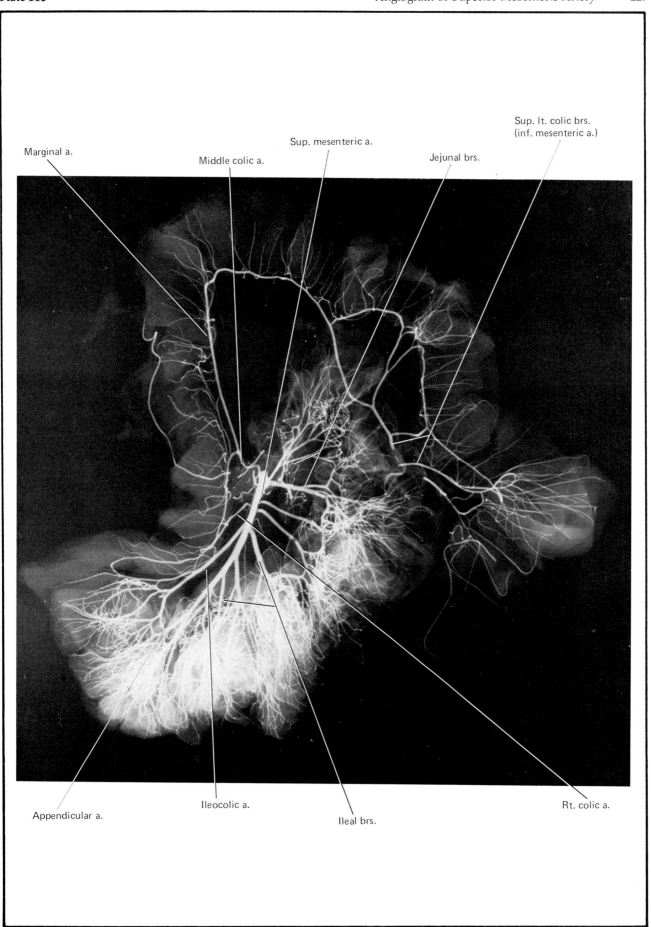

Marginal a.

Middle colic a.

Sup. mesenteric a.

Jejunal brs.

Sup. lt. colic brs.
(inf. mesenteric a.)

Appendicular a.

Ileocolic a.

Ileal brs.

Rt. colic a.

LATERAL ANGIOGRAM OF THE ABDOMINAL REGION

This is the same specimen shown in previous A-P illustrations, and its lateral aspect provides dimension to the relationships of the arteries. Of particular interest are the three visceral branches of the abdominal aorta. The most superior, the *celiac axis*, leaves the aorta between the crura of the diaphragm. Its first branches, the *inferior phrenic arteries*, are not visceral; they follow the phrenic surface upward and so define its contour over the posterior aspect of the liver. The *hepatic artery* passes posterosuperiorly, but much of its finer ramifications are lost in the network of superimposed vessels. Behind the origin of the hepatic artery, the left gastric artery arcs toward the gastric cardia, but it is the *right gastric* and *right gastroepiploic* branches of the *gastroduodenal artery* that clearly define the position of the lower part of the stomach. Realizing that the *superior mesenteric artery* passes between the pancreas and the horizontal part of the duodenum, following the *anterior superior pancreatoduodenal artery* clearly outlines this loop of the intestine. The anterior and inferior arrangements of the *jejunal* and *ileal branches* can be seen supplying their respective regions of the gut.

Just above the aortic bifurcation, the *inferior mesenteric artery* courses to the left of the ileal branches to supply the descending sigmoidal and rectal parts of the large intestine.

Plate 111　　　　　　　　　Lateral Angiogram of Abdominal Region　　　　231

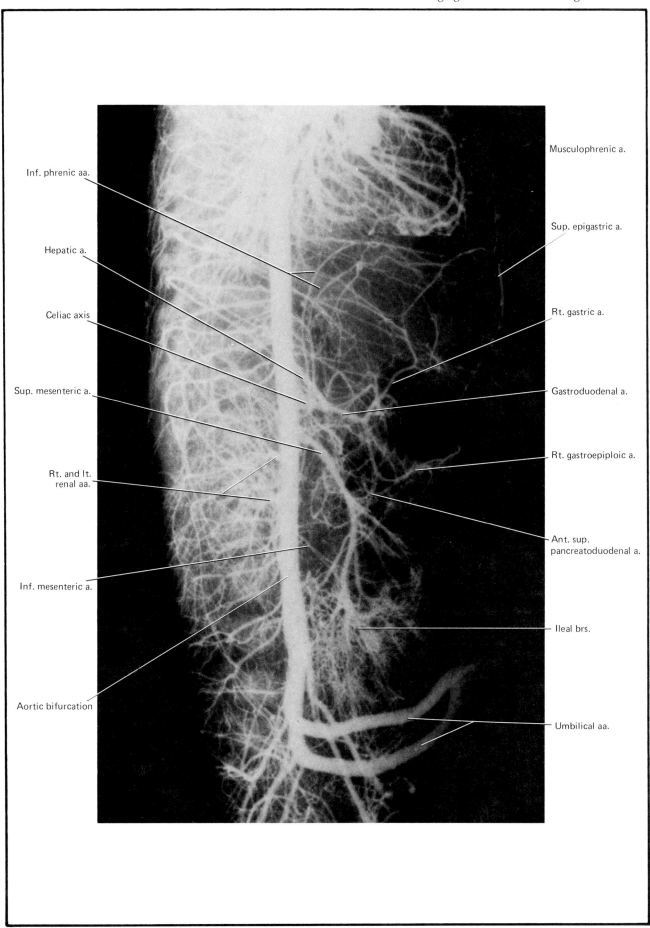

Inf. phrenic aa.

Hepatic a.

Celiac axis

Sup. mesenteric a.

Rt. and lt.
renal aa.

Inf. mesenteric a.

Aortic bifurcation

Musculophrenic a.

Sup. epigastric a.

Rt. gastric a.

Gastroduodenal a.

Rt. gastroepiploic a.

Ant. sup.
pancreatoduodenal a.

Ileal brs.

Umbilical aa.

ANGIOGRAM OF THE FETAL PORTAL AND HEPATIC VEINS

This specimen was dissected from the doubly injected fetus shown in a lateral angiogram in the introductory plates of the atlas. Here the abdominal viscera were removed in toto and radiographed in an anteroposterior view to show the portal and hepatic veins. The finely divided barium sulfate was injected via the umbilical vein and filled the portal and hepatic systems via the ductus venosus. The arterial system received the medium from the right side of the heart through the ductus arteriosus. Unfortunately, manipulation of the liver during dissection expressed some of the medium from the ductus venosus, but a sufficient amount remained to ascertain its relationships and course.

The portal system was filled primarily through the *portal sinus*, a large transverse channel that directly connects the portal vein at the hilus to the junction of *umbilical vein* and the *ductus venosus*.

The designation "portal vein" is applied only to the vessel formed by the union of the *splenic* and *superior mesenteric veins*. These veins accompany corresponding arteries throughout their courses, but the superior part of the inferior mesenteric vein must leave the company of the inferior mesenteric artery and pursue an independent course to join the splenic vein posterior to the pancreas. The confluence of the inferior mesenteric and splenic veins may occur at any point along the proximal half of the latter.

Plate 112   Angiogram of Portal and Hepatic Veins   233

Hepatic vv.

Portal sinus

Vena cava

Hepatic a.

Ductus venosus

Umbilical v.

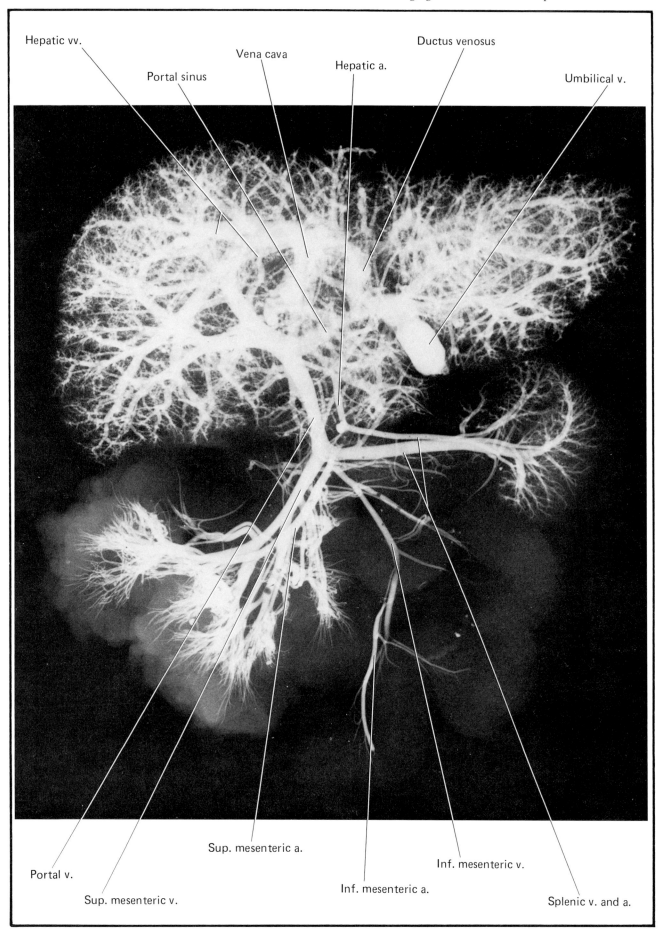

Sup. mesenteric a.

Inf. mesenteric v.

Portal v.

Inf. mesenteric a.

Sup. mesenteric v.

Splenic v. and a.

THE POSTERIOR ABDOMINAL WALL I

Because greater transparency of the posterior abdominal peritoneum and fascia were desired, a fetus younger (27 weeks) than those shown previously was prepared for this illustration. Injection of the Neoprene latex through the umbilical vein filled both the venous and arterial systems. Since the intention was to demonstrate only the major vessels, the injection pressure was low and the flow of the medium was stopped as soon as it returned through the umbilical arteries to the site of injection.

The relationships of the two great vessels of the posterior abdominal wall, the *aorta* and the *inferior vena cava*, are particularly well illustrated.

The liver has been carefully dissected away, leaving several stumps to indicate the positions of the *hepatic veins*, and the entire course of the vena cava, from the *common iliac* bifurcation to the caval hiatus of the diaphragm, is clearly visible.

Because the portal system drains the gastroenteric tract, the abdominal tributaries to the vena cava are either glandular or urogenital branches. Both the suprarenal glands and the suprarenal veins are disproportionately large in the fetus, and there is a marked asymmetry in the vessels. The *right suprarenal vein* drains directly into the vena cava just inferior to the liver, and the *left suprarenal vein* is confluent with the *left renal vein*. Since the vena cava is situated to the right of the midline, the left renal vein is longer. The *right* and *left* gonadal veins are also asymmetrical with the right vein, draining directly into the vena cava,

and with the left, joining the left renal vein. Because the gonads developed in approximation of the mesonephric region of the early posterior abdominal wall, both arteries and veins must follow their descent into the pelvic region.

The abdominal aorta is seen entering the abdomen posterior to the cardia of the stomach, and the immediate branching of the celiac axis is marked by the *left gastric* and *common hepatic arteries*. Between the celiac axis and the superior mesenteric artery, a diffuse mass of tissue represents the *celiac* and *superior mesenteric ganglia*, an accumulation of autonomic nerve fibers and synaptic junctions from which nerve plexuses follow all of the vascular branches to reach their terminal distributions.

The *superior mesenteric artery* arises from the aorta just above the left renal vein. As the artery follows the root of the mesentery downward, it bends over the left renal vein and the duodenum. The possible compression of the renal vein by the artery has been postulated as a cause of reflex hypertension.

Above the aortic bifurcation the proximal section of the severed *inferior mesenteric artery* is labeled.

The positional transition of the two great vessels is apparent. The vena cava occupies an anterior position relative to the aorta in the upper abdomen, but in the lower regions the aorta passes anterior to the vein. Scattered around the lower part of the aorta a number of paraaortic bodies are visible. Embryologically homologous to the suprarenal medulla, these structures show similar chromaffin histology. The presence of a conspicuous venous drainage suggests that they have an autonomous function prior to their involution in postnatal life.

Plate 113   Posterior Abdominal Wall I   235

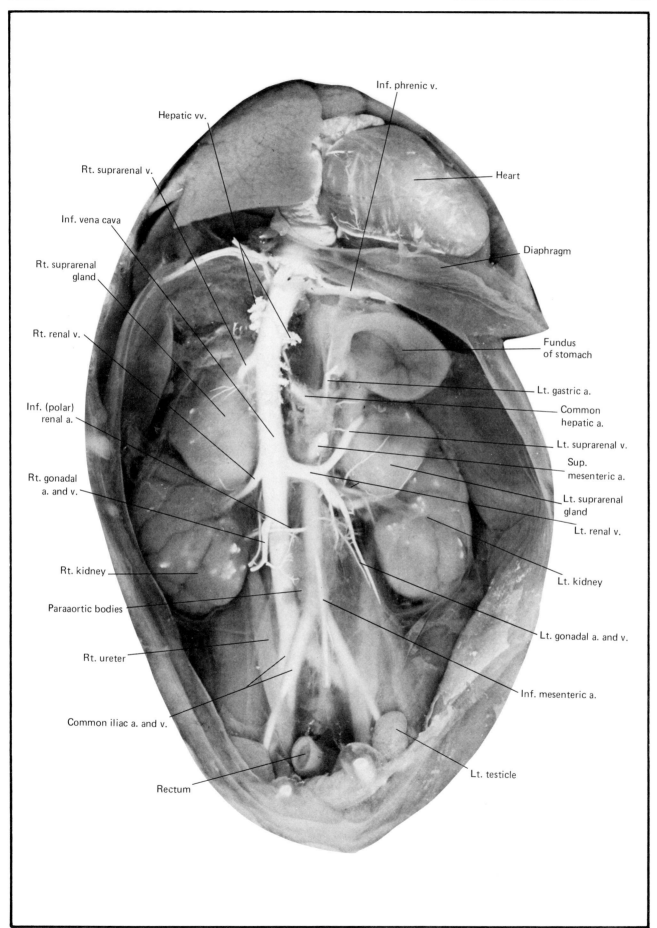

Hepatic vv.

Inf. phrenic v.

Rt. suprarenal v.

Heart

Inf. vena cava

Diaphragm

Rt. suprarenal
gland

Fundus
of stomach

Rt. renal v.

Lt. gastric a.

Common
hepatic a.

Inf. (polar)
renal a.

Lt. suprarenal v.

Sup.
mesenteric a.

Rt. gonadal
a. and v.

Lt. suprarenal
gland

Lt. renal v.

Rt. kidney

Lt. kidney

Paraaortic bodies

Rt. ureter

Lt. gonadal a. and v.

Inf. mesenteric a.

Common iliac a. and v.

Lt. testicle

Rectum

THE POSTERIOR ABDOMINAL WALL II

In this continued dissection of the previous specimen, the structures related to the lower posterior abdominal wall and pelvis are better exposed. The great vessels bifurcate anterior to the fourth lumbar vertebra at the level of the umbilicus. The resulting *common iliac* branches descend into the pelvis and redivide into the medially placed *hypogastric* (internal iliac) *arteries* and *veins* that serve pelvic and perineal structures, and the lateral *external iliac arteries* and *veins* that serve the abdominal wall and lower extremities.

The relations of the ureter to the iliac vessels are particularly well shown on the right side. Here the ureter may be traced from the hilus of the kidney down to the bladder. It crosses the iliac vessels at the bifurcation of the hypogastric and external iliac branches.

Posterior to the peritoneum and its supportive fascia, the muscles of the posterior abdominal wall are displayed. The most prominent of these is the long, thick *psoas muscle* that flexes the lumbar spine and, in combination with the iliacus, flexes the thigh. Posterior to the psoas, the unlabeled quadratus lumborum muscle forms a rectangular muscular strap between the lowest ribs and the iliac crest. It laterally flexes the spine and reinforces the posterior abdominal wall.

The external iliac artery has been followed into the leg to show its continuation as the *femoral artery.* Just superior to the superior pubic ramus, the external iliac gives off the *deep iliac circumflex artery* that supplies the lateral abdominal wall and the iliacus muscle and the *inferior epigastric artery* that is the major source of vascularity to the lower anterior abdominal wall. Note that in the retrograde injection of the caval veins, the medium was stopped by a valve proximal to the common iliac bifurcation, so that the distal vessels were left unfilled.

Plate 114   Posterior Abdominal Wall II   237

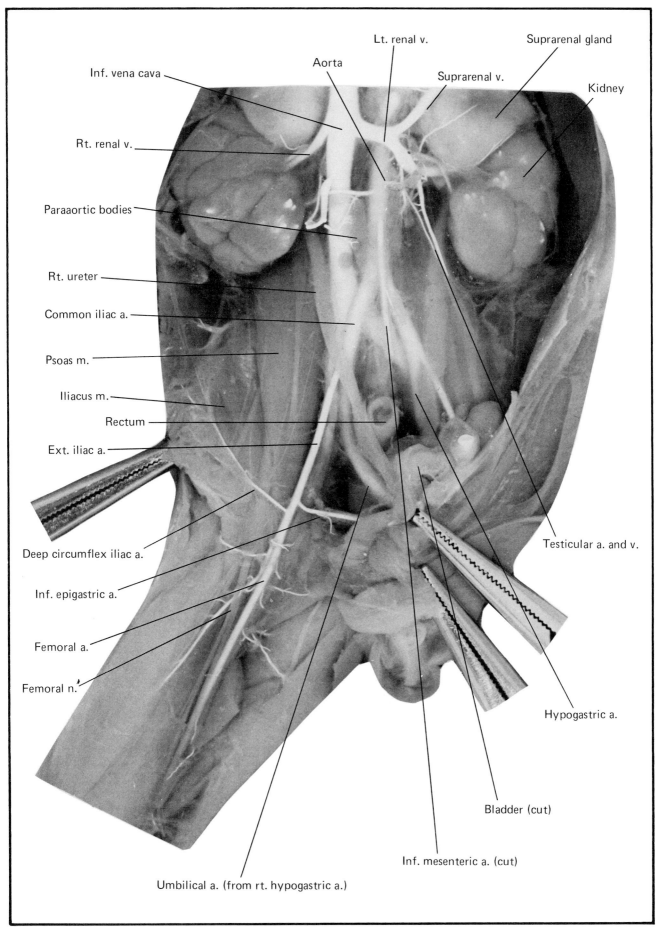

Inf. vena cava

Aorta

Lt. renal v.

Suprarenal gland

Suprarenal v.

Kidney

Rt. renal v.

Paraaortic bodies

Rt. ureter

Common iliac a.

Psoas m.

Iliacus m.

Rectum

Ext. iliac a.

Deep circumflex iliac a.

Inf. epigastric a.

Femoral a.

Femoral n.

Testicular a. and v.

Hypogastric a.

Bladder (cut)

Inf. mesenteric a. (cut)

Umbilical a. (from rt. hypogastric a.)

ARTERIOGRAM OF THE DIAPHRAGM

Shown here is the radiogram of a fetal diaphragm that has been excised and placed against an x-ray film cassette with the inferior surface facing the source of radiation.

The major ramifications of the *right* and *left inferior phrenic arteries* reveal the configuration of the central tendon and muscular areas of the diaphragm.

Each of these vessels arises on the celiac axis and ascends the anterior surface of the crura. Upon reaching the domes of each hemidiaphragm, they divide into anterior and posterior branches that form three vascular loops which outline the trefoil shape of the central tendon. The tendon seems to be relatively avascular except at the posterior part of the central leaf, where a number of small branches support the pericardium that is adherent to its superior surface. In the more peripheral muscular areas, however, fine striate arteries thread their way between the muscle fasciculi. In the extreme periphery, anastomoses with the *musculophrenic branches* anteriorly and the *intercostal branches* posteriorly are evident.

Several large structures that pass between the thorax and abdomen must pierce the diaphragm. The aorta traverses the *aortic hiatus* which is actually a muscular arch that lies between the two crura and anterior to the vertebrae. Anterior to this, the *esophageal hiatus* transmits the esophagus and is surrounded by numerous arterial contributions from the phrenic and esophageal plexuses.

To the right of this opening, the *caval hiatus* that passes the vena cava shows an arterial ring and a phrenic contribution to the pericardium, the *inferior phrenicopericardial artery*. The caval hiatus also marks the entrance of the right phrenic nerve that is distributed to the right hemidiaphragm in accordance with the arterial pattern. A small contribution of the left phrenic artery ascends the pericardium near the cardiac apex and runs along the left phrenic nerve as the left phrenicopericardial artery.

Plate 115

Arteriogram of Diaphragm

239

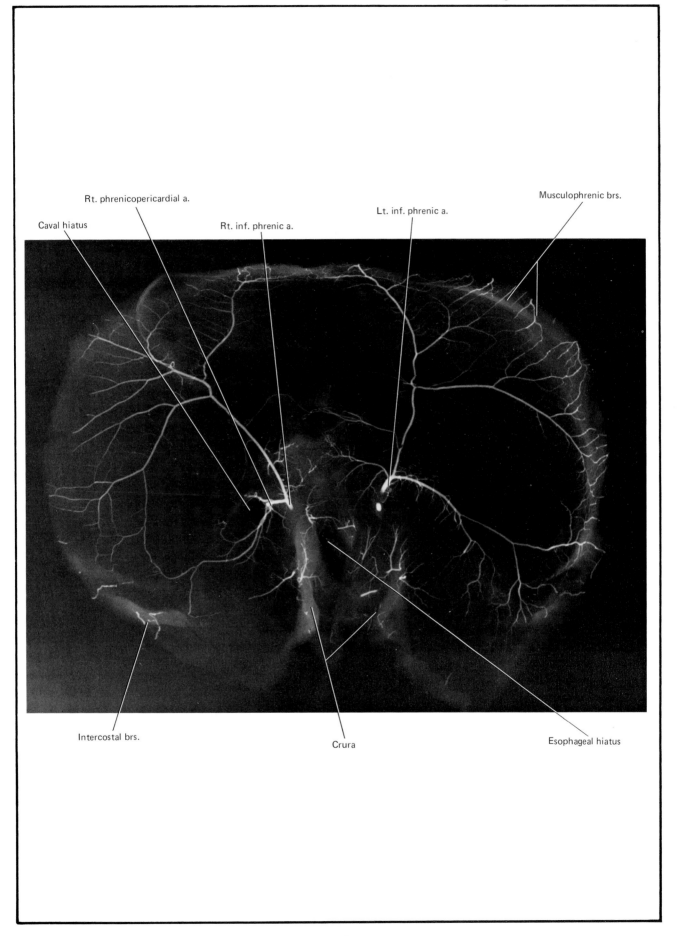

Rt. phrenicopericardial a.

Caval hiatus

Rt. inf. phrenic a.

Lt. inf. phrenic a.

Musculophrenic brs.

Intercostal brs.

Crura

Esophageal hiatus

THE KIDNEYS

This plate shows the two kidneys, their major vascular relations and the proximal ureters as they have been dissected from the posterior abdominal wall.

The fetal kidney still retains the lobulations that give external evidence of the growth of the individual pyramids. These lobulations disappear in the human postnatally, but they may be retained for life in some animals such as cattle.

The kidneys developed originally as pelvic organs from a combination of a pair of allantoic outgrowths that form the ureters and calyces, and mesodermal condensations that form the renal parenchyma. In their "ascent" from the pelvis they are associated with a variable number of lateral aortic branches (the kidneys are said to climb out of the pelvis on a ladder of aortic branches). In the definitive state, usually only a single pair of these remain as the *right* and *left renal arteries*. However, accessory aortic branches to the superior or inferior poles of the kidneys, the *polar renal arteries*, are not uncommon and simply reflect the original condition.

The kidneys are asymmetrical in regard to their positions and vascular relationships. The right kidney is lower because a greater mass of liver is interposed between it and the diaphragm, and the right renal artery is longer because the aorta is situated to the left of the midline. Conversely, the left renal vein is longer.

The urinary and vascular structures enter or leave the kidney at the renal hilus, an indentation in the medial border of each organ. At this point, the veins lie anterior to the arteries and the ureters descend posterior to the vessels. The ureters are relatively larger in the fetus, and blood supply to their proximal parts through special ureteral branches of the renal arteries is quite conspicuous.

Note here how the *celiac* and *superior mesenteric ganglia* surround the origins of the ventral splanchnic arteries.

The kidneys are supported by the renal fascia, a special split lamination of the subserous fascia that forms an inverted bag which holds both kidneys and the large vessels between them in a common container. In the late fetus and postnatal specimens, layers of fat within the renal fascia (perirenal fat) and posterior to it (pararenal fat) help fix the kidneys in position. Each organ also has its own capsule of fibrous connective tissue that may be stripped to expose the vascular cortex.

Plate 116

Kidneys   241

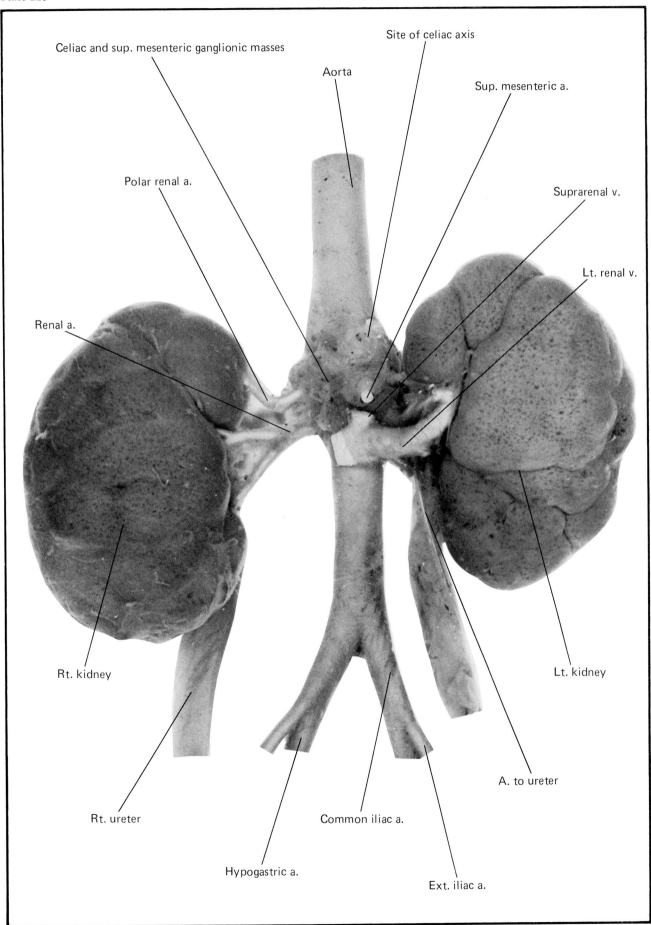

Celiac and sup. mesenteric ganglionic masses

Site of celiac axis

Aorta

Sup. mesenteric a.

Polar renal a.

Suprarenal v.

Lt. renal v.

Renal a.

Rt. kidney

Lt. kidney

A. to ureter

Rt. ureter

Common iliac a.

Hypogastric a.

Ext. iliac a.

FRONTAL SECTION THROUGH THE LEFT KIDNEY

The internal subdivisions of the kidney are easily perceived in a frontal section. The nephron is the functional unit of the kidney and consists of a glomerulus, its capsule and the distal system of convoluted tubules. Although these structures are best appreciated microscopically, their collective arrangement determines the gross structure of the kidney and accounts for the nonhomogeneous appearance of its parenchyma.

This plane of section shows the kidney to be divided into a number of subunits (varying from 8 to 18) called the *pyramids*. Each pyramid coincides with an external lobulation of the fetal kidney and consists of an aggregate of nephrons. It is actually a conical structure whose base is formed by a highly vascular layer of many glomeruli and capsules. Their systems of convoluted and collecting tubules form a striated mass that converges toward the hilus and terminates as an apical *renal papilla*. The glomerular layers of all of the pyramids constitute the *renal cortex* and the inner, less vascular striate parts collectively form the *medulla*.

The internal renal vascularity further accentuates these subdivisions. The major renal arteries branch into *interlobar arteries* that are radially dispersed in the areas between the pyramids that are called the *renal columns*. At the boundary between the medulla and the cortex, these interlobar vessels form a series of interconnecting arches, the *arcuate arteries*. From these a large number of fine *interlobular arteries* radiate out into the cortex to supply the glomeruli.

Each renal papilla discharges a number of collecting tubules into a funnel-shaped receptacle, the *minor calyx*. These structures, which may vary in number from 4 to 13, receive one or more papillae. Confluences of the minor calyces form three or four *major calyces* that empty into the expanded proximal part of the ureter, the *renal pelvis*.

The renal sinus is the space just internal to the hilus that accommodates the major vessels and the pelvis.

Plate 117   Frontal Section through Kidney   243

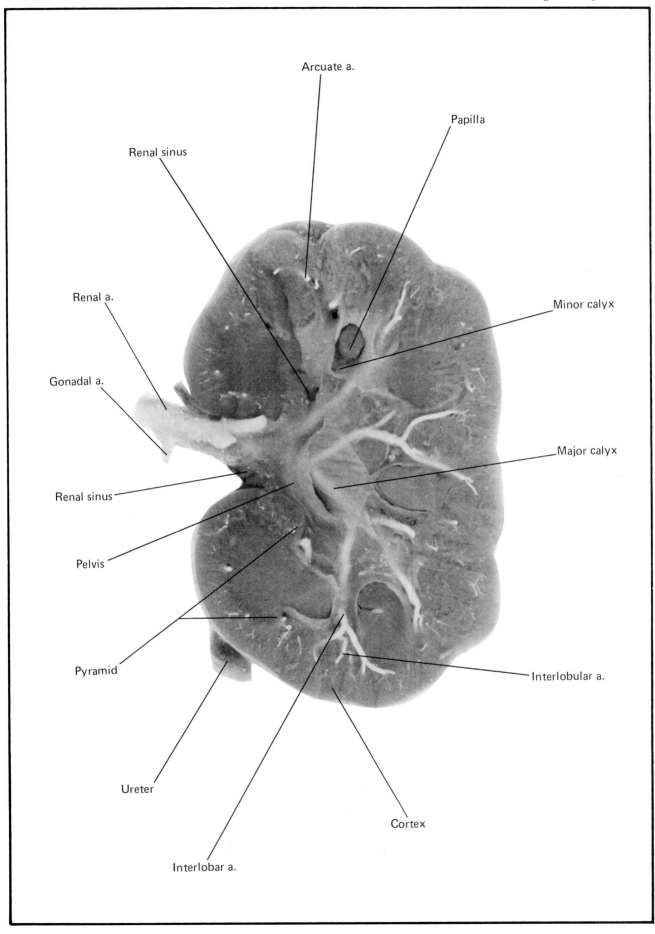

Arcuate a.

Papilla

Renal sinus

Renal a.

Minor calyx

Gonadal a.

Major calyx

Renal sinus

Pelvis

Interlobular a.

Pyramid

Ureter

Cortex

Interlobar a.

THE FINER VASCULAR RELATIONSHIPS OF THE POSTERIOR ABDOMINAL WALL

This dissection of the upper posterior abdominal region shows the finer vessels that are involved with the suprarenal glands and the gonads. On the left side, the renal fascia has been left intact except where the lower pole of the kidney has been exposed.

The fetal *suprarenal glands* are relatively massive, being almost one half the size and weight of the kidneys. However, despite their relative diminution in postnatal life, they still retain the complex vascular supply that here is seen supplying the anterior surface of the right gland. The numerous arteries of the suprarenal come from three major sources. The upper anterior and superior regions receive many branches from the *inferior phrenic arteries*, and the lower anterior and inferior areas are supplied by *renal branches*. The largest suprarenal arteries supply its posteroinferior (renal) surface and may variably arise from the proximal renal artery or the aorta.

The right *gonadal artery* may be seen arising from the junction of the right renal artery and the aorta. The sources of the gonadal arteries are usually located on the anterior surface of the aorta in the region of the renal arteries, but they may be less frequently found arising from the renal artery, particularly on the right side. These vessels are characterized by a very tortuous course as they descend retroperitoneally, entwined with their respective gonadal veins. Note the fine accessory gonadal artery from an inferior polar renal artery.

Plate 118   Vascular Relationships of Posterior Abdominal Wall   245

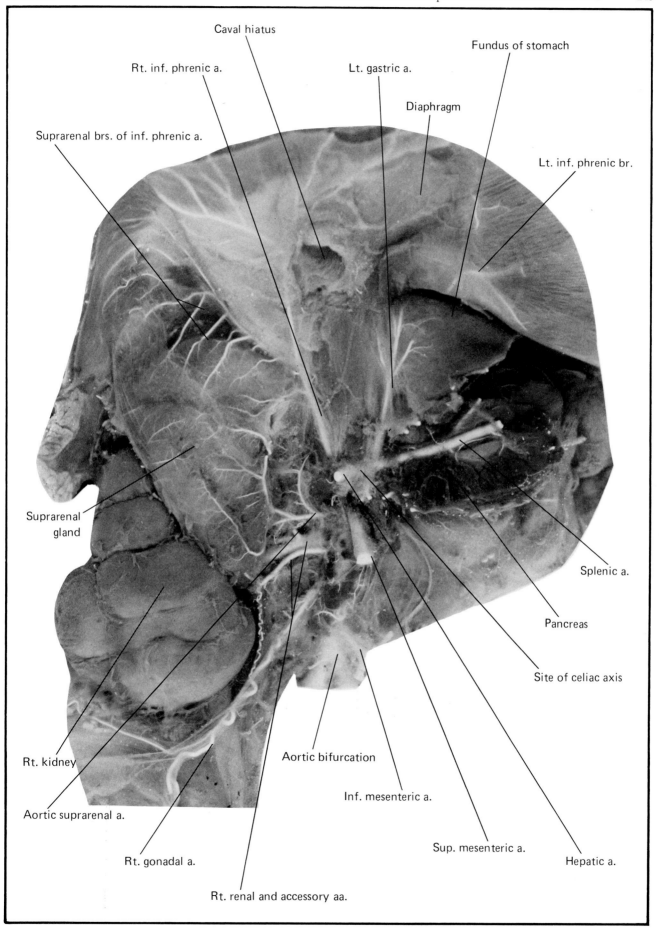

Caval hiatus

Rt. inf. phrenic a.

Lt. gastric a.

Fundus of stomach

Diaphragm

Suprarenal brs. of inf. phrenic a.

Lt. inf. phrenic br.

Suprarenal
gland

Splenic a.

Pancreas

Site of celiac axis

Rt. kidney

Aortic suprarenal a.

Aortic bifurcation

Inf. mesenteric a.

Rt. gonadal a.

Sup. mesenteric a.

Hepatic a.

Rt. renal and accessory aa.

THE SUPRARENAL GLANDS: POSTERIOR ASPECT

The suprarenal glands are endocrine organs of complex function and development. Their chromaffin-positive internal medullary cells are neuroectoderm derivatives that are homologous to the cells of the paraaortic bodies, whereas their external cortical cells are of mesodermal origin. The medullae secrete epinephrine and norepinephrine and thus reinforce the general action of the sympathetic division of the autonomic nervous system. The cortical cells secrete a series of steroid complexes that influence electrolyte balance, protein and carbohydrate metabolism, and interact with the immunologic systems.

The fetal suprarenal gland is relatively much larger than that of the adult, and at term it may be almost as large as the kidney. Much of this relative size differential is attributable to a special zone of cortical cells found only in the fetus. These cells produce dehydroxyepiandrosterone sulfate, which is utilized by the placenta in the production of estrogens for the maintenance of pregnancy.

The glands are not symmetrical in their morphology. The right one is larger and has less surface contact with the kidney. Each gland bears a rounded posterosuperior *phrenic surface*, a posteroinferior *renal impression* and an *anterior surface* that is variably related to the regional abdominal viscera. The larger arteries coursing in the renal impression are usually derived directly from the aorta on the left side because the medial border of this gland lies in close approximation to the main vessel. On the right, however, the corresponding arteries are usually branches arising from the longer right renal artery.

Plate 119   Posterior Aspect of Suprarenal Glands   247

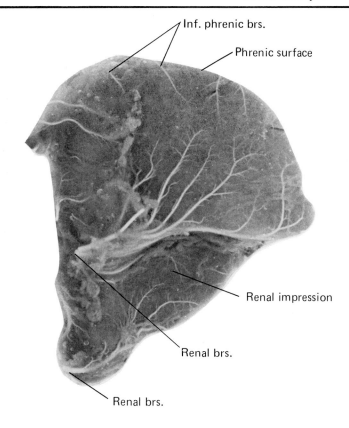

Inf. phrenic brs.

Phrenic surface

Renal impression

Renal brs.

Renal brs.

Right

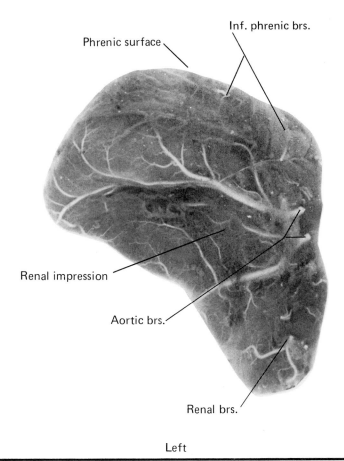

Inf. phrenic brs.

Phrenic surface

Renal impression

Aortic brs.

Renal brs.

Left

SUPERFICIAL DISSECTION OF THE LEFT LUMBAR PLEXUS

The preaxial (anterior and medial) muscle compartments of the thigh develop as extensions of the lumbar myotomes and therefore derive their innervation from anterior primary divisions of the lumbar spinal nerves. Subsequent differential growth of the lower trunk brought the inferior extremities into a more caudal position and required that these nerves take an oblique course along the musculature of the posterior abdominal wall. Removal of the peritoneum and renal fascia shows that the roots of the lumbar plexus arise posterior to the large, spindle-shaped *psoas major muscle*, but much of the plexus may be identified prior to the dissection of this structure.

In the superior part of the field, the *subcostal nerve* courses inferolaterally to innervate the abdominal muscles and skin. Being actually the 12th "intercostal" nerve (T12), it follows a dermomyotomic distribution that terminates midway between the umbilicus and the pubic symphysis. Below this, the first lumbar nerve (L1), with contributions from T12, forms a trunk that divides into the *iliohypogastric* and *ilioinguinal nerves.* The former follows a dermomyotomic strip inferior to that of the subcostal nerve, and the latter, in addition to its distribution on the abdomen, sends sensory fibers to the upper thigh and scrotum.

A fusion of fibers from L2 and L3 form the *lateral femoral cutaneous nerve* that is sensory to a long dermatomic strip down the lateral thigh.

The *genitofemoral nerve* arises from L1 and L2 and is the only nerve to pass anteriorly through the substance of the psoas muscle. It follows the surface of the muscle to the level of the internal inguinal ring. There it divides into a genital and femoral branch. The first follows the spermatic cord and supplies the cremaster muscle and the opposing skin of the scrotum and internal thigh, and the second passes deep to the inguinal ligament and innervates the skin and fascia of the upper anterior thigh.

In this plate the retraction of the aorta to the right reveals the lumbar sympathetic chain where it lies anterolateral to the bodies of the lumbar vertebrae.

Plate 120   Superficial Dissection of Lumbar Plexus   249

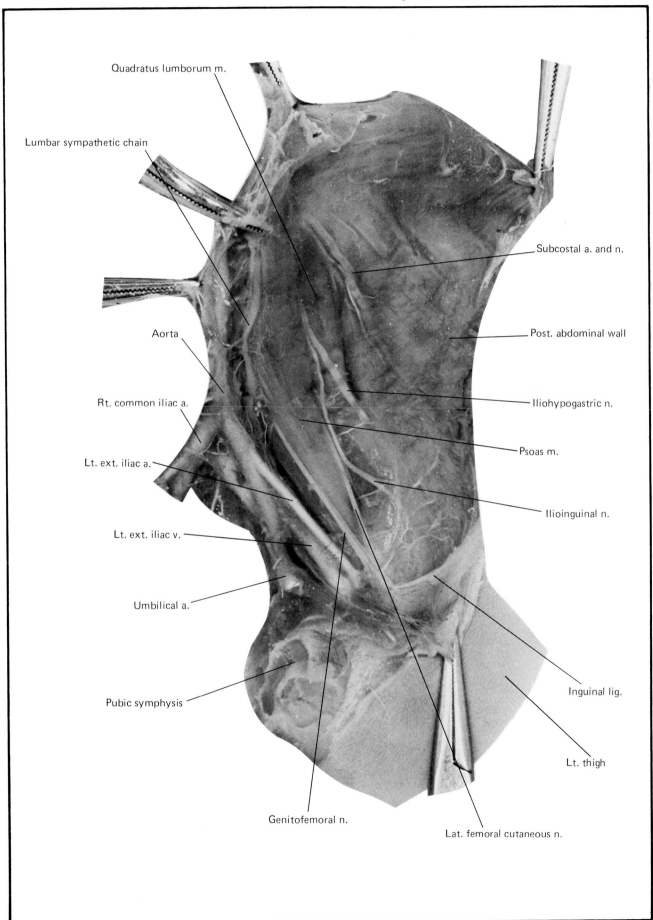

Quadratus lumborum m.

Lumbar sympathetic chain

Subcostal a. and n.

Aorta

Post. abdominal wall

Rt. common iliac a.

Iliohypogastric n.

Lt. ext. iliac a.

Psoas m.

Ilioinguinal n.

Lt. ext. iliac v.

Umbilical a.

Inguinal lig.

Pubic symphysis

Lt. thigh

Genitofemoral n.

Lat. femoral cutaneous n.

DEEP DISSECTION OF THE LEFT LUMBAR PLEXUS

In this continued dissection of the previously illustrated specimen, the central part of the psoas muscle has been removed to expose the deeper components of the lumbar plexus. The formerly discussed nerves are still visible, with the exception of the genitofemoral that has been removed with the muscle. Posterior to the psoas, the large *femoral nerve* passes inferiorly to enter the femoral triangle deep to the inguinal ligament. This nerve supplies the quadriceps femoris, the great extensor of the leg that occupies the anterior region of the thigh. Medial to the femoral nerve, the *obturator nerve* crosses the brim and internal wall of the pelvis to pass through the obturator foramen and innervate the medial adductor muscles of the thigh. Both the femoral and obturator nerves arise from L2, L3 and L4 and frequently are split into accessory branches.

The iliac vessels have been removed to reveal the deep *lumbosacral trunk* that carries thick contributions of L4 and L5 to unite with the upper sacral contributions to the sciatic nerve.

Plate 121   Deep Dissection of Lumbar Plexus   251

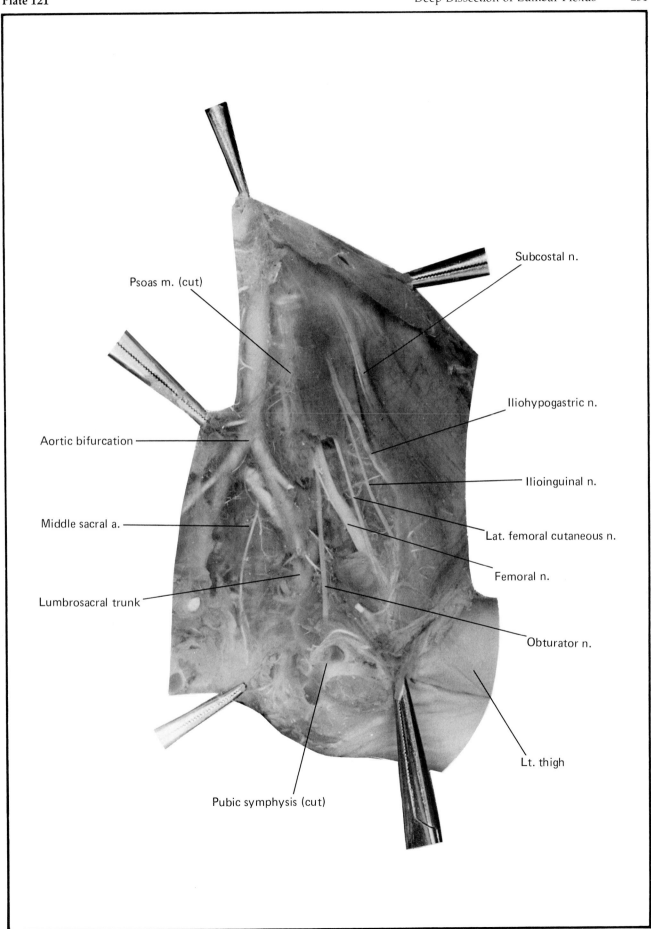

Subcostal n.

Psoas m. (cut)

Iliohypogastric n.

Aortic bifurcation

Ilioinguinal n.

Middle sacral a.

Lat. femoral cutaneous n.

Femoral n.

Lumbrosacral trunk

Obturator n.

Lt. thigh

Pubic symphysis (cut)

CROSS SECTION THROUGH THE TRANSPYLORIC REGION OF THE ABDOMEN

This cross section of a doubly injected specimen shows an interesting aspect of the visceral and vascular relationships that occurs at the transpyloric level. Opposite the first lumbar vertebra, the *aorta* can be seen giving origin to the *superior mesenteric* artery that immediately passes inferior to the *pancreas*. To the right of the aorta, the *inferior vena cava* lies against an inferior section of the right *suprarenal gland*, and the cut, superior pole of kidney demonstrates the position of this organ and its fascial coverings well.

The plane of section also includes the inferior *stomach* body and the bulb of the *duodenum*. The interposition of the pylorus as a sphincter between these two regions of the gut can be appreciated.

To the left of the stomach, the double section of the large intestine at the region of the splenic flexure shows both the *transverse colon* and the retroperitoneally fixed *descending colon* where it lies anterior to the spleen.

The right anterior region is occupied by the liver, where the *cystic duct* and *umbilical vein* may be discerned.

The posterior diaphragm may be followed along the wall of the lower rib cage, from which it is separated by a cleft of the pleural cavity, the *costophrenic sinus*. Lateral to the aorta the *diaphragmatic crura* arise from the lumbar spine.

Plate 122　　　　Cross Section through Transpyloric Region of Abdomen　　　253

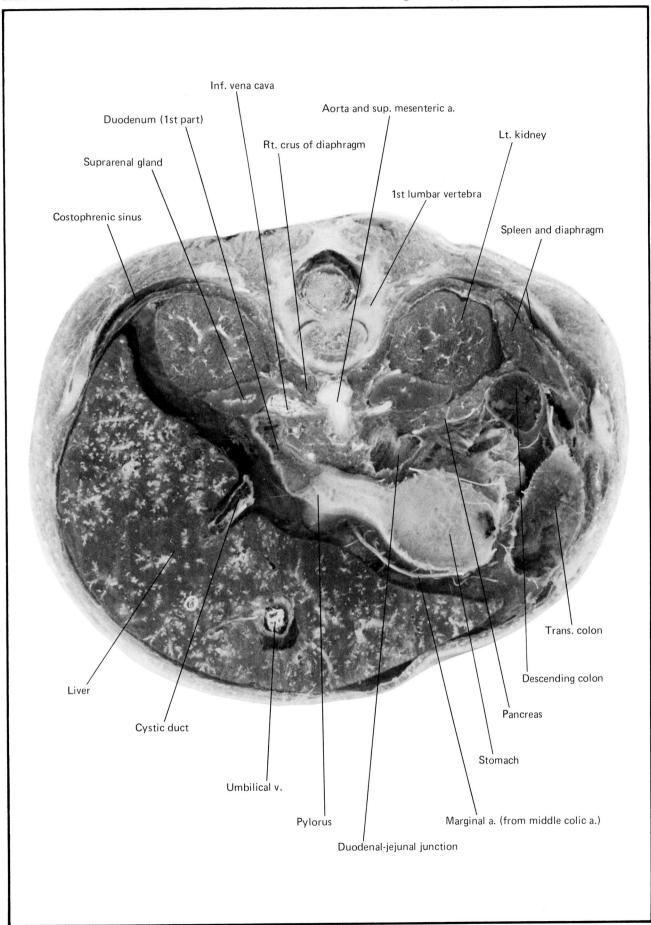

Inf. vena cava

Duodenum (1st part)

Aorta and sup. mesenteric a.

Suprarenal gland

Rt. crus of diaphragm

Lt. kidney

1st lumbar vertebra

Costophrenic sinus

Spleen and diaphragm

Liver

Cystic duct

Trans. colon

Descending colon

Pancreas

Umbilical v.

Stomach

Pylorus

Marginal a. (from middle colic a.)

Duodenal-jejunal junction

CROSS SECTION THROUGH THE ABDOMEN AT THE LEVEL OF THE THIRD LUMBAR VERTEBRA

In this lower section of the same specimen used in the preceding illustration, the renal fascia is more clearly defined and the position of the *psoas muscle* in relation to the kidney is well shown.

The lower loop of the *duodenum* cradles the inferior part of the head of the *pancreas* just anterior to the *aorta* and *inferior vena cava*. The *root of the mesentery* shows numerous intestinal branches of the superior mesenteric artery where it is surrounded by sections of the *jejunum*. The coils of the *ileum* are displayed in the right side of the cavity, and the differential character of these two parts of the small intestine is well illustrated. As in the adult, the lumen of the jejunum is larger than that of the ileum, but in the fetus the jejunal wall is thinner and the valves are not as pronounced as they become in later life.

The *ascending colon* and *descending colon* here show their typical retroperitoneal fixation to the posterior abdominal wall.

This section also demonstrates the origins of the muscles of the abdominal wall. Note that they arise from the lumbodorsal fascia that surrounds the *erector spinae muscle* complex of the back.

Plate 123   Cross Section through Abdomen at 3rd Lumbar Vertebra   255

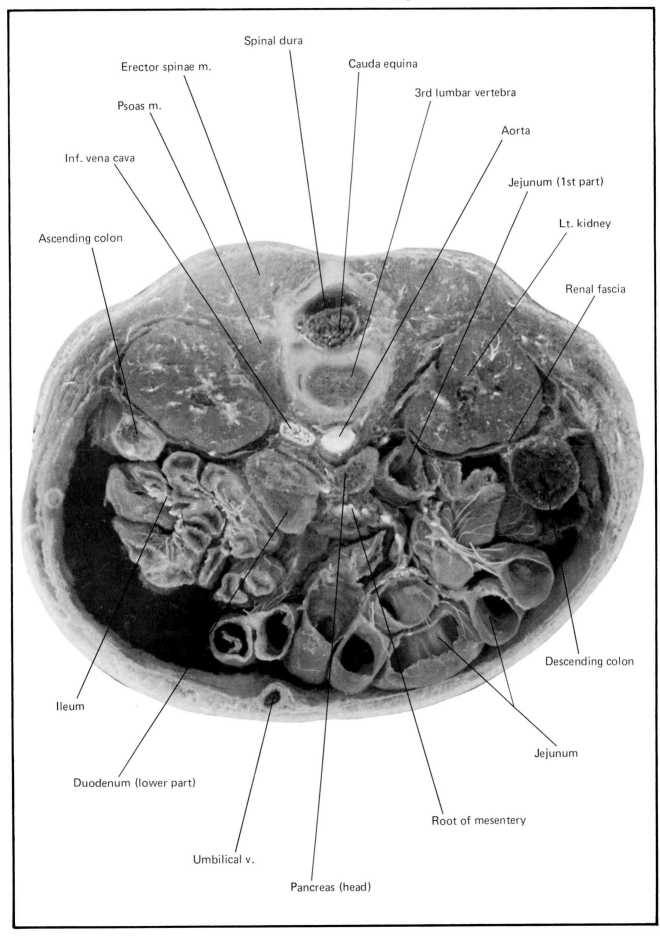

Spinal dura

Erector spinae m.

Cauda equina

Psoas m.

3rd lumbar vertebra

Inf. vena cava

Aorta

Jejunum (1st part)

Lt. kidney

Ascending colon

Renal fascia

Descending colon

Ileum

Jejunum

Duodenum (lower part)

Root of mesentery

Umbilical v.

Pancreas (head)

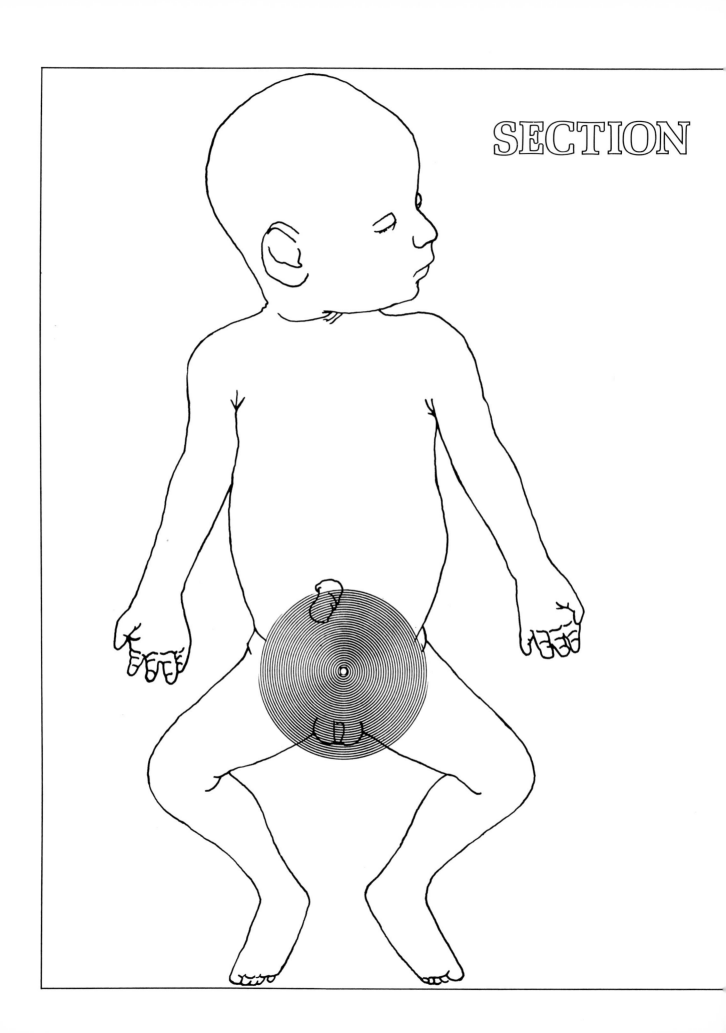

SECTION

SIX
PELVIS

RADIOGRAM OF THE FETAL PELVIS

The pelvis has the dual function of supporting and protecting the inferior enteric and urogenital viscera while transmitting forces between the spine and lower extremity that are incurred in stance and locomotion. Because the pelvis also must accommodate the birth canal, it is the skeletal component that usually shows the most pronounced sexual dimorphism. That is, the structural characteristics of the adult male and female pelvis may obviously differ; the female generally is wider and possesses a greater subpubic angle and pelvic outlet. However, in the fetus and the prepubescent child the pelvis shows no sexual differences, and the only signs of gender in the specimen illustrated here are the soft shadows of the female external genitalia.

Each half of the pelvis is formed by three bones, the *ilium*, the *ischium* and the *pubis*. All of them share in the articulation with the femur, but only the ilium articulates with the spine.

The radiologic appearance of the pelvis gives the impression that the ossified areas are "floating" without firm physical contact with the other bones, but it must be remembered that the articular areas are premodeled in radiolucent cartilage. The region of convergence of the three pelvic bones bears the deep, cuplike socket, the *acetabulum,* which receives the round, chondrous femoral head, but the actual position of the articular surfaces here may only be deduced from the relative position of the ossified part of the femoral shaft. Therefore, congenital dislocation of the hip, one of the most common dysarthroses of the newborn, is difficult to visualize radiographically. Indicative of this disorder, however, are the presence of a palpable "click" in the passive manipulation of the joint and an upward displacement of the visible part of the femoral shaft.

The elements comprising the sacrum are noticeable as five vertebral centra and the ossific centers for their neural arches. Lateral to the first, second, and later, the third sacral segments, spheroidal centers for the costal processes that form the sacral alae may be visualized. They eventually produce the sacral articular surfaces of the sacroiliac joint.

The concavity in the medial edge of each ilium indicates the *greater sciatic notch,* through which pass nerves and vessels to the gluteal and pudendal regions.

A single ossification marks the first segment of the coccyx. Often this is not radiologically visible until several months after parturition.

Plate 124   Radiogram of Fetal Pelvis   259

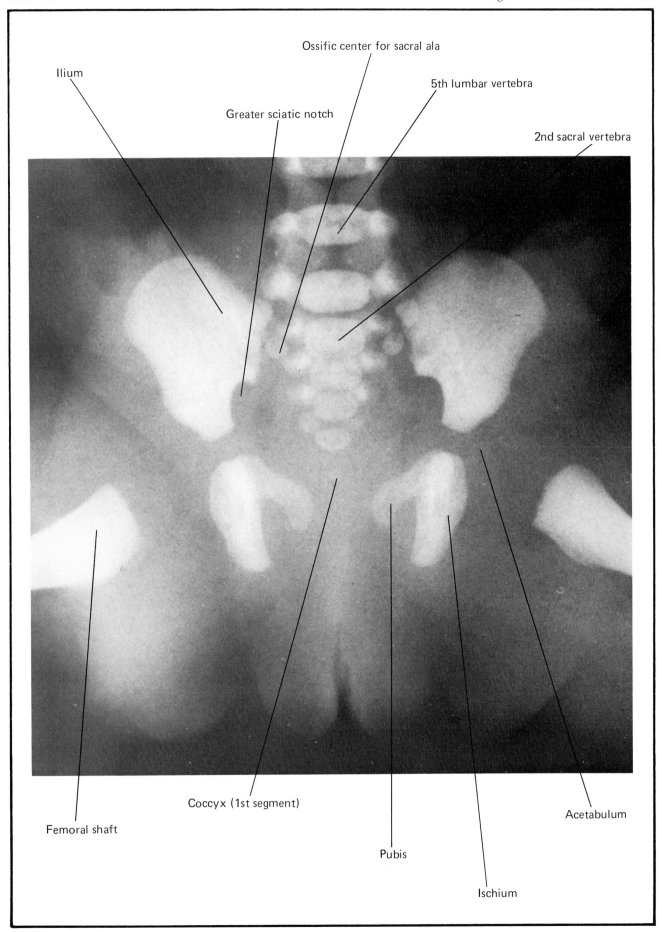

Ossific center for sacral ala

Ilium

5th lumbar vertebra

Greater sciatic notch

2nd sacral vertebra

Coccyx (1st segment)

Femoral shaft

Pubis

Ischium

Acetabulum

SUPERFICIAL ASPECT OF THE PERINEUM AND EXTERNAL GENITALIA (MALE)

The term "perineum" includes the anatomic region and structures of the pelvic outlet. In the adult, it is a rhomboidal area with its four points limited by the pubic symphysis and coccyx anteriorly and posteriorly, and the ischial tuberosities laterally. The obturation of the pelvic outlet is effected by two muscular structures, the pelvic and urogenital diaphragms. The first is a muscular sling (levator ani muscle) that is perforated by the anus, and the second, formed primarily by the deep transverse perineal muscle, bears the urethral opening and, in the female, the vagina.

The fetal pelvic outlet is very constricted in comparison with that of the adult, and the perineal structures protrude inferiorly well below the ischial tuberosities. Thus the pelvic diaphragm (levator ani) is more of a tubular structure that ensheathes the rectoanal region rather than the conical sling it will eventually become (see following frontal and cross sections of the pelvis).

Despite this distortion in the form of the perineum, the relative positions of all of the structural layers and their relations to vessels and nerves remain the same throughout life.

The superficial aspect of the fetal perineum does not reveal this distortion, however, and its external characteristics closely resemble those of the adult. In the male of approximately 30 weeks' gestation that is shown here, the only feature inconsistent with adult anatomy is the relatively longer distance between the posterior wall of the scrotum and the anus.

The inferior surface of the penis shows that the glans and urethral opening are completely covered by a redundancy of the skin and superficial fascia that forms the prepuce (foreskin), and that these layers are continuous over the scrotum. The hyperpigmentation characteristic of the skin of the external genitalia is present even at this stage and is most pronounced along the *urogenital raphe*. This cutaneous seam indicates the extent of the original orifice of the embryonic cloaca, which constituted a common opening for both the urogenital and enteric structures. The growth of the urorectal septum separated the anus from the urogenital sinus and formed the perineal body, a mass of muscular and connective tissue that is attached firmly to the anal sphincters and the urogenital diaphragm.

If the embryo were to become a female, the sinus would remain open between the swellings that give rise to either scrotal sacs or major labia, and the urethra would not be incorporated within the outgrowth of the genital tubercle, an embryonic structure that becomes either the clitoris or penis. Here is seen the end result of normal male development, where the urogenital raphe has "zippered up" the original common opening, leaving only the urethral orifice at the end of the penis and, posteriorly, the anus. Malformations involving various degrees of failure in this closure are readily envisioned. A persistent opening along the inferior surface of the penis (hypospadias) would permit urinary discharge from this area, and failure to unite the scrotal sacs would result in an opening that resembles the female vulva (pseudohermaphrodism).

Plate 125   Male Perineum and External Genitalia   261

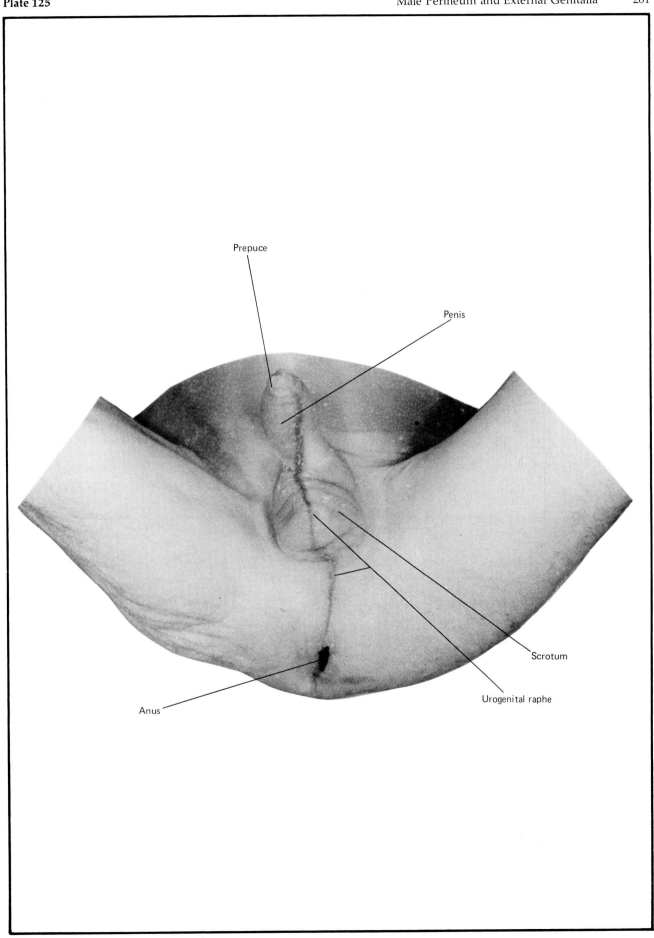

Prepuce

Penis

Scrotum

Urogenital raphe

Anus

SAGITTAL SECTION OF THE MALE PELVIS

This exposure of the male pelvis reveals visceral, perineal and urogenital structures as seen from the midline.

The urinary tract, which commences with the kidneys, enters the bladder through the *ureteral orifice* situated posterolaterally at the base of this organ. The shape of the fetal bladder is conical and its apex extends to the level of the umbilicus, but subsequent growth obliterates its superior cavity and produces the median cordlike urachus. At the base of the bladder lies the *trigone*, a nondistensible triangular area that is defined by the three bladder openings. The base of this triangle is posteriorly bounded by the *interureteric ridge*, and its apex is marked by the *internal urethral orifice*.

The urethra of the male is three to four times longer than that of the female because it must traverse the penis. Its first part, the *prostatic urethra*, lies within the prostate gland, which is located just below the base of the bladder. It is here that the ejaculatory ducts and prostatic ducts will discharge the components of the semen into the urethra. Where the urethra penetrates the urogenital diaphragm, its wall is thinnest, and it is here designated the *membranous urethra*. The part contained within the penis is surrounded by the erectile tissue of the *corpus cavernosus urethrae* (corpus spongiosum), and is called the *cavernous urethra*.

The penis with the scrotum and its contents constitute the external genitalia of the male. In this section, the *corpus cavernosum* that forms the bulk of the penile shaft can be seen containing the central artery that supplies blood to the erectile tissue. Both the corpus cavernosum and the corpus cavernosum urethrae are enclosed in a thick, white sheath of connective tissue, the *penile fascia*.

The corpus cavernosum urethrae expands terminally as the *glans* that occupies the *preputial space* under the *prepuce*.

Note that the skin and superficial fascia of the penis form a continuous layer with those of the lower abdominal wall and scrotum so that a common subcutaneous space surrounds all of these structures. Extravasated blood or urine would then tend to spread within the confines of this space.

The medial septum of the scrotum has been removed in this specimen to show the left testis contained within the *tunica vaginalis*, a peritoneal covering evaginated from the abdominal cavity. Since the testicles descend at approximately the 7th month of gestation, in this 32-week-old specimen they are in their definitive position relative to the scrotum.

Posterior to the scrotum, the *penile bulb* and the *bulbocavernosus muscle* form a prominent swelling in the fetal perineum. The superior aspect of the bulb is attached to the urogenital diaphragm, thereby marking the position of this structure, which is, unfortunately, poorly defined in this section. The erectile tissue of the bulb here reveals its cavernous nature through the amount of the injection medium that has escaped into the vascular sinuses. As the postnatal body grows, the scrotal sac will become more pendulous and will hang inferior to the penile bulb.

The section of the rectoanal region shows the anus as the constricted corrugated termination of the bowel. The raised longitudinal ridges are the *anal columns* and the intervening depressions form the *anal sinuses*. Superiorly, the more expanded *rectum* shows the constant rectal valves that protrude into its lumen. The posterior part of the *levator ani muscle* (which forms the greater part of the pelvic diaphragm) is seen descending from the coccyx along the posterior wall of the rectum, but the subdivisions of the anal sphincters are shown best in the corresponding sagittal section of the female pelvis (Plate 132).

Plate 126   Sagittal Section of Male Pelvis   263

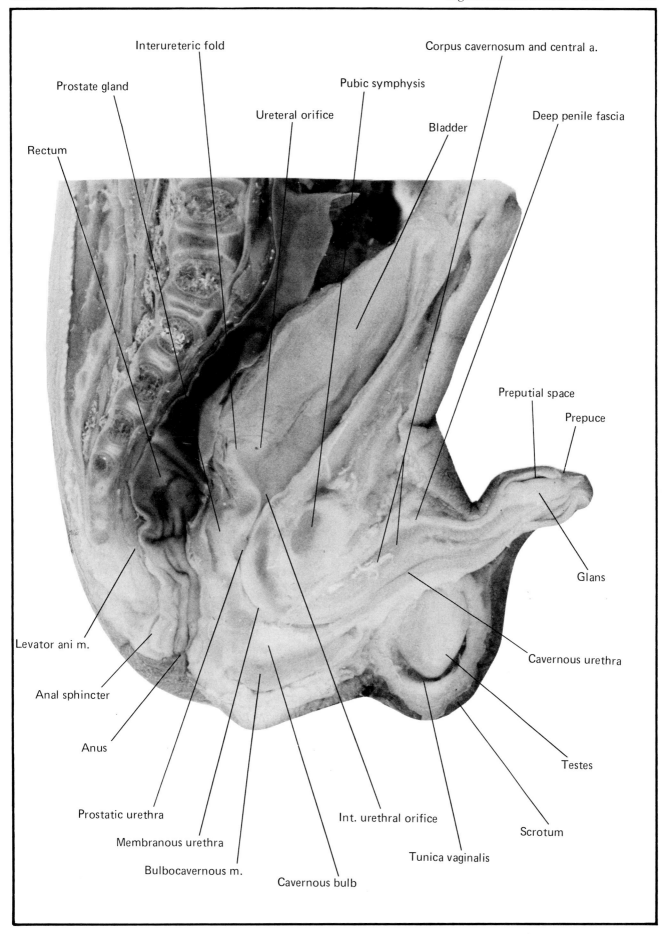

Interureteric fold

Corpus cavernosum and central a.

Prostate gland

Pubic symphysis

Ureteral orifice

Bladder

Deep penile fascia

Rectum

Preputial space

Prepuce

Glans

Levator ani m.

Cavernous urethra

Anal sphincter

Anus

Testes

Prostatic urethra

Int. urethral orifice

Scrotum

Membranous urethra

Tunica vaginalis

Bulbocavernous m.

Cavernous bulb

THE INTERNAL INGUINAL RING AND ASSOCIATED STRUCTURES

This anterosuperior view of the male internal pelvic structures has been positioned so that the left *internal inguinal ring* and its related anatomy are most fully exposed.

The anterior abdomen wall, drawn forward and downward, reveals the three landmarks of its lower internal surface: the *urachus* (superior part of bladder), *umbilical artery* and *inferior epigastric artery*. The first two become solid cords of connective tissue postnatally, but the inferior epigastric artery remains functional and constantly lies medial to the internal inguinal ring. Thus it serves as a differentiator between "direct" and "indirect" inguinal hernias. The former are forced directly through the abdomen wall medial to the artery, whereas the latter exit lateral to the artery and hence follow the indirect course of the inguinal canal.

This view of the ring clearly emphasizes the fact that the vaginal process of the scrotum is an evagination of the abdominal peritoneum. The opening is still patent and the genital structures and vessels seem to be drawn into it as if it were a vortex. However, it must be emphasized that the testicle descended posterior to the thin, transparent peritoneum, and all of the structures attached remained retroperitoneal and passed posterior to the patency of the processus vaginalis.

Again, the lack of subperitoneal fat in the preterm fetus exposes structures with a clarity umparalleled in the adult. Here, the *ductus deferens* and its artery (a branch of the inferior vesicle artery) may be traced from the inguinal ring across the umbilical artery and ureter to where they disappear into the *rectovesicle fossa* to eventually penetrate the prostate as the ejaculatory ducts.

The highly tortuous *internal spermatic artery* and *vein(s)* indicate the route of descent of the testicle from its position of origin on the posterior abdominal wall.

Plate 127   Internal Inguinal Ring and Related Anatomy   265

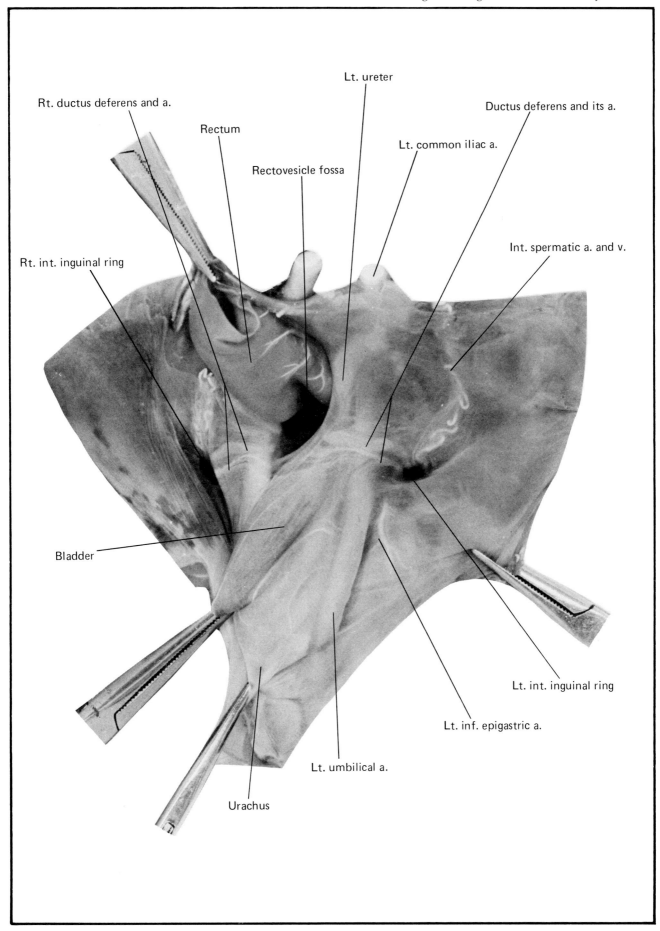

Lt. ureter

Rt. ductus deferens and a.

Ductus deferens and its a.

Rectum

Lt. common iliac a.

Rectovesicle fossa

Rt. int. inguinal ring

Int. spermatic a. and v.

Bladder

Lt. int. inguinal ring

Lt. inf. epigastric a.

Lt. umbilical a.

Urachus

EXPOSURE
OF THE
SPERMATIC CORD

This is a continued dissection of the previously illustrated specimen, and the inguinal canal and right scrotal sac have been opened to reveal the spermatic cord. In contrast to the adult situation, the inguinal canal of the fetus is a short and almost straight opening through the abdominal wall, and the internal inguinal ring lies almost immediately posterosuperior to the external ring. During the postnatal years, there is a differential growth between the three musculoaponeurotic layers of the abdomen so that the internal ring becomes more laterally displaced. This relative shift requires that the structures in the cord must abruptly course medially between the transversalis and the external oblique muscles to negotiate the discrepancy of 5 or 6 centimeters between the position of the internal and external rings. The resulting passage within the abdominal wall is called the inguinal canal.

Since the processus vaginalis is actually an extension of the abdominal cavity, it is not surprising that the spermatic cord is an extension of the three musculoaponeurotic layers that make up the abdominal wall. It is obvious, then, that as the genital ducts and vessels pass through the inguinal canal, each abdominal layer successively contributes to their sheath, so that the cord is not complete until it leaves the external inguinal ring.

In this dissection it is apparent that the transversalis fascia (subserous fascia) forms the third or innermost layer of the cord, the *internal spermatic fascia*. The thickest contribution is derived from the internal oblique layer and consists of loops of muscular fasciculae that form the cremasteric or *middle spermatic fascia*. The *external spermatic* fascia is a thin extension of the aponeurosis of the external oblique that lies under the subcutaneous fascia.

The tunica vaginalis has been opened to expose the testis and reaffirms the fact that it is a serous cavity. In the lateral wall of the scrotum, the *external pudendal artery*, a derivative of the femoral artery, may be discerned.

Plate 128

Spermatic Cord   267

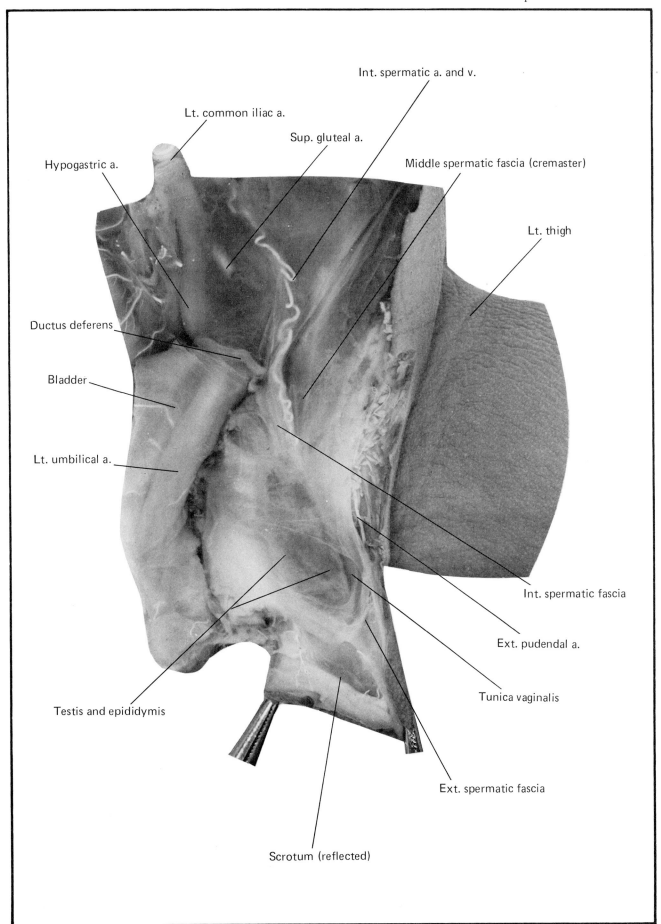

Int. spermatic a. and v.

Lt. common iliac a.

Sup. gluteal a.

Middle spermatic fascia (cremaster)

Hypogastric a.

Lt. thigh

Ductus deferens

Bladder

Lt. umbilical a.

Int. spermatic fascia

Ext. pudendal a.

Testis and epididymis

Tunica vaginalis

Ext. spermatic fascia

Scrotum (reflected)

DISSECTION OF THE SPERMATIC CORD AND EXPOSURE OF THE TESTIS

Here the *tunica vaginalis* and the layers of the cord have been slit to expose the genital ducts, vessels, the testis and its adnexa. From this view, only the internal *spermatic fascia* is visible because it is the layer that intimately surrounds the genital structures.

The *ductus deferens* is a thick-walled muscular tube that arises from the tail of the epididymis and ascends behind the testis to pass up the cord. Because of its firmness, the ductus can be readily palpated in the postnatal scrotal sac. The *internal spermatic artery* runs down beside the ductus and is here filled with the white injection medium. This artery, which supplies the testis and epididymis, arises on the anterior surface of the aorta near the renal arteries in approximation to where the gonadal tissue embryonically originated. The associated veins form the intricate *pampiniform plexus*, which eventually drains into either the renal veins or their adjacent part of the inferior vena cava.

The *epididymis* is a C-shaped structure that embraces the testis in its curvature. The head of the epididymis surmounts the upper pole of the testis while the *body* descends along its posterior aspect and terminates in the tail at the inferior testicular pole. The cleft between the two structures is the epididymal *sinus*. Internally, the epididymis consists of a highly convoluted tubule that, like the ductus, was derived from the mesonephric duct. The tubule receives sperm from a number of efferent vasa in the head and transports them to the commencement of the ductus in the tail. Near the epididymal head, a small pedunculated lobe, the *appendix of the testis*, represents a remnant of the proximal end of the paramesonephric (Müllerian) duct.

The *inferior testicular ligament* that connects the gonad to the bottom of the scrotal sac is the much attenuated remnant of the *gubernaculum*, a developmental structure that "guides" the descent of the testis into the scrotum. Its homologue in the female is representated by the ovarian and round ligaments.

The peritoneal connection between the tunica vaginalis and the abdominal cavity is usually obliterated, but an occasional remnant may persist and has the potential of forming a fluid-filled cyst (hydrocele).

Plate 129   Dissection of Spermatic Cord and Exposure of Testis   269

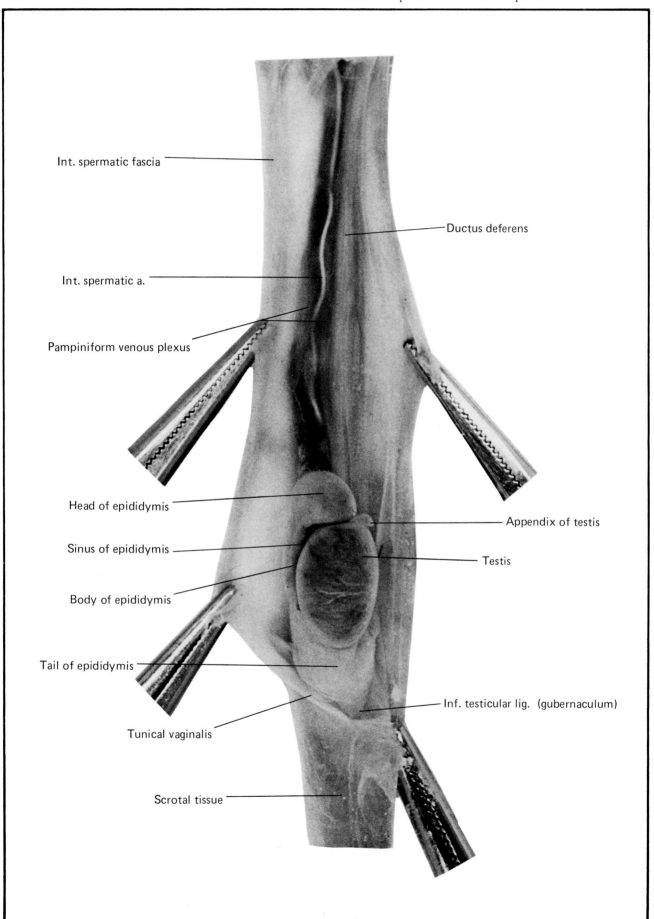

Int. spermatic fascia

Ductus deferens

Int. spermatic a.

Pampiniform venous plexus

Head of epididymis

Appendix of testis

Sinus of epididymis

Testis

Body of epididymis

Tail of epididymis

Inf. testicular lig. (gubernaculum)

Tunical vaginalis

Scrotal tissue

ARTERIOGRAM OF THE FETAL PELVIS (MALE)

The major blood supply to the pelvis and its viscera is derived from the *hypogastric* (internal iliac) *artery* through a series of branches that show considerable variation in their sequence and site of origin. Because of the functional significance of the umbilical branch of the hypogastric in the fetus, the caliber of the main stem of the hypogastric artery is roughly three times that of the external iliac, a situation that is reversed in the adult.

The first large pelvic branch is usually the *superior gluteal artery*, which is here shown curving dorsally to pass through the greater sciatic notch. Once in the gluteal region, this artery forms a number of radiating branches that anastomose with those of the *inferior gluteal artery* and circumflex branches of the *deep femoral artery*.

Descending from the hypogastric, a common stem here gives rise to the *internal pudendal*, inferior gluteal and *obturator arteries*. The first of these passes posteriorly around the sacrospinous ligament to reenter the pelvis inferior to the pelvic diaphragm. It gives off *inferior hemorrhoidal* branches to the anus and continues toward the urogenital diaphragm where two medial branches pierce the crura of the penis as the *deep* (central) *arteries*. The terminal branches of both pudendals indicate the position of the penis as they ascend and pass down its dorsum as the two *dorsal arteries* of the penis.

In the middle of the specimen, both the *middle sacral* and *superior rectal* (hemorrhoidal) arteries descend anterior to the sacrum, and lateral to these the superior and inferior vesicle branches may be discerned.

Plate 130   Arteriogram of Male Pelvis   271

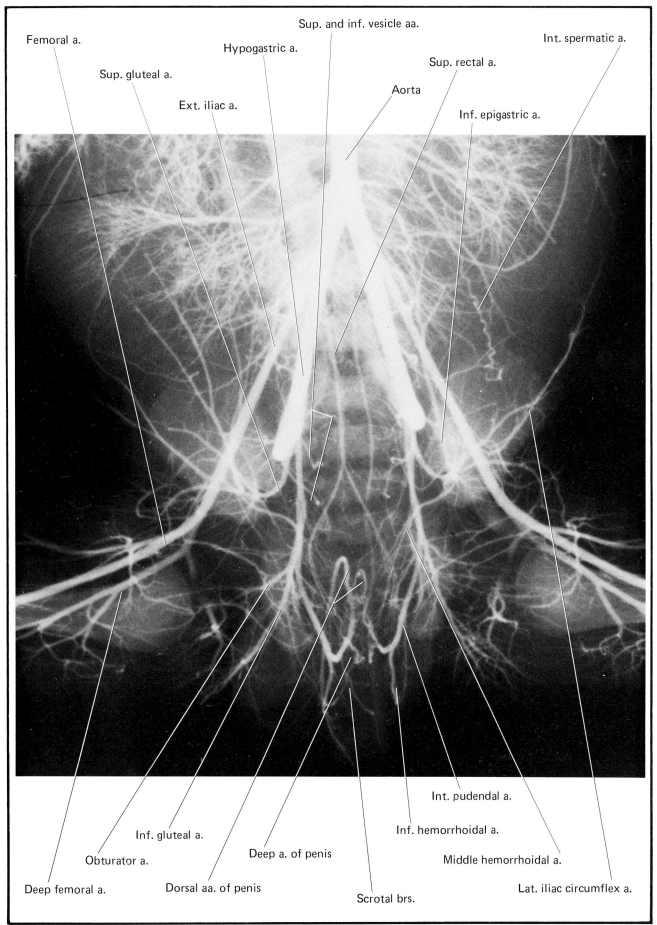

Femoral a.

Sup. gluteal a.

Ext. iliac a.

Hypogastric a.

Sup. and inf. vesicle aa.

Aorta

Sup. rectal a.

Inf. epigastric a.

Int. spermatic a.

Int. pudendal a.

Inf. hemorrhoidal a.

Middle hemorrhoidal a.

Lat. iliac circumflex a.

Inf. gluteal a.

Obturator a.

Deep femoral a.

Dorsal aa. of penis

Deep a. of penis

Scrotal brs.

SUPERFICIAL ASPECT OF THE PERINEUM AND EXTERNAL GENITALIA (FEMALE)

This plate should be compared with the previous illustration showing the corresponding view of the male perineum (Plate 125). The essential difference lies in the fact that the urogenital sinus remains open and exposes both the urinary and genital orifices in a common fissure, the vulva. Superior to the vulva, a fatty tumescence over the pubic symphysis forms the *mons pubis*, and laterally the *major labia* produce swellings homologous to the scrotal sacs. Within the vulva the homologue of the penis, the *clitoris*, may be seen where its glans protrudes between the *prepuce* and *frenulum*. Both of these latter structures are derived from the urethral folds that lie on both sides of the embryonic urogenital sinus. In the male the urethral folds closed and incorporated the urethra within the ventral part of the erectile body to form the penis, whereas in the female they remain unfused and the urethral meatus persists as an independent opening inferior to the clitoris. The inferior extensions of the urethral folds form the *minor labia* that lie on both sides of the *vaginal orifice* (introitus). The smooth posterior margin of the vulva is formed by the pudendal frenulum that separates the vulva from the perineal body. This last structure is a firm mass of connective and muscular tissue in the female, and unfortunately is often referred to as "the" perineum in gynecologic literature.

Plate 131   Female Perineum and External Genitalia   273

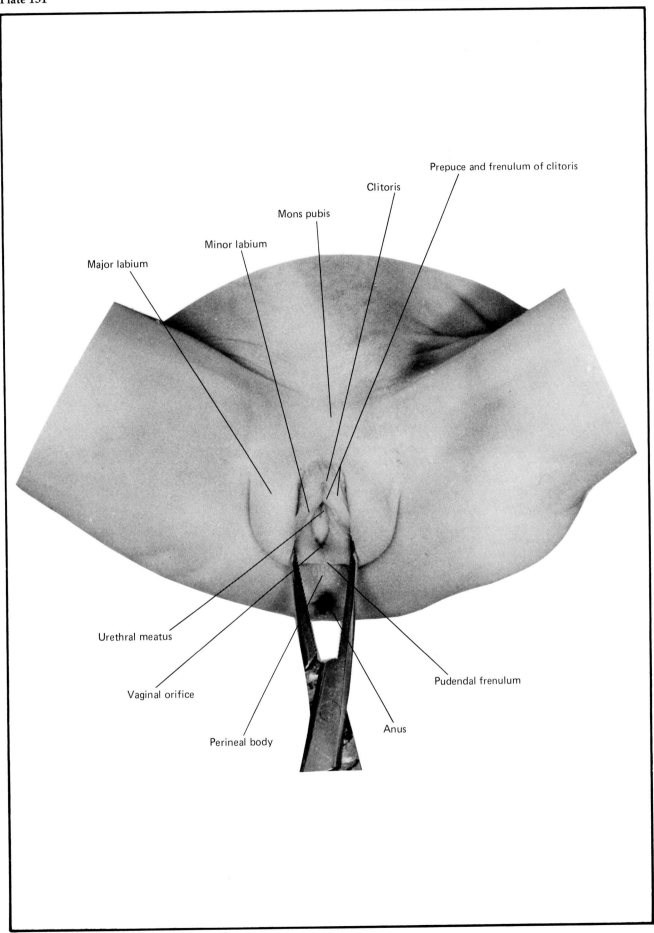

Prepuce and frenulum of clitoris

Clitoris

Mons pubis

Minor labium

Major labium

Urethral meatus

Vaginal orifice

Perineal body

Anus

Pudendal frenulum

SAGITTAL SECTION OF THE FEMALE PELVIS

This section shows the female counterpart of the midline exposurer of the male pelvis shown in Plate 126. It is immediately apparent that the distal urinary tract of the female is shorter and less complicated than in the male. The *urethra* commences as the *internal urethral orifice* at the base of the bladder and terminates at the urethral meatus in the anterosuperior part of the vulva. It seems to be of fairly uniform construction throughout its course, having no prostatic or cavernous regions. The fact that the female is more easily catheterized and more prone to urinary tract infections is anatomically obvious.

Anterior to the urethral meatus, the entire body of the *clitoris* is shown in section. This structure is far more extensive than the superficial appearance of its glans would indicate. As a miniature version of the penis (without urethra) it also arises from two crura along the inferior borders of each pubis and ischium. These unite below the pelvic symphysis and form the shaft of the clitoris that, like the penis, abruptly turns inferiorly. The termination of the internal pudendal arteries as the paired *dorsal arteries of the clitoris* further complete the homologous image.

The female genital tract is interposed between the urinary and enteric tracts. In the midline it shows the split body of the *uterus* communicating with the *vagina* through a conical *cervix*. The cervix is bounded by four fornices. The two lateral fornices are not visible here but the *anterior* and *posterior fornix* can be identified. The anterior fornix of the fetus is relatively much deeper than in the adult because of the conical extension of the cervix.

The posterior fornix, however, shows the same relative depth it will have in later life. Its superior posterior wall is covered by the peritoneum of the *rectouterine fossa* (pouch of Douglas), and at the point where it joins the posterior part of the cervix it is very thin. Because of this, the posterior fornix may be readily perforated in the adult for instrumental optical examination of the internal pelvis (culdoscopy).

The fetal vagina is quite rugose, bearing many transverse ridges on its internal surface, and it terminates (in preterm specimens) as a conical projection in the vulva. This projection will form the more transverse hymenal membrane.

At this point it is appropriate to mention that all fetal pelvic and perineal structures seem to be protracted. This is especially true of those that are more transversely situated in the adult. Thus the hymenal membrane, the pelvic and urogenital diaphragms as well as the cervix are of a more conical or tubular form than when the perineum assumes its definitive position and is retracted into the pelvic outlet. This rule should be kept in mind when contemplating digital anorectal examination of the newborn, because the constricted pelvic outlet restricts lateral distension of the organs.

This section again shows the pelvic diaphragm (levator ani) as a tubular structure ensheathing the rectum, and the distance from the coccyx to the anus indicates the extent of protrusion. Particularly well defined are the anal sphincters. The *external sphincters* are a muscular complex derived from the levator ani, whereas the *internal sphincter* is an extension of the circular muscle of the bowel.

The perineal body is more pronounced in the female, and in this figure the transverse fibers of the deep *transverse perinei*, its largest component, can be identified.

Plate 132 Sagittal Section of Female Pelvis 275

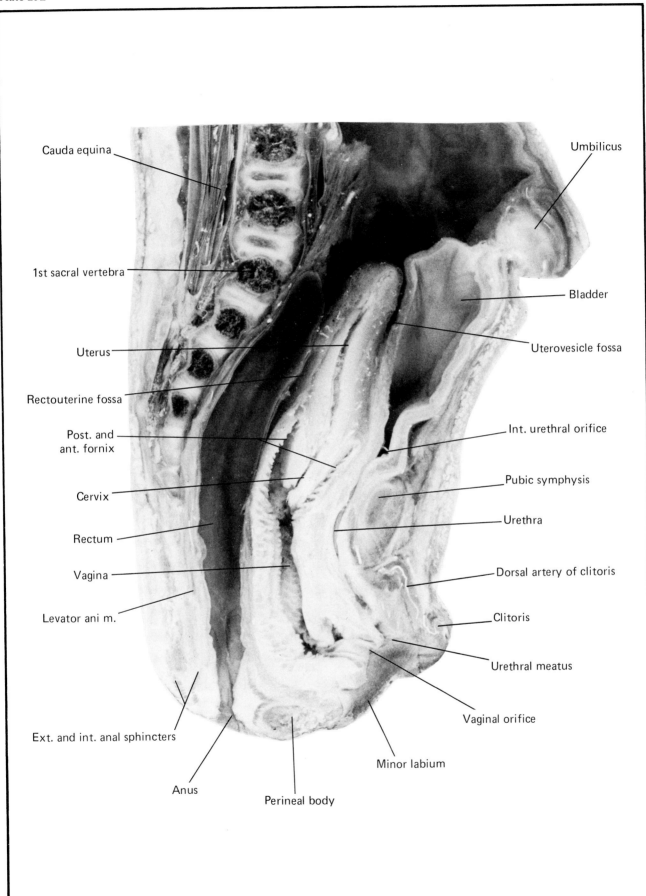

Cauda equina

Umbilicus

1st sacral vertebra

Bladder

Uterus

Uterovesicle fossa

Rectouterine fossa

Post. and
ant. fornix

Int. urethral orifice

Pubic symphysis

Cervix

Urethra

Rectum

Vagina

Dorsal artery of clitoris

Levator ani m.

Clitoris

Urethral meatus

Ext. and int. anal sphincters

Vaginal orifice

Anus

Minor labium

Perineal body

ANTEROSUPERIOR ASPECT OF THE INTERNAL ORGANS OF THE FEMALE FETUS

The lower anterior abdominal wall has been retracted forward and downward and positioned to favor the left internal inguinal ring for comparison with a similar exposure of the male in a previous plate (Plate 127).

The structures on the internal surface of the abdominal wall are again well displayed. The bladder, showing a branch of its *superior vesicle artery*, lies between the two massive *umbilical arteries*. These, in turn, are flanked by the *inferior epigastric arteries* made prominent by the latex injection.

In contrast to the male pelvis, the *uterus* is interposed between the rectum and the bladder, and the peritoneal lining of the abdominopelvic structures follows the contours of the organs. What was simply the rectovesicle fossa of the male pelvis is now divided into a posterior *rectouterine fossa* and an anterior *uterovesicle fossa*. The separation is completed not only by the uterus itself, but also by the peritoneal membranes that ensheath the organ. The *oviducts* are retracted from each side of the pelvic wall in the broad ligaments and thus effect a complex transverse intrapelvic septum.

The ovary, the female gonadal gland, is irregularly shaped in the fetus and is here best seen on the left side where it shows its attachment to the posterior surface of the broad ligament. It is suspended by its superior pole from the *suspensory ligament of the ovary* that contains the ovarian artery and vein. Its inferior pole is attached to the *ovarian ligament* that is affixed to the lateral wall of the uterus, but it continues anterolaterally as the *round ligament of the uterus* (ligamentum teres).

Plate 133   Anterosuperior Aspect of Female Internal Organs   277

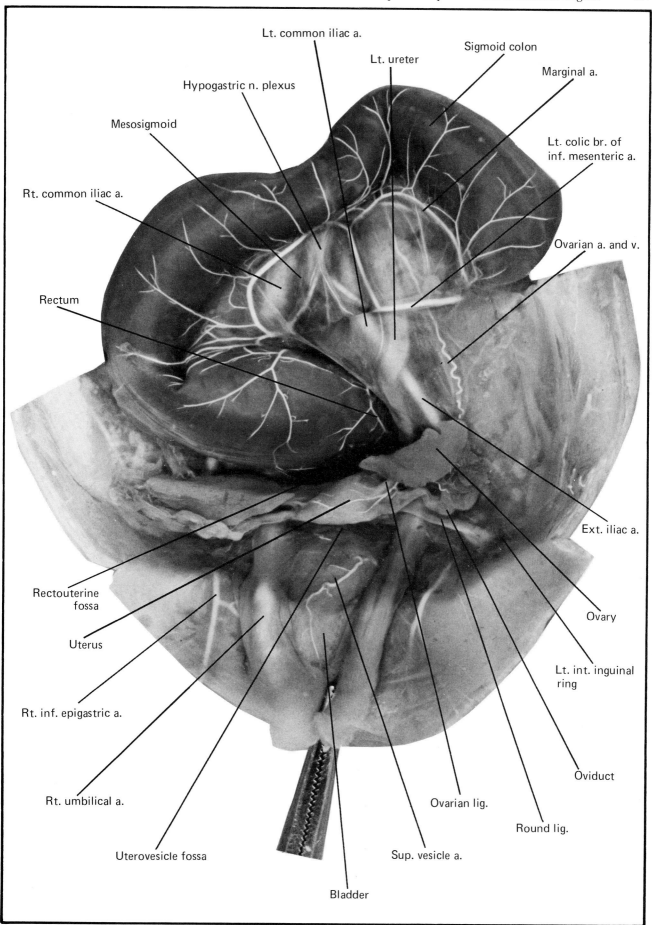

Lt. common iliac a.

Lt. ureter

Sigmoid colon

Marginal a.

Hypogastric n. plexus

Lt. colic br. of
inf. mesenteric a.

Mesosigmoid

Rt. common iliac a.

Ovarian a. and v.

Rectum

Rectouterine
fossa

Ext. iliac a.

Uterus

Ovary

Rt. inf. epigastric a.

Lt. int. inguinal
ring

Rt. umbilical a.

Oviduct

Uterovesicle fossa

Ovarian lig.

Round lig.

Sup. vesicle a.

Bladder

SUPERFICIAL FRONTAL DISSECTION OF THE FEMALE PELVIS

In this progressive dissection of the previously illustrated specimen, the anterior abdominal wall has been cut away, exposing sections of the superior part of the *bladder* and the *umbilical* and *inferior epigastric arteries*.

The *ligamentum teres* can be traced from the lateral wall of the uterus to the internal inguinal ring, and from there down the anterior surface of the abdominal wall to disappear in the tissue of the major labium. In this route it imitates the course of the spermatic cord, and the passage through the abdominal wall that corresponds to the inguinal canal is known as the canal of Nuck in the female.

In the external genitalia the tissue has been pared away to show the paired *dorsal arteries of the clitoris* anterosuperior to the *urethral meatus*. Lateral to these structures the major labia have been sectioned, exposing their internal musculature, the bulbocavernosus, which has a weak sphincter-like action on the vulva. On the left side, ramifications of the *external pudendal artery* can be traced into the major labium.

Plate 134   Superficial Frontal Section of Female Pelvis   279

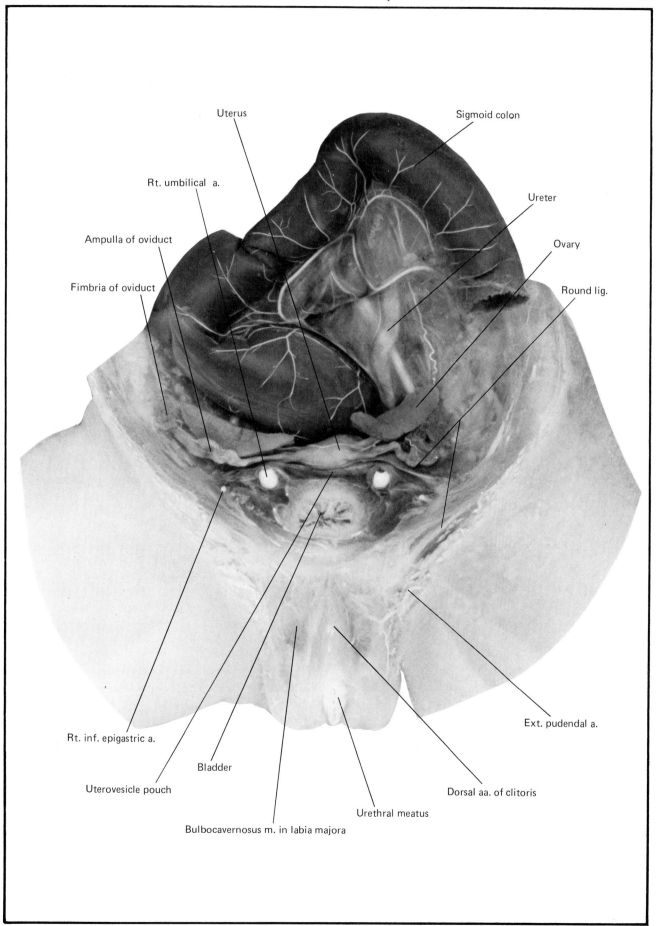

Uterus

Sigmoid colon

Rt. umbilical a.

Ureter

Ampulla of oviduct

Ovary

Fimbria of oviduct

Round lig.

Ext. pudendal a.

Rt. inf. epigastric a.

Bladder

Dorsal aa. of clitoris

Uterovesicle pouch

Urethral meatus

Bulbocavernosus m. in labia majora

FRONTAL SECTION THROUGH THE LOWER URINARY TRACT OF THE FEMALE PELVIS

This section has exposed the *bladder trigone* and the entire *urethra.* The orifice of the ureters may be seen at the base of the trigone, and its apex is formed by the *internal urethral orifice.* The distensible parts of the bladder are marked by many infolding ridges, whereas the nondistensible trigone is quite smooth.

The relation of the body of the uterus to the superoposterior surface of the bladder is well shown, as is the extent of the two paravesicle spaces.

The level of the pelvic outlet is marked by sections of the cartilaginous parts of the pubic rami, and of particular interest is this view of the most anterior part of the pelvic diaphragm. This structure is here represented by the slinglike membrane lateral to the midportion of the urethra. Where the most anterior parts of the pelvic diaphragm attach to the inner sides of the pubis, they extend forward over the urogenital diaphragm so that the *anterior recess* of the *ischiorectal fossa* intervenes as a space between the two structures.

The urogenital diaphragm is the thick, musculomembranous complex occluding the anteroinferior part of the outlet where it is stretched between the inferior rami of the pubic cartilages. Attached to its lateral edges, the sectioned ends of the *crura of the clitoris* can be seen containing the branches of the internal pudendal arteries.

It is anatomically apparent that the diaphragm contributes a sphincter action to the urethra.

Plate 135

Frontal Section through Female Urinary Tract   281

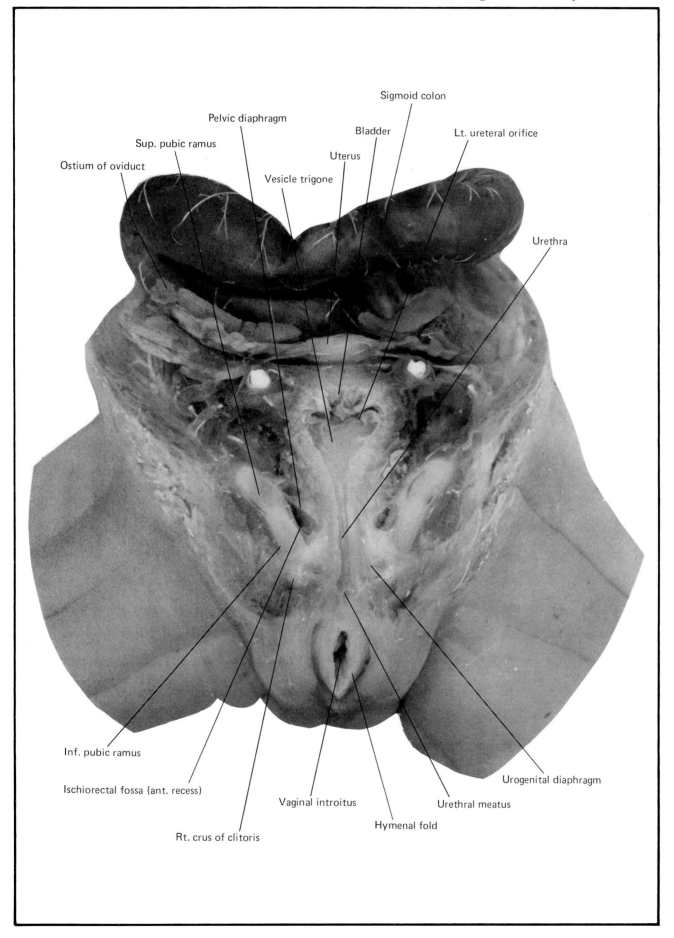

Sigmoid colon

Pelvic diaphragm

Bladder

Sup. pubic ramus

Uterus

Lt. ureteral orifice

Ostium of oviduct

Vesicle trigone

Urethra

Inf. pubic ramus

Ischiorectal fossa (ant. recess)

Urogenital diaphragm

Vaginal introitus

Urethral meatus

Rt. crus of clitoris

Hymenal fold

FRONTAL SECTION THROUGH THE LOWER GENITAL TRACT OF THE FEMALE PELVIS

In this last illustration from a series of progressive dissections of the same specimen, the anterosuperior wall of the vagina has been removed to expose its lumen and junction with the uterus at the cervix.

Superiorly, the uterus still occupies its typical position in which the cervical os is directed downward and slightly forward and the body is anteflexed at the cervix and projects forward over the bladder. For some unexplained reason, the uterus most frequently does not occupy a precisely midline position but is usually deflected to the left. This displacement advantageously displays the relations of the structures laterally related to the uterus and vagina. The *uterine artery*, a branch of the hypogastric, passes superior to the ureter as it approaches the uterocervical junction. Just before reaching the ureter, this vessel gives off a large vaginal branch that passes inferior to the ureter so that this structure is embraced by two major vessels at this point. The mass of connective tissue at the base of the broad ligament through which the ureter and the surrounding vessels pass is called the *cardinal ligament*. It

has complex and ill defined fibrous connections with the rectum posteriorly and the bladder arteriorly, but its greater mass attaches laterally to the pelvic wall. This ligament provides a main support of the uterus, and when damaged in later life, uterine prolapse may result.

This specimen shows the conical projection of the future hymenal membranes characteristic of the preterm fetus.

The *ligamentum teres* (round ligament of the uterus) is attached to the uterine wall near the entrance of the oviduct and extends through the internal inguinal ring as the homologue of the male gubernaculum testis. This structure assists in keeping the uterus in its normal anteflexed position.

Superior to the uterus in the left posterior abdominal wall, the retroperitoneal structures are displayed through the transparent *mesosigmoid* and peritoneal membrane. The ureter descends over the point where the *external iliac* and *hypogastric* arteries divide from the common iliac. It is accompanied by a ureteral artery derived from the *left colic branch* of the inferior mesenteric that crosses the anterior surface of the ureter. Lateral to these structures, the *internal ovarian artery* descends in a course identical to the gonadal artery of the male, but the fixation of the ligamentum teres to the uterus prevents the continued descent of the ovary through the internal inguinal ring.

Plate 136   Frontal Section through Female Genital Tract   283

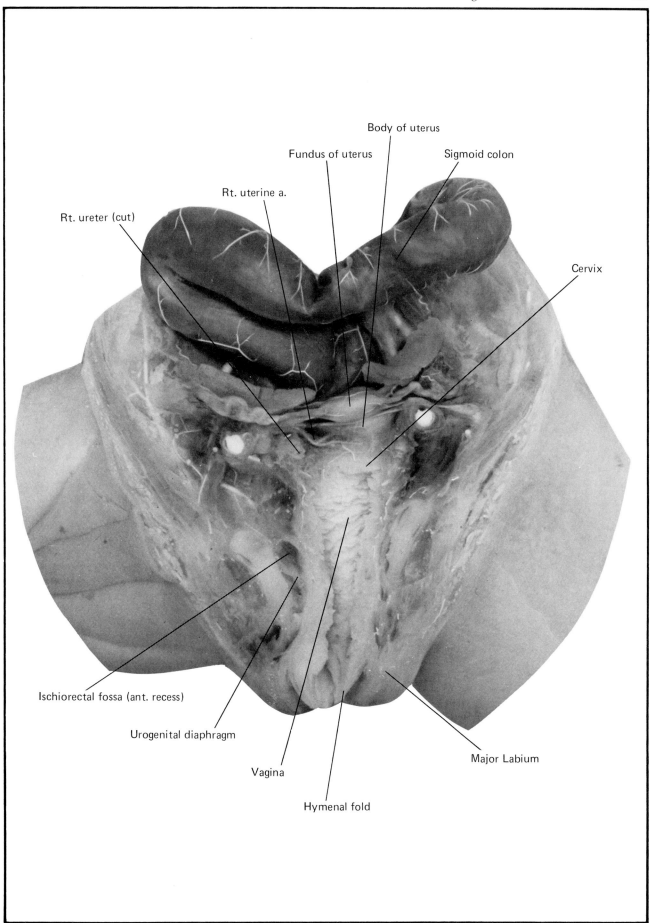

Body of uterus

Fundus of uterus

Sigmoid colon

Rt. uterine a.

Rt. ureter (cut)

Cervix

Ischiorectal fossa (ant. recess)

Urogenital diaphragm

Vagina

Major Labium

Hymenal fold

THE FETAL UTERUS

The uterus with its pelvic adnexa and the upper part of the vagina were removed and photographed. Since the *ureters* and *umbilical arteries* are retroperitoneal structures lying deep to the endopelvic fascia that supports the pelvic peritoneum, it is apparent that the entire broad ligament is included in the specimen.

The uterus is formed by the fusion of the inferior parts of the paramesonephric ducts, and the oviducts represent the unfused bilateral superior portions. As these structures arose from the posterolateral wall of the abdominopelvic region, they elevated the peritoneum over their surfaces and thus raised the broad ligament. It can be seen that the ligament extends upward to ensheath the oviducts, and its subdivisions take specific names according to the structures they support. Therefore, the major part which lies lateral to the body of the uterus is called the *mesometrium* and the lateral parts from which the oviducts are suspended are designated the *mesotubaria*. As with all mesenteries, the broad ligament is a double peritoneal fold that passes the nerves and vessels between its layers. The anterior layer is pulled forward to enshroud the conspicuous *ligamentum teres* that passes from the lateral uterine wall to the internal inguinal ring. A similar fold, extended from the posterior layer to enclose and support the ovaries, is called the *mesovarium*.

The oviducts are not simple tubes of uniform caliber, but progressively expand as they extend laterally. The narrowest parts of their lumina are within and just lateral to the wall of the uterus. Here the narrow first part of the free duct is called the *isthmus*, which gradually expands to form the *ampulla*. The terminal flare of the duct ends around the *atrium*, which is surrounded by fronds of tissue forming the *fimbria*.

Here it should be noted that the peritoneal membrane of the male is never perforated under normal circumstances, whereas that of the female is perforated in two cases. The ostia of the oviducts maintain a constant opening between the peritoneal cavity and the external environment through the ramifications of the genital tract, and the peritoneal covering of the ovary eventually disappears forming a second normal discontinuity of the female peritoneal membrane.

The position and course of the uterine arteries is well illustrated and their relation to the sectioned ureters is obvious. The normal anteflexed posture of the uterus shows the paired fundic branches that supply the *fundus*.

The *cervix* is directed inferiorly and covers the posterior fornix, and the lateral rugae of the fetal vaginal mucosa are very conspicuous. Note that the blood supply to the upper vagina is derived from the vaginal branches of the uterine artery.

Plate 137

Uterus 285

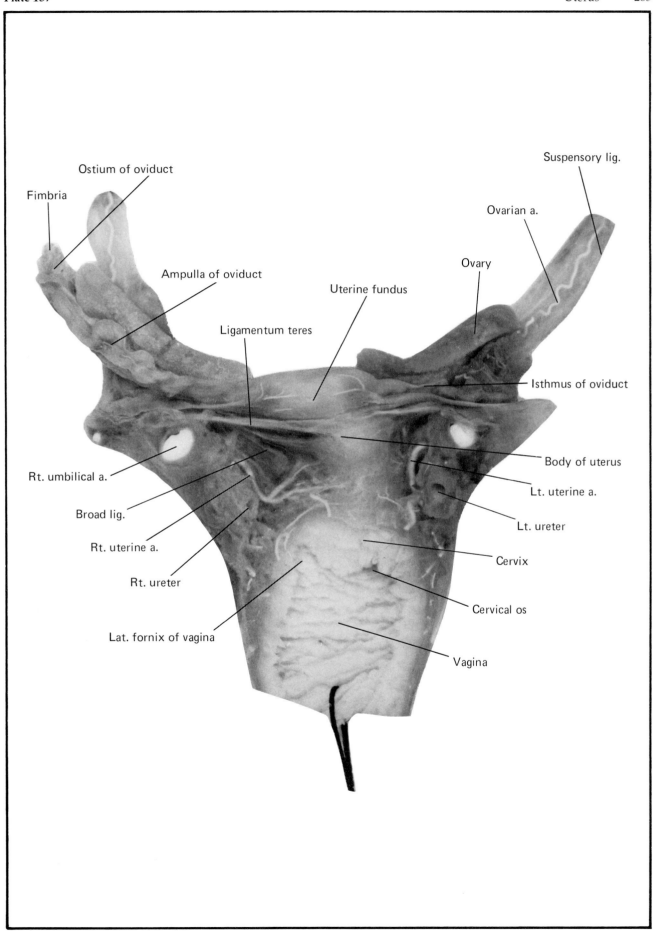

Ostium of oviduct

Fimbria

Suspensory lig.

Ovarian a.

Ovary

Ampulla of oviduct

Uterine fundus

Ligamentum teres

Isthmus of oviduct

Body of uterus

Rt. umbilical a.

Lt. uterine a.

Broad lig.

Lt. ureter

Rt. uterine a.

Cervix

Rt. ureter

Cervical os

Lat. fornix of vagina

Vagina

ARTERIOGRAM OF THE FETAL UTERUS AND PROXIMAL VAGINA

The dual vascularity of the uterus can be readily appreciated from this P-A radiogram, which shows the prominent anastomotic arcades formed bilaterally between the *ovarian* and *uterine* arteries. The anticipated multifold increase in the size of the uterus during pregnancy provides a functional rationale for this highly efficient system of vessels.

Assuming that the point of anatomic junction between the two major arteries occurs just interior to the isthmus of the oviduct, the vascular territory of the ovarian artery includes the ovary and the tubes. Here the faint shadows of the soft structures indicate both ovarian and tubal branches arising at irregular intervals along the artery as it approximates these organs.

The uterine artery, particularly on the left side, can be traced passing through the cardinal ligament to divide into the proper *uterine* and *cervical branches* at the junction between these two regions. The uterine branch sends numerous vessels into the myometrium as it passes upward along the side of the body. The derivation of the larger *branches of the fundus* indicate the point of its inosculation with the ovarian artery.

The midsagittal plane of the uterus is an area of relative hypovascularity, and incisions along this line would produce the least bleeding during hysterotomies.

The cervial branches form a ring of vessels around the proximal part of the cervix that elaborates a conspicuous corona of fine arteries down into the conical lips of the cervix. The relative size of the cervix becomes much reduced in the adult, as does its vascularity. The functional reason for this profusion of cervical arteries in the fetus is obscure.

The proximal part of the vagina is supplied by branches of the uterine artery that here have been cut distal to their origin. Often a large single vessel, called the *azygos* (meaning unpaired) *artery,* runs down the posterior wall of the vagina. The distal part of the vagina that lies below the urogenital diaphragm is supplied by branches of the internal pudendal artery.

Plate 138

Arteriogram of Uterus and Proximal Vagina 287

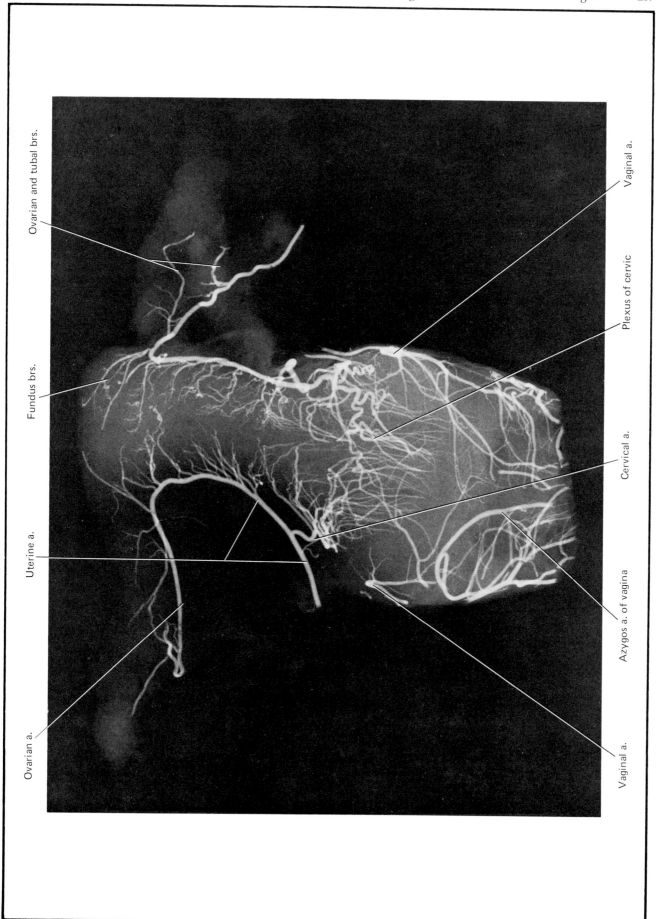

Ovarian and tubal brs.

Vaginal a.

Plexus of cervic

Fundus brs.

Cervical a.

Uterine a.

Azygos a. of vagina

Ovarian a.

Vaginal a.

ARTERIOGRAM OF THE FETAL PELVIS (FEMALE)

This A-P radiogram of the injected vessels of a fetal female pelvis should be compared with its male counterpart shown in Plate 130. The most outstanding features not common to both sexes and not discussed in the previous plate are the prominent *labial branches* derived from the *internal pudendal arteries*. The intricate plexus formed from these branches is sufficiently dense to show the configurations of the labia. Just proximal to the labial plexus, two vessels converge toward the midline as the paired *dorsal arteries of the clitoris*. Deep to these, the pudendal contributions to the lower vagina form a fine longitudinal plexus that anastomoses with vaginal branches of the *uterine artery*. Atypically, the uterus here (the same shown excised in the preceding plate) deviates to the right so that the left *uterine* and *ovarian arteries* occupy an almost midline position, seen just below the shadow of the bifurcation of the superior rectal artery.

Plate 139   Arteriogram of Female Pelvis   289

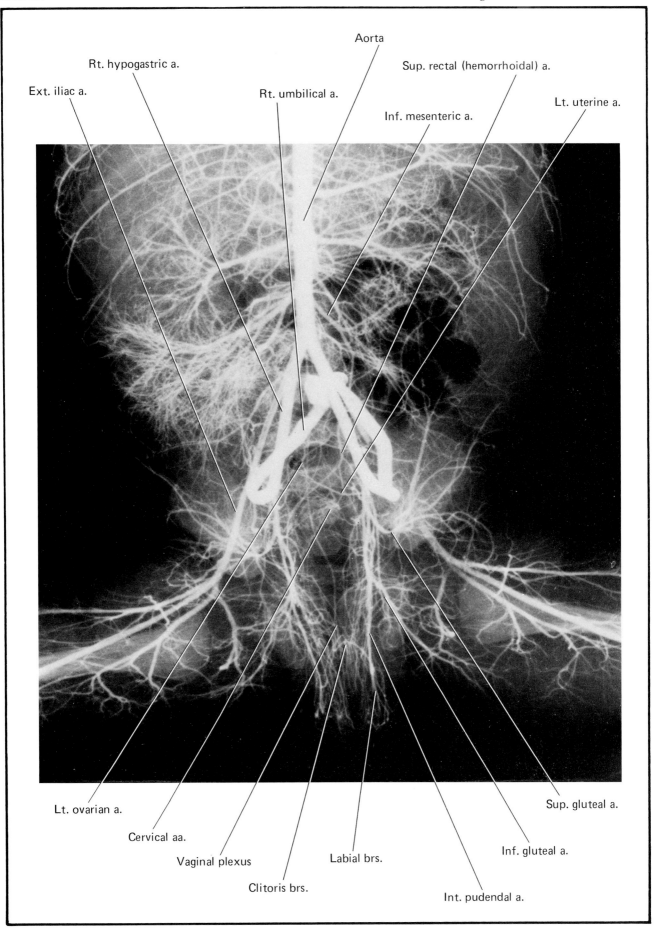

Aorta

Rt. hypogastric a.

Sup. rectal (hemorrhoidal) a.

Ext. iliac a.

Rt. umbilical a.

Lt. uterine a.

Inf. mesenteric a.

Lt. ovarian a.

Sup. gluteal a.

Cervical aa.

Inf. gluteal a.

Vaginal plexus

Labial brs.

Clitoris brs.

Int. pudendal a.

EXPOSURE OF THE INTERNAL PELVIC WALL

In this dissection a female fetal pelvis has been entirely eviscerated to show the vasculature and major nerves of its posterolateral wall.

The *common iliac artery* descends from the aortic bifurcation just superior to the origin of the *middle sacral artery* and shortly divides into the lateral *external iliac artery* and the *hypogastric artery* that dominates the upper anterior aspect of the specimen. The proximal hypogastric is much larger than the external iliac because it supplies the umbilical artery, but with the postnatal occlusion of the latter, the hypogastric becomes the smaller of the two.

The first major branch of the hypogastric is the *superior gluteal artery* that immediately gives rise to the lateral *sacral artery*. The continuation of the first passes back between the lumbosacral trunk and first root of the sacral plexus to enter the gluteal region, and the second runs down the anterior surface of the sacrum to send branches into the anterior sacral foramina. The second major branch is what will be the direct continuation of the postnatal hypogastric, and the point just distal to its origin marks the commencement of the umbilical artery. This descending, relatively "normal"-sized part of the hypogastric first gives off anteriorly the *uterine artery* with its *cervical branch*. Its next anterior branch is the *obturator artery* that leaves the pelvis through the obturator foramen with the *obturator nerve*. Inferiorly, the hypogastric then gives off a posterior branch, the *inferior gluteal artery,* and continues to pass through the greater sciatic foramen as the *internal pudendal artery*. Below the pelvic diaphragm it is seen reentering the pelvis with the pudendal nerve within a duplication of the fascia (pudendal canal) of the obturatorius internus muscle. It is there distributed to the perineum and external genital structures. The elevated cut edge of the *levator ani* shows that the lateral parts of this muscle arise from the fascia of the obturatorius internus.

Postnatally, the umbilical artery atrophies except for the proximal small branches that form the inferior and superior vesicle arteries of the bladder.

Plate 140   Internal Pelvic Wall   291

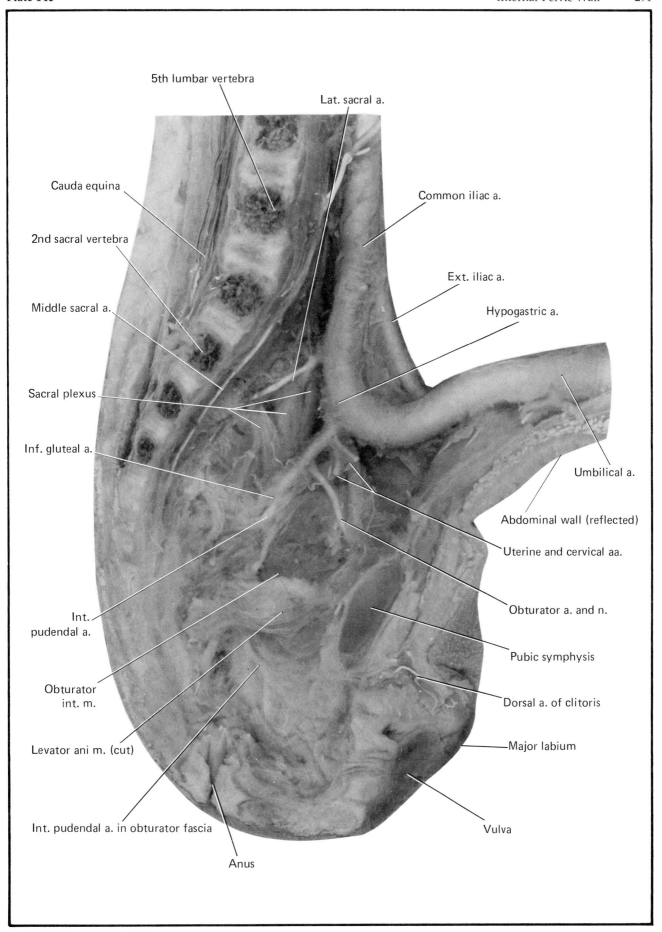

5th lumbar vertebra

Lat. sacral a.

Cauda equina

Common iliac a.

2nd sacral vertebra

Middle sacral a.

Ext. iliac a.

Hypogastric a.

Sacral plexus

Inf. gluteal a.

Umbilical a.

Abdominal wall (reflected)

Uterine and cervical aa.

Int.
pudendal a.

Obturator a. and n.

Pubic symphysis

Obturator
int. m.

Dorsal a. of clitoris

Levator ani m. (cut)

Major labium

Int. pudendal a. in obturator fascia

Vulva

Anus

LATERAL ANGIOGRAM OF THE FETAL PELVIS (FEMALE)

In this lateral view of a doubly injected specimen, the major veins received retrograde filling by the medium only as far peripherally as the first competent valves. These were located just distal to the union of the external iliac and hypogastric veins. The valvular block of the external iliac can be seen as a rounded mass lying posterior to the midsection of the corresponding artery. In the *hypogastric vein,* the first valve was encountered below the ostium of the superior gluteal vein so that its tributaries accompanying the superior gluteal artery received some of the medium.

Since this is a view of the entire pelvis, vessels of both right and left sides may often be visualized as duplicated arteries running parallel courses. As in the preceding figure, the origin of the pelvic part of the *hypogastric artery* marks the commencement of the umbilical artery, which, until parturition, is the major derivative of the proximal hypogastric artery and seems to be its direct continuation.

The distal part of the hypogastric is discerned as the doubly represented vessels curving posteriorly to give origin to the *inferior gluteal* and *internal pudendal arteries.* The perineal branches of the latter are quite conspicuous, and the forward course of the vessels to the urogenital diaphragm and external genitalia indicates the relative position of the pudendal canal.

In the middle pelvic field of this radiogram, the *uterine* and *obturator arteries* arise from the proximal part of the pelvic hypogastric. Because the uterus is anteflexed, the tortuous *ovarian arteries* descend anterior to the uterine vessels.

Branches of the *superior rectal artery* descend along the bowel to anastomose with the inferior rectal branches of the pudendal artery. Also well illustrated are the anastomotic relations of the femoral circumflex branches with the inferior gluteals to supply the hip joint and the adjacent soft structures.

Plate 141   Lateral Angiogram of Female Pelvis   293

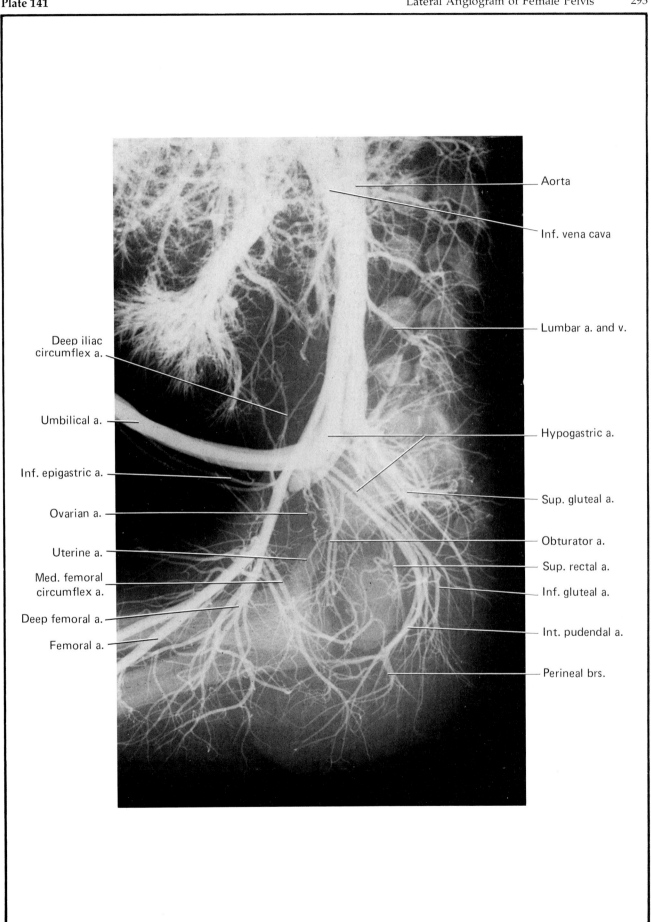

Deep iliac
circumflex a.

Umbilical a.

Inf. epigastric a.

Ovarian a.

Uterine a.

Med. femoral
circumflex a.

Deep femoral a.

Femoral a.

Aorta

Inf. vena cava

Lumbar a. and v.

Hypogastric a.

Sup. gluteal a.

Obturator a.

Sup. rectal a.

Inf. gluteal a.

Int. pudendal a.

Perineal brs.

FRONTAL SECTION OF THE FETAL PELVIS

This pelvis has been sectioned through the pelvic diaphragm and rectum to emphasize the narrowness of the fetal pelvic outlet and the protracted nature of the perineal structures. The section is slightly oblique so that different planes of the hip joint are presented. The more posterior representation lies to the left side of the illustration.

The centrally located rectum is filled with dark meconium, the fetal fecal material that is composed of exfoliated mucosal cells and some material resulting from the swallowing of amniotic fluid. The *rectal valves* and constriction identifying the *anus* are quite conspicuous. On the right side of the section (left side of fetus) the *obturator muscle* lines the lateral pelvic wall, and its medial fascia serves as an origin for the lateral part of the *levator ani muscle,* which constitutes the pelvic diaphragm. Here it seems to be virtually part of the rectum because it closely approximates this structure until its lower fibers form the external sphincters. To conceptualize the adult condition, imagine a widened pelvic outlet. The anus is then retracted into the outlet as the levator ani muscle suspends it in a more conical and less tubular sling. The sphincters then lie at the level of the ischial tuberosities. The fat of the ischiorectal fossae then comes to lie medial to the tuberosities rather than below them as seen here. The pudendal canals which will lie lateral to the ischiorectal fossae in the adult are pressed between the obturatorius internus and the levator ani muscles in the fetus. Their position here is revealed by the end sections of the *internal pudendal arteries* and nerves encased in the sheath of obturator fascia that forms the canal.

The complexity of the anal sphincter is well displayed, and the fact that the internal sphincter is an extension of the rectal circular muscle is obvious.

The sectional views of the hip joints and their related muscles in two planes should be correlated with the illustrations in the previous section on the lower extremity.

Plate 142

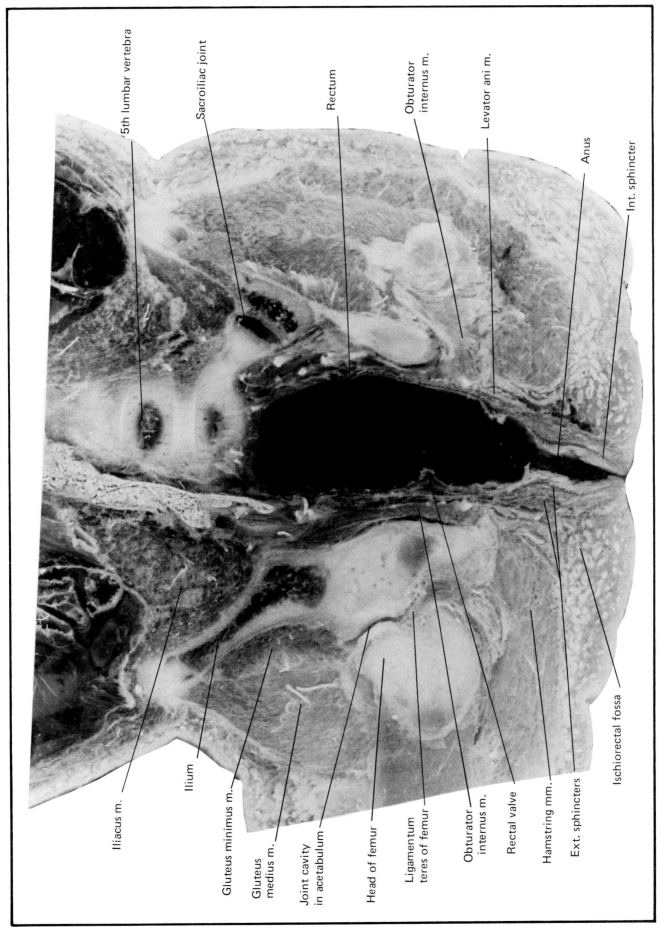

5th lumbar vertebra

Sacroiliac joint

Rectum

Obturator internus m.

Levator ani m.

Anus

Int. sphincter

Iliacus m.

Ilium

Gluteus minimus m.

Gluteus medius m.

Joint cavity in acetabulum

Head of femur

Ligamentum teres of femur

Obturator internus m.

Rectal valve

Hamstring mm.

Ext. sphincters

Ischiorectal fossa

CROSS SECTION OF THE FETAL PELVIS AT THE LEVEL OF THE FOURTH SACRAL FIBROCARTILAGE

The functional and structural relations of both the *obturatorius internus* and *externus muscles* are difficult to explain or to demonstrate by dissection. This section of the pelvis, however, displays the origin, course, and therefore, the action of the obturatorius internus, which cannot be revealed by any other approach. This muscle lines both sides of the pelvis as it originates from the internal surface of both the superior and inferior ischiopubic rami and the intervening obturator membrane. It converges into a tendon that bends around the lesser sciatic notch at an angle greater than 90 degrees to insert (with the gemelli) into the trochanteric fossa of the femur. It is apparent, then, that the contraction of the obturatorius internus pulls the trochanter posteriorly, laterally rotates the hip when the leg is extended and abducts the hip when it is flexed as in the normal fetal position. The tendon is protected by a bursa where it slides around the sciatic notch.

The fortunate obliquity of this section also shows the origin and functional position of the obturatorius externus on the left side of the illustration. This muscle arises from the external surface of the pelvis that roughly corresponds to the extent of origin of the internus on the internal surface of the same side. It passes posteriorly under the neck of the femur to insert into the inferior part of the trochanteric fossa. Thus, like the internus, it is also a lateral rotator of the femur; but being innervated by the obturator nerve, it is a muscle of the adductor group of the thigh.

The muscular lamina that forms the *levator ani* originates from, and here lies against, the internal surface of the obturatorius internus. The extent of its origin from the anterior pubic rami to the coccyx may be traced as it passes around the vagina and rectum. The pelvic diaphragm that is formed by this muscle is incomplete anteriorly where the fibers of pubic origin pass above the urogenital diaphragm, where it presents an open interval for the passage of the urethra and vagina.

Again it is shown that the urogenital and enteric structures almost completely fill the fetal pelvic outlet and have little room for lateral expansion.

The exceptionally good representation of the hip joint on the left side of the figure should be compared with the plates presented in the section on the lower extremity. The extent of the joint capsule and the connection of the *ligamentum teres* to the head of the femur is particularly well shown.

Plate 143   Cross Section at Level of 4th Sacral Fibrocartilage   297

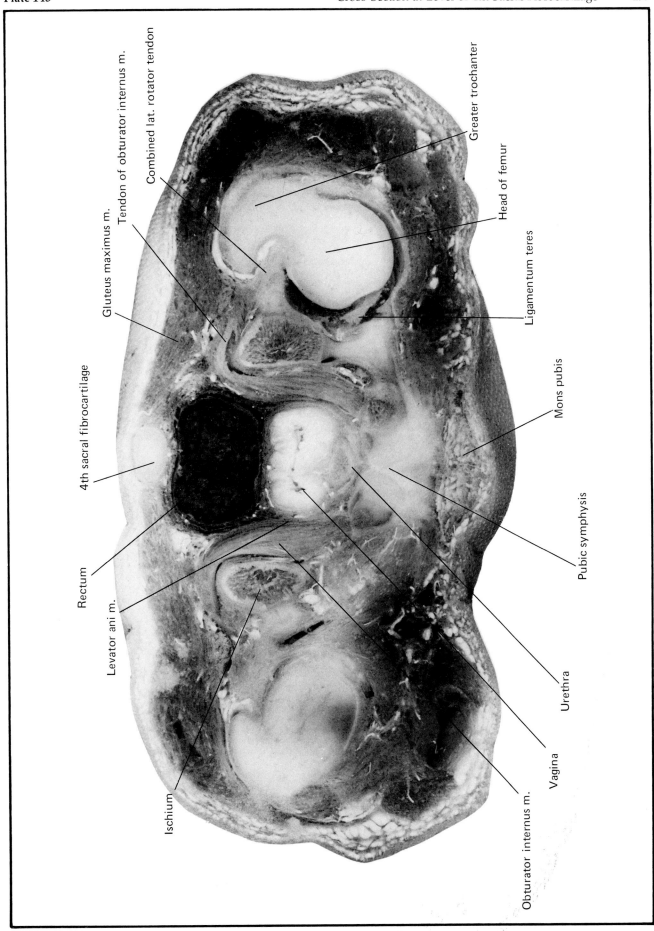

Tendon of obturator internus m.

Combined lat. rotator tendon

Gluteus maximus m.

Greater trochanter

Head of femur

Ligamentum teres

4th sacral fibrocartilage

Mons pubis

Rectum

Levator ani m.

Pubic symphysis

Ischium

Urethra

Obturator internus m.

Vagina

CROSS SECTION OF THE FETAL PELVIS AT THE LEVEL OF THE UROGENITAL DIAPHRAGM

The rhomboidal shape of the pelvic outlet, and the boundaries of the two perineal triangles that lie within it are well defined in this section. The base of the posterior perineal triangle is formed by a line connecting the most inferior parts of the two *ischial tuberosities*, and its apex is the *coccyx*. The triangle contains the anorectal structures and the fat of the posterior ischiorectal fossae. The anterior perineal triangle shares a common base with the posterior, but its apex lies at the pubic symphysis. At this level the anterior triangle is completely filled by the urogenital diaphragm and the lumina of the structures which pierce it. Here, the cartilaginous inferior rami of both the pubic and ischiac components form the lateral borders of the diaphragm and serve as the origin of its main muscular component, the *transverse perinei profundus muscle.* Only a small part of this muscle can be discerned in the

female fetus where the urethra and vagina occupy most of the anterior perineal triangle, but it is reenforced by a thick superior and inferior layer of investing fasciae which form, respectively, the deep and superficial perineal membranes.

The ischiocavernosus and its muscular cover, which together form the crus of the clitoris, lie attached to the ischiopubic ramus and the lateral margin of the diaphragm, and here may be seen conducting the anterior parts of the *internal pudendal arteries.* Where the two crura converge, they form the shaft of the clitoris that arched up under the pubic symphysis and then descended toward the vulva. The course of these structures is well marked by the sectioned ends of the pudendal arteries and their reappearance in the shaft of the clitoris as the paired *dorsal arteries* of the clitoris.

The large opening anterior to the vagina (the smaller eccentric foramina are veins) is the section of the urethra that penetrates the diaphragm.

It is apparent that the musculature of the diaphragm surrounding this structure can function as a urethral sphincter.

The large muscle mass seen arising from the inferior puboischiac rami is mostly formed by the *adductor magnus* muscle, whose insertion to the posterior border (linea aspera) of the femur may be followed on the right side of the figure.

Plate 144   Cross Section at Level of Urogenital Diaphragm   299

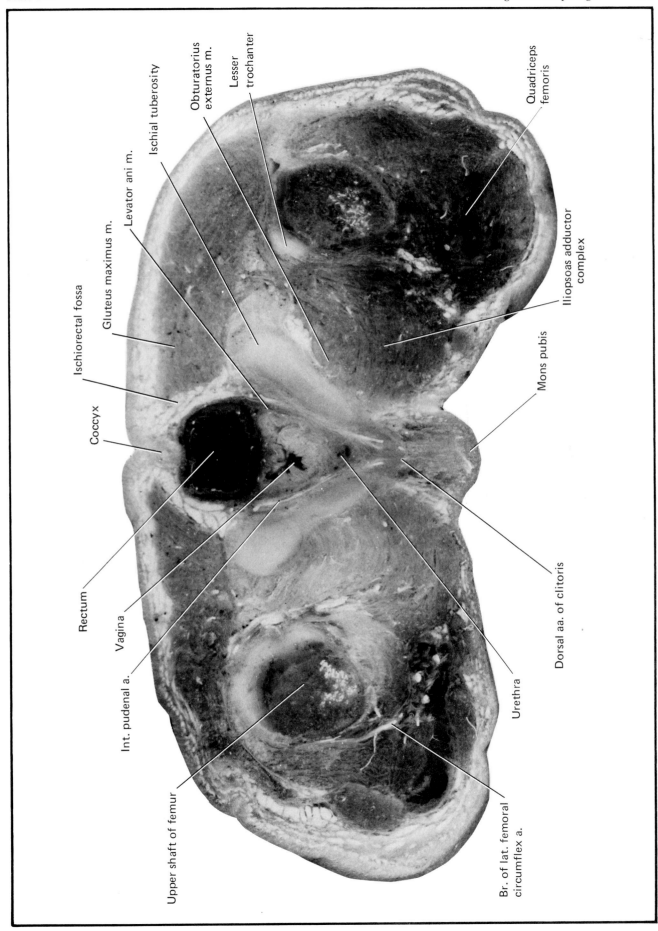

Quadriceps femoris

Lesser trochanter

Obturatorius externus m.

Ischial tuberosity

Levator ani m.

Gluteus maximus m.

Ischiorectal fossa

Coccyx

Iliopsoas adductor complex

Mons pubis

Dorsal aa. of clitoris

Urethra

Rectum

Vagina

Int. pudenal a.

Upper shaft of femur

Br. of lat. femoral circumflex a.

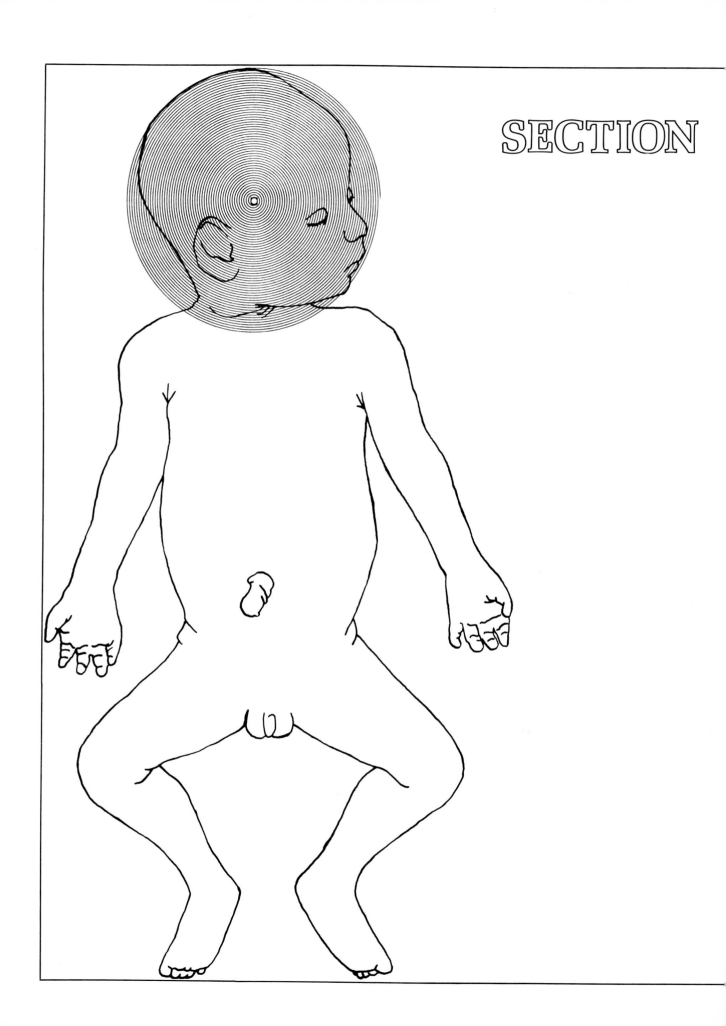

SECTION

SEVEN

HEAD AND NECK

LATERAL ASPECT OF THE FETAL SKULL

The skull consists of a number of bony enclosures that contain and protect the brain and its major sensory outgrowths. Because the olfactory and visual organs primarily serve to orient the organism for feeding or fighting, the entranceways of the digestive and respiratory tracts are also enclosed by skeletal elements of the head.

Structurally, the skull may be subdivided into the cranium and the face. The first is the closed ovoid container of the brain that is formed from a number of bony plates and the skull base. These are joined together by irregular joints called sutures. The thinner bones that cover the top and circumference of the cranium form the calvaria and are unique in that they develop by intramembranous rather than endochondrous ossification. The skull base is chiefly comprised of irregular, thick bones of endochondrous origin that bear numerous foramina for the passage of nerves and vessels. The superior part of the face includes a series of bones that are joined to the cranium and each other by sutures. They enclose the orbital cavities for the eyes and the nasal cavity for olfaction and respiration, and they provide the superior skeletal structures of the oral cavity. The lower part of the face consists of a single, tooth-bearing bone, the mandible, which is joined to the cranium by the only freely moving diathrodial joint in the skull, excluding those of the ear ossicles.

As the postnatal skull increases in size, some of the bones of the face and cranium become thicker, so that their weight is reduced by the invasion of epithelium-lined cavities from the nasopharynx. The total function of these paranasal sinuses is not yet understood, but the discomfort attending their inflammation is well known. Only simple, shallow concavities in the maxillae represent the sinuses of the nasal cavity in the term fetus, and these structures do not attain their full relative proportions until puberty.

In the illustrated lateral aspect of the fetal skull of approximately 32-week gestation, the cranium is represented by *frontal, parietal* and *occipital bones* and the squamous part of the *temporal bone.* The frontal and parietal bones are separated by the *coronal suture,* and the *lambdoidal suture* lies between the parietal and occipital bones. A horizontal *squamous suture* delineates the temporal bone and intersects those previously mentioned.

The sutures in the adult are, for the most part, immovable joints that are separated by a thin membrane of connective tissue and tend to become obliterated with age. In the late fetus, however, the sutures are of variable width and permit a degree of movement between the bones of the skull. Thus they are more like syndesmotic joints than the accepted definition of true sutures. Where the sutures intersect, large triangular or rhomboidal spaces, called fontanelles, are evident. Here only the external and internal periostia and dura protect the brain.

The lateral view shows the *sphenoid* and *mastoid fontanelles,* which tend to close earlier than those at the top of the calvaria.

At the base of the temporal bone, the *tympanic ring* outlines the position of the external auditory meatus. The form of this ring becomes more tubular with postnatal age.

The relatively small size of the face in proportion to the fetal cranium is one of the most striking characteristics of the fetal skull. Much of this disparity is related to the edentulous condition of the fetal jaws. With the growth of alveolar ridges and the eruption of the dentition, the maxillae become more elongated inferiorly, and the angle and *ramus* of the *mandible* become more pronounced. The increase in the size of the postnatal skull is an excellent example of heterogonic growth. That is, the growth is not simply an enlargement of preexisting structures but consists of differential rates of expansion in various directions.

Plate 145   Lateral Aspect of Skull   303

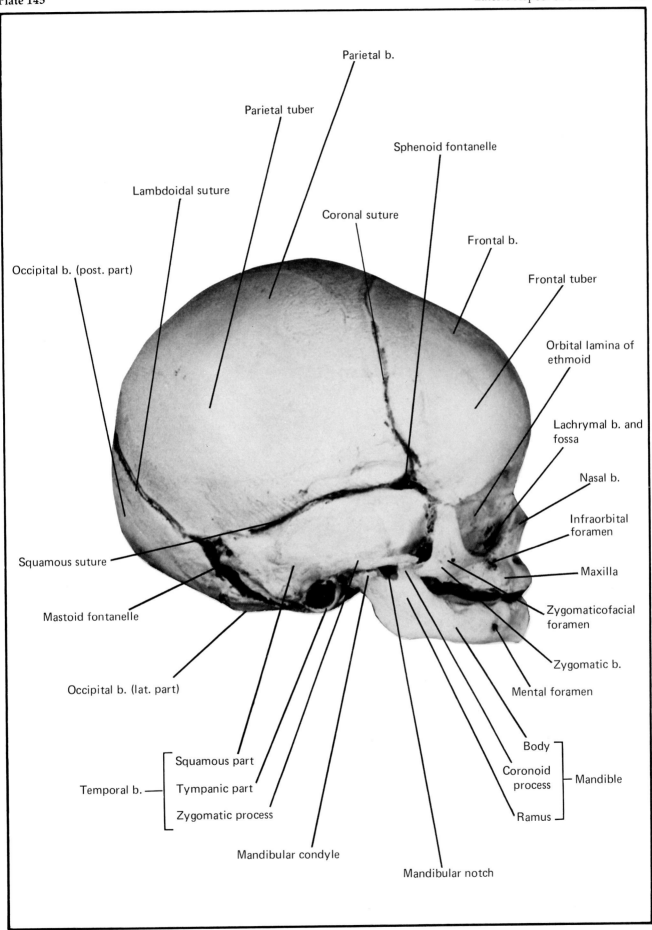

Parietal b.

Parietal tuber

Sphenoid fontanelle

Lambdoidal suture

Coronal suture

Frontal b.

Occipital b. (post. part)

Frontal tuber

Orbital lamina of ethmoid

Lachrymal b. and fossa

Nasal b.

Infraorbital foramen

Maxilla

Squamous suture

Zygomaticofacial foramen

Mastoid fontanelle

Zygomatic b.

Mental foramen

Occipital b. (lat. part)

Body

Coronoid process

Mandible

Temporal b. — Squamous part

Tympanic part

Zygomatic process

Ramus

Mandibular condyle

Mandibular notch

FRONTAL ASPECT OF THE FETAL SKULL

In this view of the same skull shown in the preceding plate, the anterior bones of the cranium and face may be discerned.

The *frontal bones* constitute the major anterior part of the cranium and form the roofs of the orbits. The *metopic suture* is a transient feature and usually obliterates without a trace after the second decade. On each bone the *frontal tuber,* a bullous eminence, indicates the center where the intramembranous ossification commenced, and transillumination would show a pattern of ossification radiating from these points.

The *maxillae* and *zygomatic bones* are the most visible parts of the upper face. Both give substantial contributions to the orbit. The *ethmoid,* which forms the medial wall of the orbit, surrounds the superior part of the nasal cavity and contributes the *perpendicular plate* to the septum. The *inferior conchae* are independent ossifications seen on the inferolateral walls of the cavity.

It is again evident that the compressed character of the fetal face is primarily caused by lack of teeth and the bone growth that supports them. Although the buds of the deciduate (and some permanent) dentition already lie within the gingival surface of the maxillae and mandible, their eruption will be accompanied by growth of the alveolar processes.

The three sensory foramina of the face are arrayed in a nearly vertical line on each side, and each gives exit to superficial sensory branches of the three divisions of the *trigeminal nerve* (CNV) (CN, cranial nerve). The supraorbital foramen passes sensory branches of the ophthalmic division to the forehead and scalp, and the *infraorbital foramen* passes fibers of the maxillary divisions to the superior labial, nasal and cheek area. Through the *mental foramen* exit the sensory nerves of the mandibular division that are distributed to the lower lip and chin.

Plate 146   Frontal Aspect of Skull   305

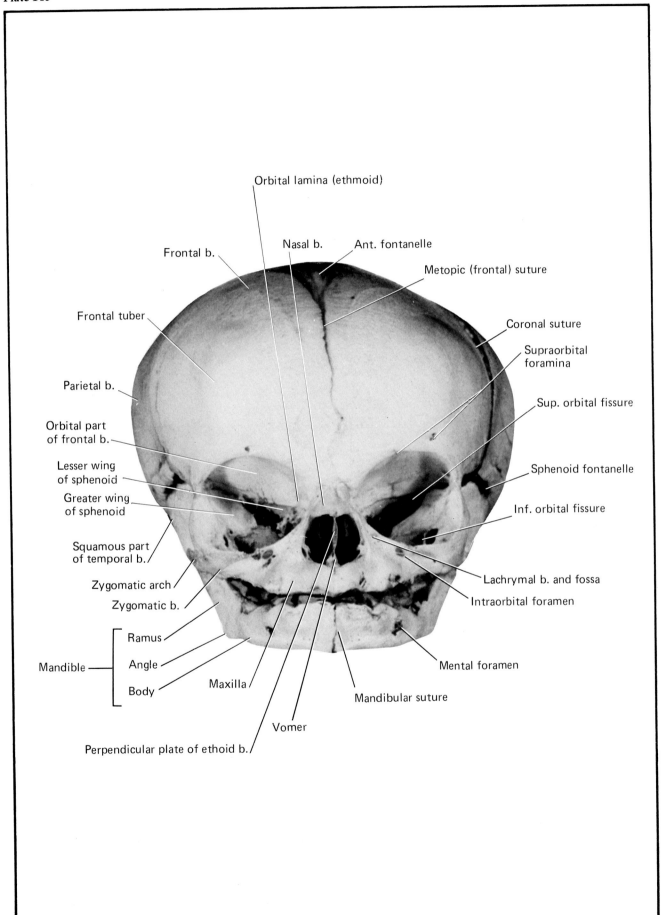

Orbital lamina (ethmoid)

Nasal b.   Ant. fontanelle

Frontal b.   Metopic (frontal) suture

Frontal tuber   Coronal suture

Supraorbital
foramina

Parietal b.

Sup. orbital fissure

Orbital part
of frontal b.

Lesser wing
of sphenoid   Sphenoid fontanelle

Greater wing
of sphenoid   Inf. orbital fissure

Squamous part
of temporal b.

Lachrymal b. and fossa

Zygomatic arch
Intraorbital foramen
Zygomatic b.

Ramus

Mandible —   Angle   Mental foramen

Body

Maxilla

Mandibular suture

Vomer

Perpendicular plate of ethoid b.

SUPERIOR ASPECT OF THE FETAL CALVARIA

The *parietal bones* form the greater part of the superior calvaria, where they are separated from each other by the midline *sagittal suture*. In the fetus each of these bones bears a prominent tuber that, as in the frontal bone, indicates the center from which the radiating intramembranous ossification commenced.

The *coronal* and *lambdoidal sutures* separate the parietal bones from the *frontal* and *occipital bones*, respectively. Where the coronal suture intersects with the sagittal and metopic (frontal) sutures, the large *anterior fontanelle* is evident. Its distinctive rhomboidal shape, as opposed to the triangular shape of the *posterior fontanelle*, enables the palpating finger of the obstetrician to determine the position of the face while the head is yet in the birth canal.

As previously mentioned, the sutures of the perinatal skull are actually movable syndesmotic joints that permit a certain amount of deformation of the cranium at parturition. Excessive motion, however, is undesirable, for in some cases the skull compression may cause an overlapping of the parietal bones at the sagittal suture, resulting in a rupture of the underlying superior sagittal epidural sinus with unpleasant consequences.

Plate 147   Superior Aspect of Calvaria   307

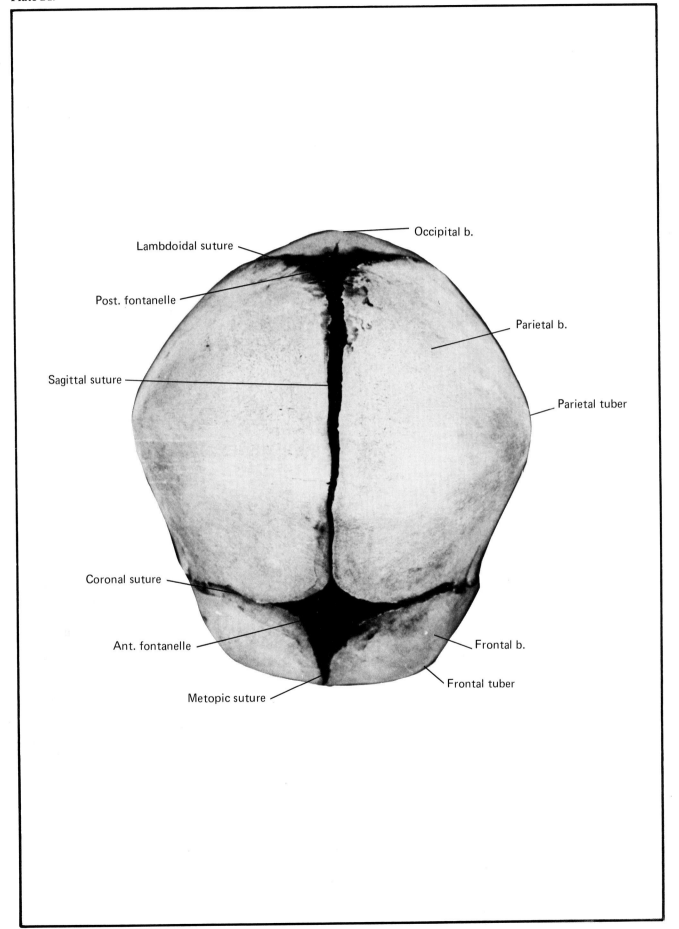

Occipital b.

Lambdoidal suture

Post. fontanelle

Parietal b.

Sagittal suture

Parietal tuber

Coronal suture

Ant. fontanelle

Frontal b.

Frontal tuber

Metopic suture

THE BASE OF THE FETAL SKULL: INFERIOR ASPECT

The bones of the base of the skull are irregular in thickness and contour, and except for the squamous parts of the more peripheral bone complexes, they are derived from endochondrous ossification.

In this specimen, the inferior view of the facial bones is presented at the anterior part of the skull, and although they may obscure some of the skull base, most of the essential bones and foramina may be identified.

The *hard palate,* which lies within the dental arch, is composed mostly of the *palatine processes* of the *maxillae,* but its posterior edge is formed by the *palatine bones.* These are separated from the maxillae by a fine suture that laterally intersects the *palatine foramina,* which pass the palatine nerves and arteries to the roof of the mouth. The bones directly posterior to the palate are the *pterygoid processes* of the *sphenoid,* each of which bears a hooked extension, the *hamulus.* The sphenoid is one of the most complex bones of the skull. When disarticulated from the rest of the cranium it roughly resembles a disorganized butterfly. Its lateral processes, which are aptly named wings, form the posterior part of the orbit and the greater part of the middle cranial fossa superiorly and infratemporal fossa inferiorly. It is the *greater wings* that can be seen to extend laterally toward the *zygomatic arches* and which bear a number of foramina. These wings arise from the central body of the *sphenoid,* which also bears an inferior set of winglike processes, the *pterygoid laminae,* that encompass a depression, the pterygoid fossa.

In the posterior edge of the greater wings, the *foramen ovale* and *foramen spinosum* provide passage for the mandibular division of the trigeminal nerve and middle meningeal artery, respectively. Lateral to these, a depressed part of the temporal bone forms the *mandibular fossa* for the articulation of the mandibular condyles. An irregular suture posteriorly separates the sphenoid from the petrous part of the temporal bone. The lateral part of this suture leads into the tympanic cavity as the *auditory tube,* and its most medial part joins a large, irregular opening, the *foramen lacerum,* that in life is mostly occluded by fibrocartilage.

The *petrous part* of the *temporal bone* contains the auditory and vestibular organs, and the lateral opening surrounded by the *tympanic ring* bears the tympanum or ear drum. Medial to this an obliquely directed foramen marks the entrance to the *carotid canal,* through which the internal carotid artery gains access to the cranial cavity. Posterior to the tympanic ring, the sharp *styloid process* projects before the *stylomastoid foramen* that passes the facial nerve to the muscles of expression.

The large depression between the petrous bone and the occipital complex is a persistent sutural opening, the *jugular fossa,* that gives exit to the jugular vein and the glossopharyngeal, vagus and accessory cranial nerves.

The four subdivisions of the fetal *occipital bone* that surround the *foramen magnum* become fused into a single bone in later life. The basal and lateral parts, and the inferior segment of the posterior part, evidently are derived from vertebral elements in earlier vertebral evolution. The lateral parts bear the thickened *occipital condyles* that articulate with the lateral masses of the atlas and permit the flexion-extension of the craniovertebral joint.

Plate 148   Inferior Aspect of Skull Base   309

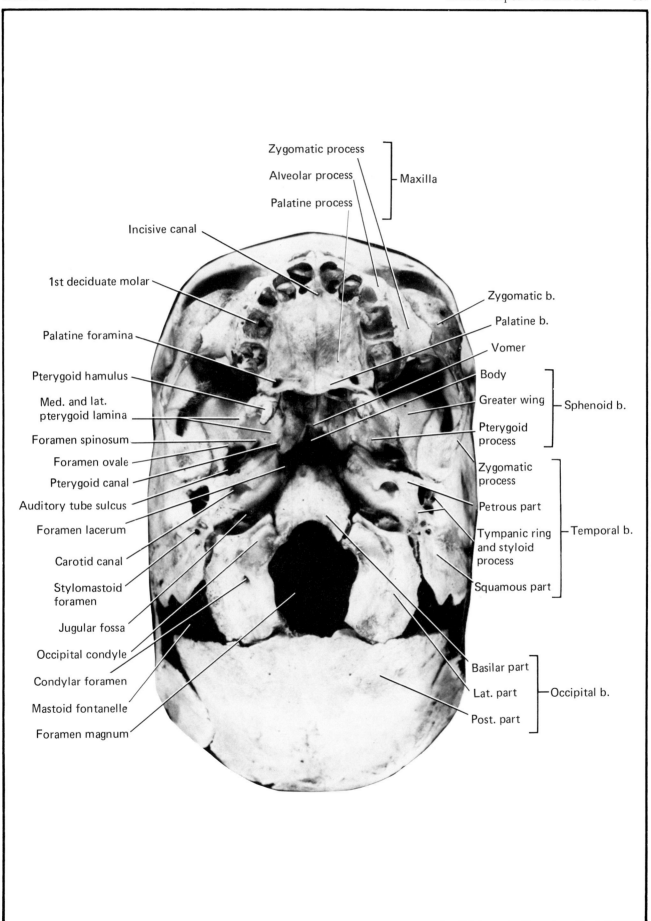

Zygomatic process

Alveolar process

Palatine process

⎤
⎥ Maxilla
⎦

Incisive canal

1st deciduate molar

Palatine foramina

Pterygoid hamulus

Med. and lat.
pterygoid lamina

Foramen spinosum

Foramen ovale

Pterygoid canal

Auditory tube sulcus

Foramen lacerum

Carotid canal

Stylomastoid
foramen

Jugular fossa

Occipital condyle

Condylar foramen

Mastoid fontanelle

Foramen magnum

Zygomatic b.

Palatine b.

Vomer

Body

Greater wing

Pterygoid
process

⎤
⎥ Sphenoid b.
⎦

Zygomatic
process

Petrous part

Tympanic ring
and styloid
process

Squamous part

⎤
⎥
⎥ Temporal b.
⎥
⎦

Basilar part

Lat. part

Post. part

⎤
⎥ Occipital b.
⎦

THE BASE OF THE FETAL SKULL: SUPERIOR ASPECT

From the interior, the base of the skull is divided into three depressions, the anterior, middle and posterior cranial fossae, which accommodate the frontal, temporal and cerebellar parts of the brain, respectively. The frontal fossa is floored primarily by the *orbital plates* of the *frontal bone*. In the center of the anterior fossa, the *cribriform plate* indicates where the *ethmoid bone* forms the floor of the olfactory fossa. In the fetus this plate is incompletely ossified and the central part is cartilaginous. The numerous perforations, which give the plate its name, pass olfactory nerves to the sensory epithelium in the superior nasal meatus.

The posterior central part of the anterior fossa includes the *lesser wing* of the *sphenoid,* whose sharp posterior edge forms the medial part of the border between the anterior and middle fossae. The lesser wing bears two posterior projections, the *anterior clinoid processes,* which bracket the *optic canals* that pass the optic tracts to the orbits. Just posterior to the optic canals, the *carotid grooves* in the sides of the sphenoid body guide the internal carotid arteries to the base of the brain.

The *hypophyseal fossa* straddles the superior surface of the sphenoid body and is posteriorly bordered by the *dorsum sellae,* which bears the blunt *posterior clinoid processes*. These processes serve as attachments for the dural folds supporting the tentorium cerebelli.

The greater wings of the sphenoid bone provide most of the floor of the middle cranial fossa. Posterior to the orbit, the greater wing is separated from the lesser wing by the superior orbital fissure (not visible in this view) that passes cranial nerves III, IV, VI and part of V into the orbit. Close to the medial end of the fissure, the *foramen rotundum* indicates the exit of the maxillary division of the trigeminal (CNV) nerve. In the medial end of the suture separating the greater wing from the petrous bone, a jagged opening, the *foramen lacerum,* is visible. The carotid artery passes over the superior aspect of this foramen, but only small emissary veins pass through it.

The *foramen ovale* lies lateral to the lacerum and anterior to the *foramen spinosum*. The former transmits the mandibular division of the trigeminal (CNV) nerve, and through the latter the middle meningeal artery gains access to the cranium.

The petrous part of the temporal complex is a wedge-shaped bone that intervenes between the greater wing of the sphenoid and the occipital complex and contains the cochlear and vestibular apparatus of the inner ear. Its most superior part (the petrous ridge of the adult skull) divides the middle and posterior cranial fossae and serves as the anterolateral attachment of the tentorium. In the fetus, however, the exaggerated *arcuate eminence* and the *subarcuate fossa* render the ridge less distinct.

Medial to the arcuate eminence the *internal auditory meatus* conducts the auditory (CNVIII) and facial (CNVII) nerves into the petrous bone. The auditory nerve terminates within the petrous bone, but the facial nerve passes through it and out the stylomastoid foramen to reach the muscles of the face. A branch carrying autonomic fibers forms the greater petrous nerve, which leaves the facial nerve through the *hiatus of the facial canal* located anterior to the arcuate eminence.

A large section of the suture between the petrous bone and the lateral part of the occipital complex remains open as the *jugular foramen*. This irregular and indirect opening (called the jugular fossa on the inferior side) passes the glossopharyngeal (CNIX), vagus (CNX) and accessory (CNXI) nerves in conjunction with the jugular vein.

The components of the occipital complex surround the *foramen magnum,* which transmits the spinal medulla and its meningeal coverings as well as the vertebral arteries and the ascending spinal roots of the accessory nerve. Each lateral part of the occipital complex is perforated on its medial edge by the *hypoglossal canal,* which transmits the hypoglossal (CNXII) nerve to the muscles of the tongue.

Plate 149   Superior Aspect of Skull Base   311

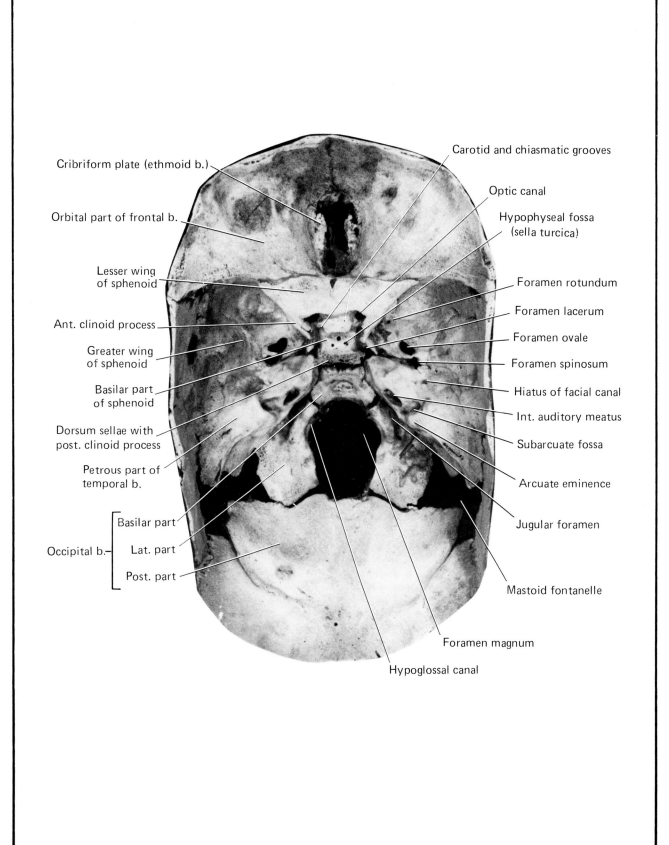

Cribriform plate (ethmoid b.)

Carotid and chiasmatic grooves

Optic canal

Orbital part of frontal b.

Hypophyseal fossa
(sella turcica)

Lesser wing
of sphenoid

Foramen rotundum

Foramen lacerum

Ant. clinoid process

Foramen ovale

Greater wing
of sphenoid

Foramen spinosum

Hiatus of facial canal

Basilar part
of sphenoid

Int. auditory meatus

Dorsum sellae with
post. clinoid process

Subarcuate fossa

Petrous part of
temporal b.

Arcuate eminence

Occipital b.— Basilar part

Lat. part

Jugular foramen

Post. part

Mastoid fontanelle

Foramen magnum

Hypoglossal canal

OSTEOLOGY OF THE FACE: ORBITAL DETAIL

In this plate the face has been sheared from the cranium and positioned so that the composite view of both orbits reveals their entire osseous structure. The contributions of the frontal bones to both the visage and the orbit are well shown on the right side of the face, as are the zygomatic and sphenoidal parts of the lateral orbital wall.

On the left side the medial and posterior components of the orbit are revealed. The thin *orbital lamina* of the *ethmoid,* the *lachrymal* and parts of the *frontal* and *maxillary bones* make up the medial wall of the orbit. The *ethmoidal foramina* pass the ethmoidal branches of the ophthalmic artery into the nasal cavity, and the sac of the lachrymal apparatus rests in the *lachrymal fossa,* from where it sends its duct inferiorly to the inferior nasal meatus.

The posterior orbit shows a variety of foramina and fissures. The *superior orbital fissure* is a cleft between the lesser and greater wings of the sphenoid. It transmits the ophthalmic division of the trigeminal nerve (CNV) along with the oculomotor (CNIII), trochlear (CNIV) and abducens (CNVII) that innervate the muscles of the bulb and levator of the eyelid. Medial to the fis-

sure, the *optic canal* penetrates the sphenoid to pass the optic tract (CNII) and its dural sheath to the orbit.

The *inferior orbital fissure* occurs between the greater wing of the sphenoid and the orbital part of the maxilla. Visible in its medial end is the *foramen rotundum* that transmits the maxillary division of the trigeminal nerve (CNV), which traverses the fissure to pass through the infraorbital canal and foramen to distribute sensory branches to the nose, upper lip and cheek.

In the medial depths of the fissure a small wedge of the palatine bone makes its orbital contribution.

On the right wall of the nasal cavity, the *inferior nasal concha* is separated by a circumferential suture that shows it to be an independent bone of the face.

The superior aspect of the *mandible* shows the alveolar sockets containing the tooth buds. In the vital specimen these are covered by the gingival membrane and are visible only upon eruption. The *ramus* is an indistinct extension of the body and lacks the pronounced angle acquired in later life (see lateral view of mandible in Plate 145). On the medial surface of the ramus distal to the *condyle,* the *mandibular foramen* receives the inferior alveolar branch of the mandibular division of the trigeminal (CNV) just medial to the *lingular process,* to which is attached the sphenomandibular ligament.

Plate 150   Orbital Detail of Face   313

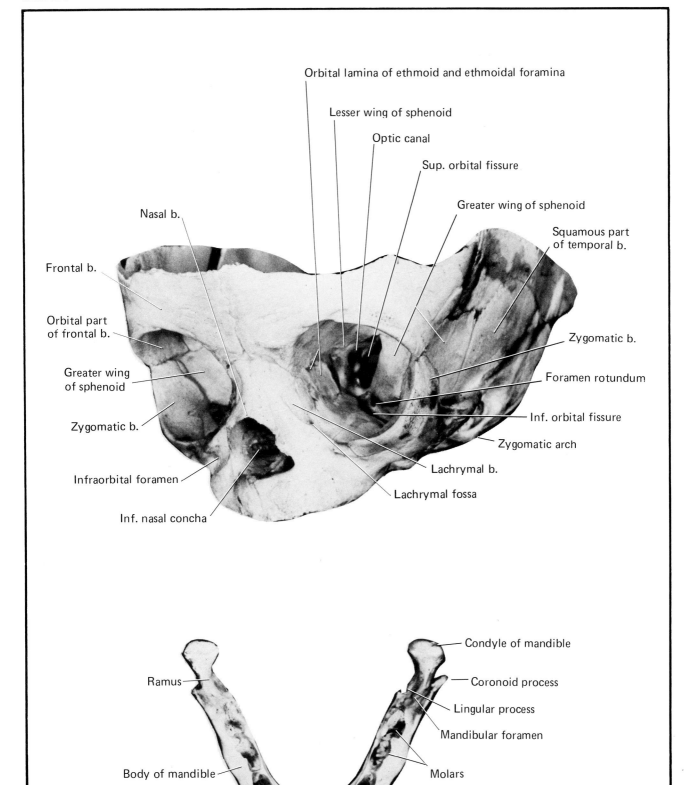

Orbital lamina of ethmoid and ethmoidal foramina

Lesser wing of sphenoid

Optic canal

Sup. orbital fissure

Greater wing of sphenoid

Squamous part
of temporal b.

Nasal b.

Frontal b.

Orbital part
of frontal b.

Greater wing
of sphenoid

Zygomatic b.

Zygomatic b.

Foramen rotundum

Infraorbital foramen

Inf. orbital fissure

Zygomatic arch

Lachrymal b.

Lachrymal fossa

Inf. nasal concha

Condyle of mandible

Ramus

Coronoid process

Lingular process

Mandibular foramen

Body of mandible

Molars

Canine

Incisors

SAGITTAL SECTION OF THE FETAL SKULL

This section particularly emphasizes the diminutive size of the fetal face in relation to the cranial cavity. The inferior and middle nasal meatus are well delineated by the *inferior nasal concha*. Superior to this the *labyrinthine part of the ethmoid* overhangs the *semilunar hiatus*, which bears the foramina that eventually will communicate with the maxillary, frontal and ethmoidal sinuses. At this stage both frontal and ethmoidal sinuses are deficient, and the openings lead to shallow depressions that represent the maxillary sinus. Eventually, the body of the sphenoid becomes pneumatized by a pair of sinuses that will open into the superior nasal meatus.

Posterior to the ethmoid is the *pterygopalatine fossa* that contained the pterygopalatine ganglion, and superior to this an ephemeral communication to the orbit is evident. This latter fact should emphasize that throughout life, only thin ethmoidal bone and epithelium separate the nasal cavity from the orbital contents.

This section also gives a good view of the superior configurations of the fetal petrous bone. The *arcuate eminence* which houses the posterior semicircular canal is very evident. Postnatally, the eminence becomes less pronounced and the subarcuate fossa disappears.

Plate 151

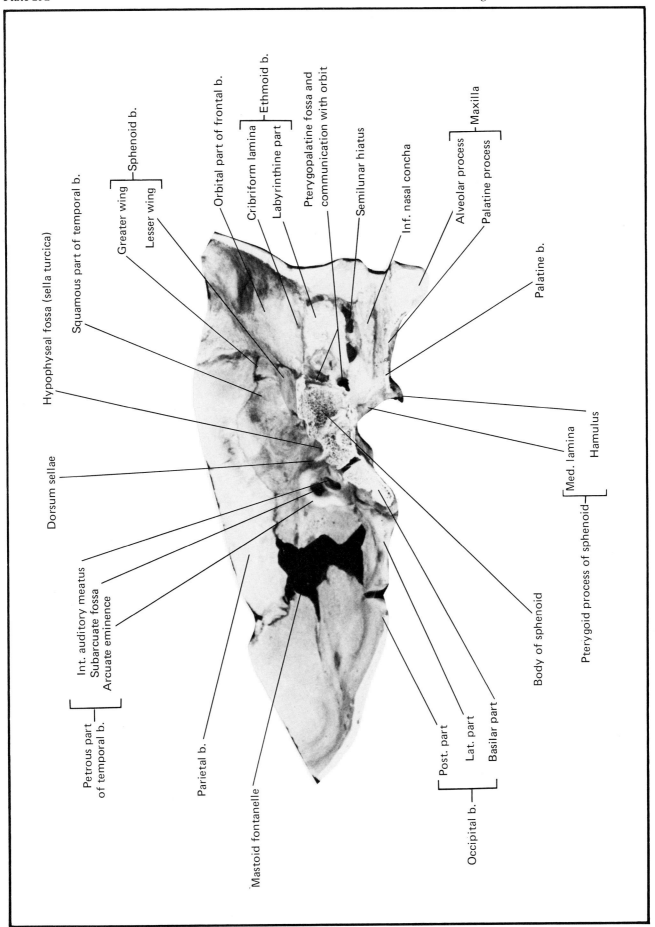

Hypophyseal fossa (sella turcica)

Squamous part of temporal b.

Greater wing
Lesser wing — Sphenoid b.

Orbital part of frontal b.

Cribriform lamina
Labyrinthine part — Ethmoid b.

Pterygopalatine fossa and
communication with orbit

Semilunar hiatus

Inf. nasal concha

Alveolar process
Palatine process — Maxilla

Palatine b.

Med. lamina
Hamulus — Pterygoid process of sphenoid

Body of sphenoid

Dorsum sellae

Int. auditory meatus
Subarcuate fossa
Arcuate eminence — Petrous part of temporal b.

Parietal b.

Mastoid fontanelle

Post. part
Lat. part
Basilar part — Occipital b.

LATERAL RADIOGRAM OF THE FETAL SKULL

This and the following two x-rays are from the same skull used in Plates 145, 146 and 147.

The lateral view emphasizes the density and irregularity of the bones in the base of the skull. The *body of the sphenoid* can be identified by its relation to the hypophyseal fossa, and the role of the anterior sphenoid processes in buttressing the bones of the face can be appreciated. The facial bones, although relatively thin in themselves, seem to be denser because they are bilaterally represented and their combined density is cumulative. The particular radiopacity of the *petrous bone* is not only because of its thickness, but also, as its name implies, it is an extremely compact bone, being the hardest substance in the body except tooth enamel. The *internal auditory meatus* and *subarcuate fossa* can be identified by the radiolucency they provide.

In the tuber of the frontal bone, the radiating streaks of lower density indicate the venous channels developing between the external and internal laminar plates. These are the precursors of the *diploic veins* that course between the compact layers of the adult calvaria.

Plate 152

Lateral Radiogram of Skull   317

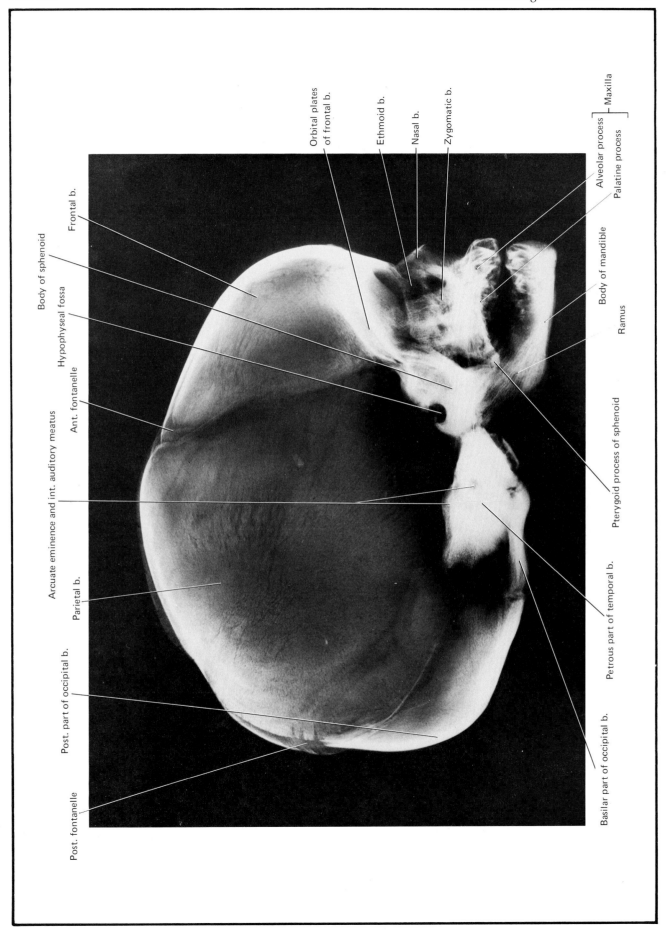

Orbital plates
of frontal b.

Ethmoid b.

Nasal b.

Zygomatic b.

Maxilla

Alveolar process

Palatine process

Frontal b.

Body of sphenoid

Hypophyseal fossa

Ant. fontanelle

Body of mandible

Ramus

Arcuate eminence and int. auditory meatus

Parietal b.

Pterygoid process of sphenoid

Post. part of occipital b.

Petrous part of temporal b.

Basilar part of occipital b.

Post. fontanelle

ANTEROPOSTERIOR RADIOGRAM OF THE FETAL SKULL

This radiographic view again emphasizes the relative disparity between the fetal cranium and face. The expanded bones of the cranium display the development of the diploic veins radiating from nutritive foramina. It is obvious that the frontal and parietal bones are thicker at their tuberal prominences, and venous channels are more profuse at these points.

The coronal suture and *anterior fontanelle* are well marked, and although this is a dried specimen, the potential overlapping of the parietal bones at the sagittal suture indicates the danger of shearing that may occur with compression of the cranium.

The radiographic detail of the orbit is quite revealing. The orbital plate of the frontal bone is paper thin at its medial part and hence appears as a slanted radiolucent slit. The thicker lateral parts of the sphenoid body surround the optic canal before they extend out to the lesser wings. The maxillary and zygomatic parts of the orbit show greater density as they are viewed edgewise, but the position of the infraorbital canal is well marked.

The edge views of the ethmoidal laminae and the nasal septum further illustrate that very thin bones can be quite radiopaque when their greater dimensions are positioned parallel to the direction of radiation.

Because the solid maxillae are posteriorly reinforced by the pterygoid process of the sphenoid, considerable cumulative shadow is produced by these bones.

Plate 153   Anteroposterior Radiogram of Skull   319

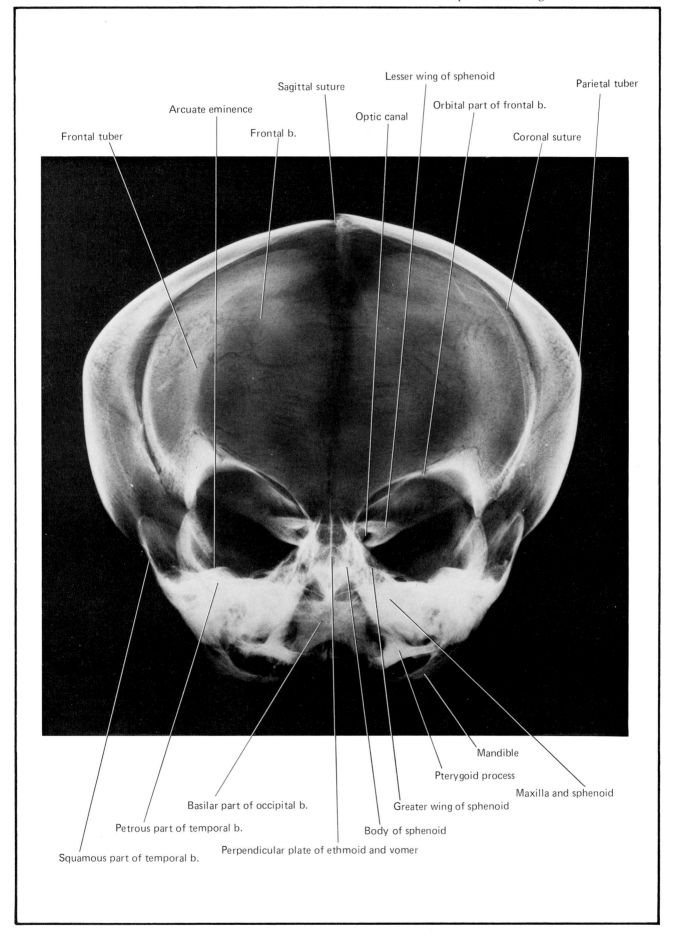

Frontal tuber

Arcuate eminence

Frontal b.

Sagittal suture

Optic canal

Lesser wing of sphenoid

Orbital part of frontal b.

Parietal tuber

Coronal suture

Squamous part of temporal b.

Petrous part of temporal b.

Basilar part of occipital b.

Perpendicular plate of ethmoid and vomer

Body of sphenoid

Greater wing of sphenoid

Pterygoid process

Mandible

Maxilla and sphenoid

RADIOGRAM
OF THE
FETAL SKULL BASE

This plate provides more radiographic detail of the fetal skull structure than the two preceding plates have shown.

The inferior view of the face shows the mandible and articulation with the temporal bone just medial to the temporal base of the zygomatic arch. Framed by the mandibular arch, the nasal cavity shows the cumulative shadows of the middle and inferior nasal conchae with the perpendicular plate of the *ethmoid* and the *vomer* lying in the sagittal plane. The radiolucent areas lateral to the ethmoids are the deeper parts of the orbits.

The combined shadows of the *lesser* and *greater wings* of the *sphenoid* extend laterally from the body and from the posterior orbital wall. The area between the *anterior clinoid process* and *hypophyseal fossa* contains the carotid groove that passes the artery to the base of the brain. Between the *basilar part* of the *occipital* bone and the hypophyseal fossa, the *dorsum sellae* forms a transverse ridge of a greater density.

Within the dense mass of the petrous bone, the *vestibular* and *cochlear ducts* show numerous radiolucent points, and medial to these the *internal auditory meatus* and *carotid canal* may be discerned. The ossicles of the middle ear are easily defined as they approximate their definitive sizes in the perinatal skull.

Plate 154

Radiogram of Skull Base   321

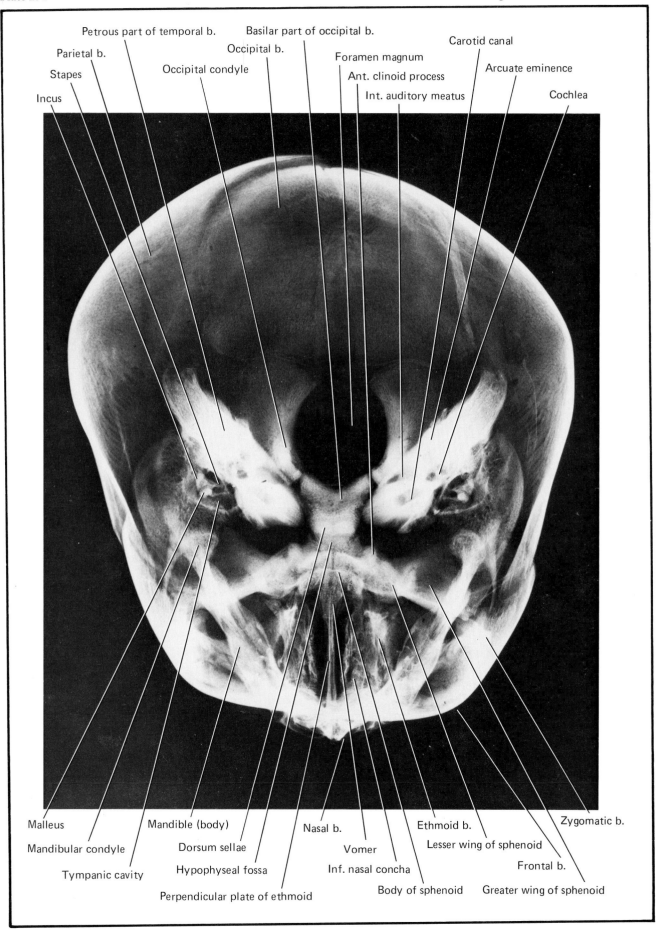

Petrous part of temporal b.

Parietal b.

Stapes

Incus

Occipital condyle

Basilar part of occipital b.

Occipital b.

Foramen magnum

Ant. clinoid process

Int. auditory meatus

Carotid canal

Arcuate eminence

Cochlea

Malleus

Mandibular condyle

Tympanic cavity

Mandible (body)

Dorsum sellae

Hypophyseal fossa

Perpendicular plate of ethmoid

Nasal b.

Vomer

Inf. nasal concha

Body of sphenoid

Ethmoid b.

Lesser wing of sphenoid

Frontal b.

Greater wing of sphenoid

Zygomatic b.

THE INTRACRANIAL DURAL FOLDS

The dura is the external and thickest of the three meningeal layers that ensheath the central nervous system. Within the skull it is intimately bound to the internal cranial periosteum, but in the spine where it surrounds the cord, a layer of epidural fat intervenes between the dura and the enclosing bone. However, in certain intracranial areas the dura leaves the periosteum and invaginates as a double layered fold to provide support between the major cleavages of the brain. The venous drainage of the brain and skull flows into a complex system of channels that run between the double layers of a fold or between the dura and periosteum. The larger of these epidural venous sinuses are found along the attachments and intersections of the folds or in their free edges. They are lined only with a thin endothelium that is supported by the dura, and they have no valves. Through a number of villous invaginations from the arachnoid, the epidural sinuses receive the effluent cerebrospinal fluid from the subarachnoid space.

The largest dural fold, the *falx cerebri,* is situated between the cerebral hemispheres. It arises from the inner surface of the calvaria along the midsagittal line and extends from the tentorium to the crista galli with its free edge passing over the corpus callosum. The large *superior sagittal sinus* runs within the attached edge of the fold and the smaller *inferior sagittal sinus* runs in its free edge.

The other major dural fold, the *tentorium cerebelli,* forms a sling between the cerebral and cerebellar regions and supports the posterior parts of the cerebral hemispheres. It is attached anteriorly at the clinoid processes and along the petrous ridge. Posteriorly, it is attached transversely across the occipital bone and intersects the falx cerebri at the midline. The free edge of the tentorium provides an opening, the *tentorial incisure,* that gives the brain stem access to the supratentorial cerebral hemispheres.

The posterior attachment of the tentorium contains the transverse sinuses. These receive the sagittal and straight sinuses (the latter runs in the intersection of the falx and tentorium) and course laterally around the occiput toward the petrous bones. Here they take a tortuous turn inferiorly as the sigmoidal sinuses and drain into the jugular veins at the jugular foramen. A number of minor sinus complexes run beneath the dura of the floors of the cranial fossae. These have numerous communications with veins of the orbit and face through virtually all of the skull foramina. Most of the minor sinuses also communicate with a pair of irregular *cavernous sinuses* located on either side of the sphenoid body; these in turn drain toward the jugular system through the petrous sinuses.

In the temporal region of this specimen, the dura has been elevated from the skull to show the potential epidural space that carries the *middle meningeal artery.* Rupture of this vessel may produce dissecting hematomas that elevate the dura.

Plate 155

Intracranial Dural Folds   323

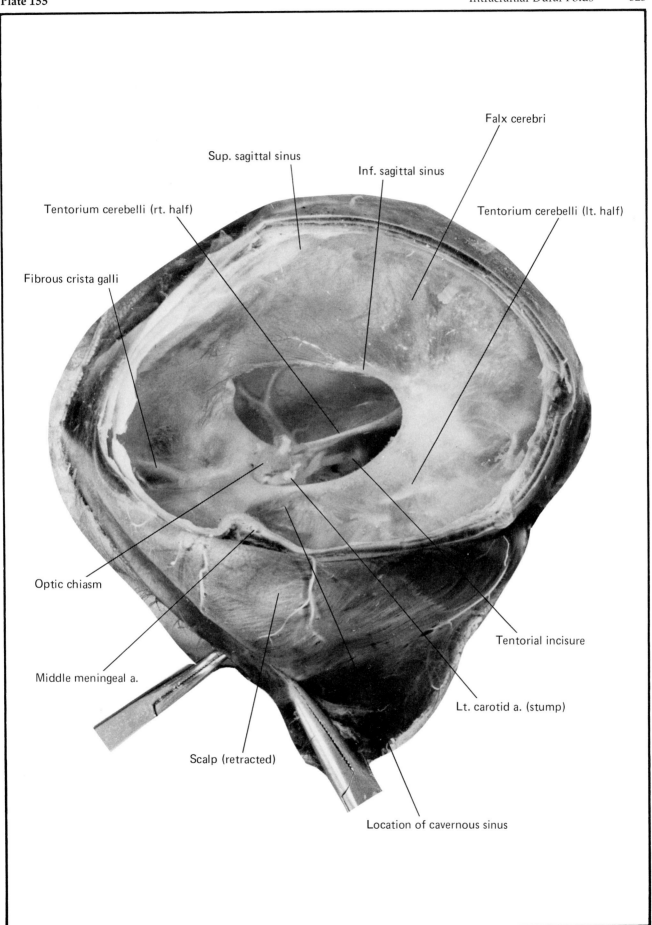

Falx cerebri

Sup. sagittal sinus

Inf. sagittal sinus

Tentorium cerebelli (rt. half)

Tentorium cerebelli (lt. half)

Fibrous crista galli

Optic chiasm

Tentorial incisure

Middle meningeal a.

Lt. carotid a. (stump)

Scalp (retracted)

Location of cavernous sinus

SAGITTAL SECTION OF THE FETAL HEAD

The essential value of this section of a full term fetal head is not in its detail but in the display of the topographic relations of the various structures in the head.

The manner in which the brain occupies the cranium is particularly well shown. The large *cerebral hemisphere* fills the cavity from the tentorium to the anterior fossa. On its medial surface the intact *falx cerebri* is displayed as a transparent double fold of dura. Its free edge may be followed from the level of the tentorium to the *crista galli,* and the *inferior sagittal sinus* can be seen in its free edge. Posteriorly, part of the *superior sagittal sinus* has been opened and its *confluence* with the *transverse* and *straight sinuses* indicates the level of the tentorium.

A less pronounced *falx cerebelli* lies between the lobes of the cerebellum. It can be seen that the tentorium covers the posterior cranial fossa, which contains the cerebellum, pons and medulla oblongata. The cerebral peduncles and *corpora quadrigemina* of the midbrain lie encircled by the *tentorial incisure,* and the diencephalon with its *thalamic* and *hypothalamic regions* lies superior to the tentorium. The *corpus callosum,* which connects the two cerebral hemispheres, is situated in close relation to the free edge of the falx.

Inferior to the hypothalamus the *hypophysis* and its *stalk* are evident just posterior to a section of the *optic chiasm.* The *olfactory bulb* lies in the olfactory fossa of the cribriform plate, and its close proximity to the olfactory epithelium of the superior nasal meatus can be appreciated.

Plate 156

Sagittal Section of Head   325

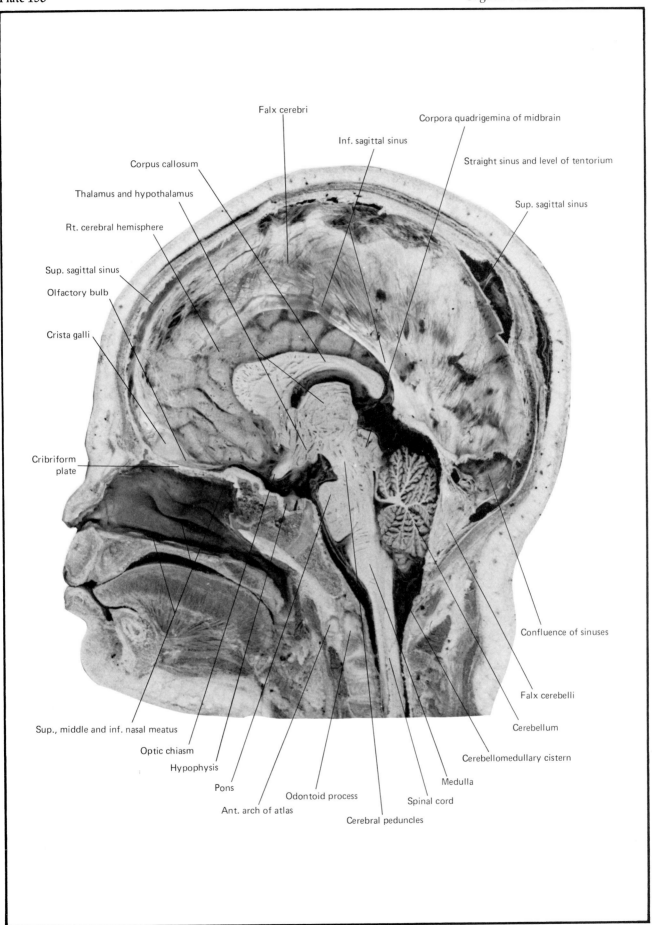

Falx cerebri

Corpora quadrigemina of midbrain

Inf. sagittal sinus

Straight sinus and level of tentorium

Corpus callosum

Thalamus and hypothalamus

Sup. sagittal sinus

Rt. cerebral hemisphere

Sup. sagittal sinus

Olfactory bulb

Crista galli

Cribriform plate

Confluence of sinuses

Falx cerebelli

Cerebellum

Sup., middle and inf. nasal meatus

Cerebellomedullary cistern

Optic chiasm

Hypophysis

Medulla

Pons

Odontoid process

Spinal cord

Ant. arch of atlas

Cerebral peduncles

THE CRANIAL FOSSAE

For this view the calvaria of a 33-week-old fetus was removed and the exposed brain extirpated, leaving the stumps of the cranial nerves, the dura and the vessels of the cranial fossae intact.

The lateral expanses of the anterior fossa show the bulging of the subadjacent orbits but have little other interesting detail. In the medial region, however, the two *fossae of the olfactory bulbs* lie on both sides of the *crista galli.* In the lateral limits of these fossae, the *anterior* and *posterior ethmoidal arteries* (from the ophthalmic artery) supply much of the dura and bone of the medial anterior cranial fossa.

The sharp ridges of the lesser wing of the sphenoid separate the anterior and middle fossae. The lateral depressions of the middle cranial fossae accommodate the temporal lobes of the cerebral hemispheres. In the center of these depressions, the *middle meningeal artery* enters the cranium through the foramen spinosum and abruptly divides into *frontal* and *parietal branches.* The arteries run an epidural course supplying the dura and bone of the skull. Should a skull fracture shear one of the branches of the middle meningeal artery, an epidural hematoma dissects the dura from the periosteum and compresses the brain. A slight swelling on the medial wall of the middle fossa marks the position of the cavernous sinus which surrounds a segment of the carotid artery and several cranial nerve elements entering the orbit.

The body of the sphenoid lies between the two middle cranial fossae. The *hypophyseal fossa* lies in its central region and the contained *hypophysis* is covered by a dural fold, the *sellar diaphragm,* which bears a perforation that passes the hypophyseal stalk. Anterior to this the chiasmatic groove contains the stumps of the optic tracts (CNII). Between these and the *anterior clinoid processes,* the carotid arteries rise to reach the brain.

Both the anterior and posterior clinoid processes support a dural fold that is the commencement of the

tentorium. The cut edge of the tentorium shows its anterior attachment to the petrous ridge, which also serves to separate the middle and posterior cranial fossae. The attachment extends posteriorly to the transverse sinuses, indicating that the tentorium roofed the entire posterior fossa and its contents. The small *superior* and *inferior* petrous sinuses that course posterolaterally along the petrous bone connect the cavernous sinus to the sigmoid sinus and jugular vein.

Except the optic tract, all of the cranial nerves to the orbit pierce the dura near the anterior folds of the tentorium and run a subdural course along the cavernous sinus to reach the superior orbital fissure. The *oculomotor nerve* (CNIII) pierces the dural fold lateral to the dorsum sellae and anterior to the site of penetration of the fine *trochlear nerve* (CNIV). Just inferior to the cut edge of the tentorium, the *trigeminal nerve* (CNV) enters the dura, and the *abducens nerve* (CNVI) penetrates the dura more medially where it overlies the base of the occipital bone.

On the posteromedial aspect of the petrous bone, the dura evaginates into the internal auditory meatus to pass the *facial* (CNVII) and *auditory* (CNVIII) nerves. The former lies anterosuperior to the latter and usually can be separated where the two enter the meatus.

Inferior to the above nerves, another large opening indicates the dural evagination into the jugular foramen, which passes the *glossopharyngeal* (CNIX), *vagus* (CNX) and *accessory* (CNXI) *nerves.* These can be separated into distinct bundles of rootlets, and the *spinal root* to the accessory is readily identified where it ascends through the foramen magnum to exit via the jugular foramen.

The *hypoglossal nerve* (CNXII) pierces the dura in the hypoglossal canal located on the medial surface of the edge of the foramen magnum inferior to the dural opening of the three previous cranial nerves.

Deep within the foramen magnum the rootlets of the upper cervical nerves can be seen.

Plate 157   Cranial Fossae   327

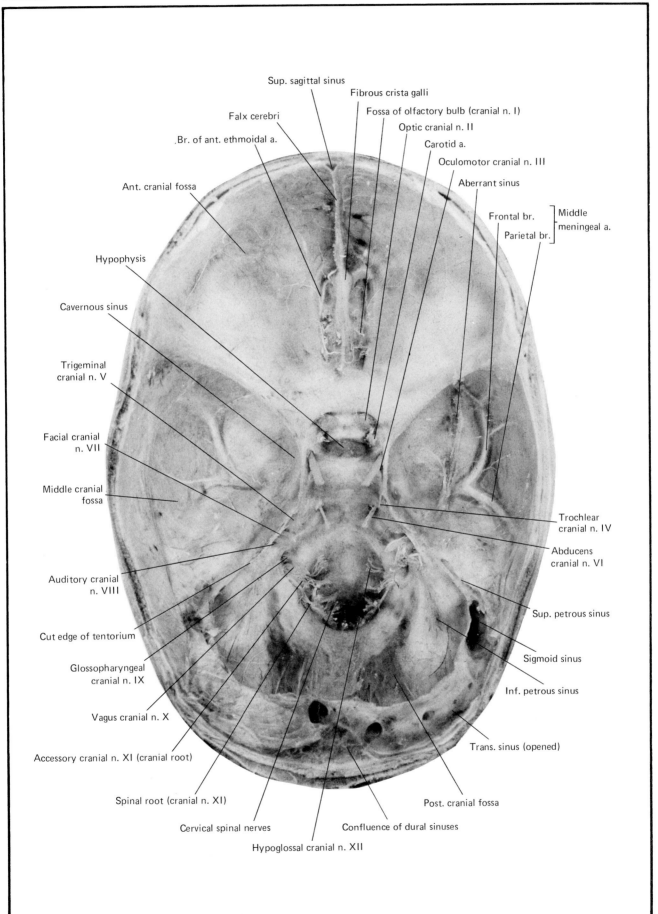

Sup. sagittal sinus

Fibrous crista galli

Falx cerebri

Fossa of olfactory bulb (cranial n. I)

Optic cranial n. II

Br. of ant. ethmoidal a.

Carotid a.

Oculomotor cranial n. III

Ant. cranial fossa

Aberrant sinus

Frontal br.

Parietal br.

Middle meningeal a.

Hypophysis

Cavernous sinus

Trigeminal cranial n. V

Facial cranial n. VII

Middle cranial fossa

Trochlear cranial n. IV

Abducens cranial n. VI

Auditory cranial n. VIII

Sup. petrous sinus

Cut edge of tentorium

Sigmoid sinus

Glossopharyngeal cranial n. IX

Inf. petrous sinus

Vagus cranial n. X

Accessory cranial n. XI (cranial root)

Trans. sinus (opened)

Spinal root (cranial n. XI)

Cervical spinal nerves

Confluence of dural sinuses

Post. cranial fossa

Hypoglossal cranial n. XII

LATERAL ASPECT OF THE FETAL BRAIN

Traditionally, atlases of the gross morphology of the body treat the brain simply as the viscus of the cranial cavity and leave the wealth of its structural detail to the specialized texts and atlases of neuroanatomy. In keeping with this convention, this and the following two illustrations serve primarily to relate the brain to the internal structure of the skull and depict its vascularity, and to facilitate the interpretation of the cranial angiograms.

Here is shown the lateral view of the brain of a term fetus. The gyri and sulci appear late in the fetal period, for the brain surface of a 7-month fetus is smooth and shows only the major sulci. During the later weeks of gestation the gyri and sulci develop rapidly, so that by term they have aquired their definitive complexity and relative proportions.

The cerebral hemisphere is divided into lobes, whose names correspond to the bone of the cranium that is externally related to them.

The *central* and *lateral sulci* separate three of the lobes. Thus the part of the hemisphere anterior to the central sulcus and superior to the lateral is the *frontal lobe,* which abuts the frontal bone, and its anteroinferior part occupies the anterior fossa. The region posterior to the central sulcus and superior to the lat-

eral is the *parietal lobe.* Inferior to the lateral sulcus lies the *temporal lobe,* whose anterior part occupies the middle cranial fossa. A line intersecting the *parietooccipital sulcus* with a more arbitrarily positioned *occipital* notch separates the *occipital lobe* from the temporal and parietal regions.

In situ the tentorium occupied the fissure between the inferior surface of the cerebrum and the cerebellum and supported the posterior cerebral regions. The *cerebellum* and the more anterior *pons* and *medulla oblongata* occupied the posterior cranial fossa.

In this specimen the middle meningeal layer, the arachnoid, was left intact, for it supports the superficial vascularity of the brain. A latex injection has emphasized the cortical arterial branches, and the dark, blood-filled spaces in the sulci indicate the cerebral venous channels. The middle and *anterior cerebral arteries* supply all of the frontal lobe and most of the temporal and parietal lobes. The distribution of the posterior *cerebral artery* lies in the inferior regions of the temporal and occipital lobes.

On the lateral surface of the cerebellum, the *posterior superior* and *inferior cerebellar arteries* of vertebral and basilar origins can be seen in addition to the *pontine branches* of the *basilar artery.*

There are a number of arteriovenous anastomoses in the vasculature of the brain, and often cerebral veins are found partially filled from arterial injections. A good example of a partially injected vein lies near the labeled posterior cerebral artery branch in the inferior temporal region.

Plate 158
Lateral Aspect of Brain
329

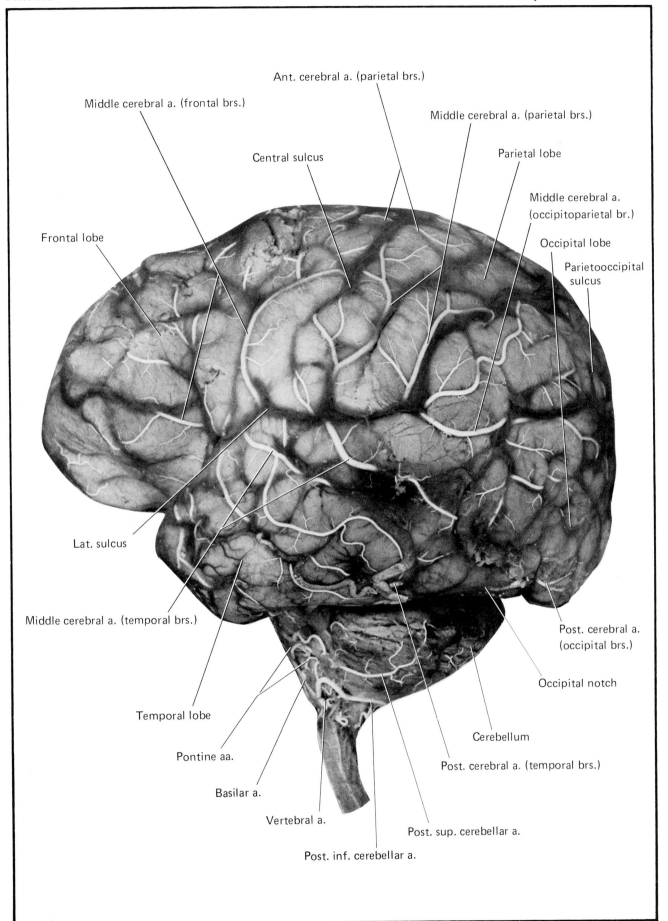

Ant. cerebral a. (parietal brs.)

Middle cerebral a. (frontal brs.)

Middle cerebral a. (parietal brs.)

Central sulcus

Parietal lobe

Middle cerebral a. (occipitoparietal br.)

Frontal lobe

Occipital lobe

Parietooccipital sulcus

Lat. sulcus

Middle cerebral a. (temporal brs.)

Post. cerebral a. (occipital brs.)

Occipital notch

Temporal lobe

Pontine aa.

Cerebellum

Post. cerebral a. (temporal brs.)

Basilar a.

Vertebral a.

Post. sup. cerebellar a.

Post. inf. cerebellar a.

SAGITTAL ASPECT OF THE FETAL BRAIN

This view shows the extensive vascular domain of the *anterior cerebral artery*. The major channel follows the superior contour of the great cerebral commissure, the *corpus callosum,* and distributes branches to the frontal, parietal and occipital lobes. Most of these branches supply not only the medial area of the hemisphere but also a substantial part of its superior surface as well.

The *posterior cerebral artery* is represented by a number of *cortical branches* on the occipital lobe and the significant *posterior choroidal artery*.

The sagittal section of the diencephalon and brain stem shows *striate* branches of the *middle cerebral artery* penetrating the cerebral peduncle to reach the striate regions, and branches of the *basilar artery* penetrating the pons and medulla to supply these vital areas.

Plate 159   Sagittal Aspect of Brain   331

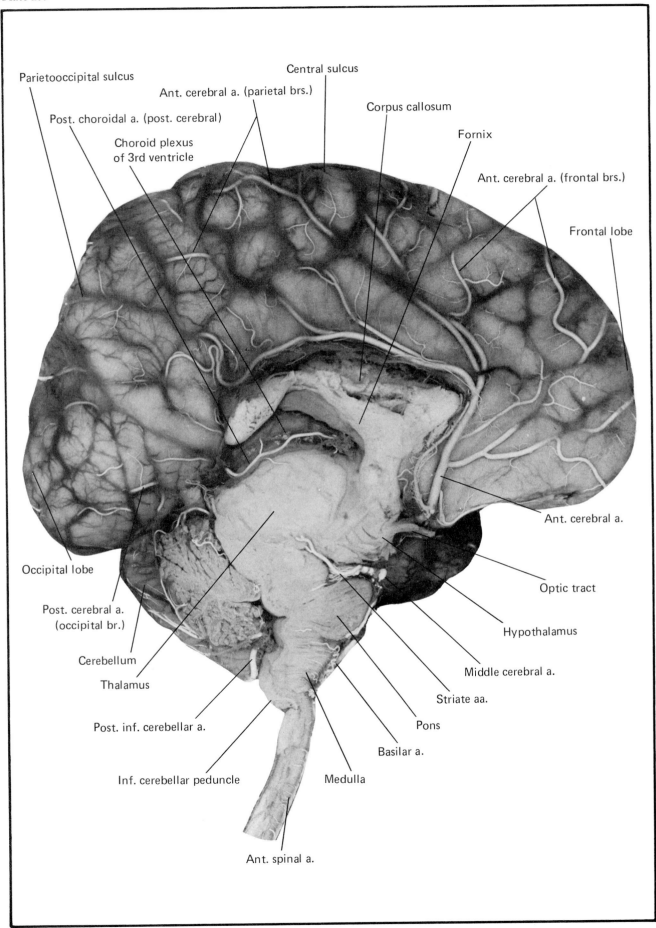

Parietooccipital sulcus

Central sulcus

Ant. cerebral a. (parietal brs.)

Post. choroidal a. (post. cerebral)

Corpus callosum

Choroid plexus
of 3rd ventricle

Fornix

Ant. cerebral a. (frontal brs.)

Frontal lobe

Ant. cerebral a.

Occipital lobe

Optic tract

Post. cerebral a.
(occipital br.)

Hypothalamus

Cerebellum

Middle cerebral a.

Thalamus

Striate aa.

Post. inf. cerebellar a.

Pons

Basilar a.

Inf. cerebellar peduncle

Medulla

Ant. spinal a.

INFERIOR ASPECT OF THE FETAL BRAIN

This view shows the surfaces of the brain that are in direct contact with the floors of the cranial fossae.

The orbital gyri of the *frontal lobe* lie directly against the orbital plates of the frontal bone, and the rounded anteroinferior surfaces of the *temporal lobes* fill the depressions of the middle cranial fossae. The cerebellum and its regional parts of the brain stem occupy the posterior cranial fossa.

Frontal branches of the anterior *cerebral arteries* and *middle cerebral* arteries supply an approximately equal share of inferior surfaces of the frontal lobes. The anterior and lateral areas of the inferior surfaces of the temporal lobes are supplied by middle cerebral branches, but temporal branches of the *posterior cerebral arteries* supply the medial inferior areas.

The main trunks of all three cerebral arteries arise from the *cerebral arterial circle,* a ring of intercommunicating vessels that surround the inferior part of the hypothalamus and the optic chiasm. It receives the internal carotid arteries near the site where the middle and anterior cerebral arteries arise, and a bifurcation on the basilar artery gives rise to the posterior cerebral arteries. The *posterior communicating arteries* form anastomotic channels between the carotid and basilar sources, and an interconnecting channel between the converging proximal sections of the anterior cerebral arteries completes the circle anteriorly.

On the anterior surface of the medulla the *vertebral arteries* converge to form the *basilar artery.* The first give rise to the posteroinferior cerebellar arteries, and the second is the source of the *anteroinferior cerebellar artery* and the *superior cerebellar artery.* Medial branches of the converging vertebral arteries form the *anterior spinal artery* that provides the major vascularity of the spine.

Again, the partially injected cerebral vein (posterior anastomotic vein) that drained into the transverse sinus can be seen on the right inferior surface of the temporal lobe.

The roots of all of the cranial nerves, except the very fine trochlear nerve, can be identified in this view. The *olfactory tracts* (CNI) run along the medial orbital surface of the frontal lobes, and the *optic tracts* (CNII) diverge from the chiasm medial to the stumps of the carotid arteries. Lateral to the posterior communicating arteries, the *oculomotor* (CNIII) and *trigeminal* (CNV) roots course along the medial surface of the temporal lobe after arising near the superior border of the pons. Between the pons and cerebellum the *facial* (CNVII) and *auditory* (CNVIII) arise, and the *abducens* (CNVI) nerve leaves the stem near the inferior border of the pons and runs along its anterior surface.

Posterior to the olive, the main roots of the glossopharygeal (CNIX), vagus (CNX) and *accessory* (CNXI) nerves can be identified. Near the vertebral artery at the ventral part of the olive the hypoglossal (CNXII) rootlets leave the brain stem.

Plate 160

Inferior Aspect of Brain

333

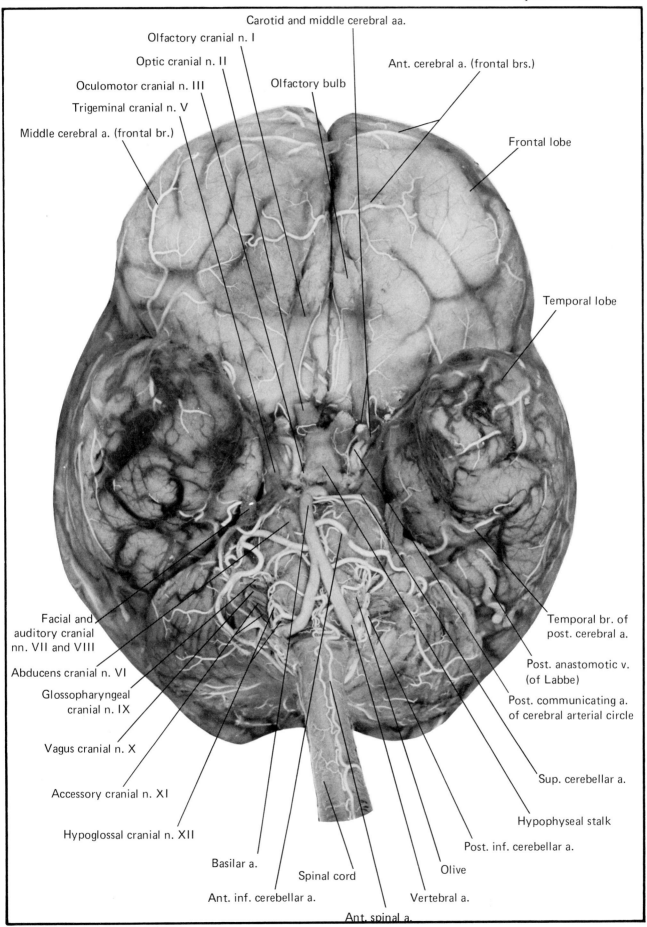

Carotid and middle cerebral aa.

Olfactory cranial n. I

Optic cranial n. II

Oculomotor cranial n. III

Trigeminal cranial n. V

Middle cerebral a. (frontal br.)

Olfactory bulb

Ant. cerebral a. (frontal brs.)

Frontal lobe

Temporal lobe

Facial and
auditory cranial
nn. VII and VIII

Abducens cranial n. VI

Glossopharyngeal
cranial n. IX

Vagus cranial n. X

Accessory cranial n. XI

Hypoglossal cranial n. XII

Basilar a.

Ant. inf. cerebellar a.

Spinal cord

Olive

Vertebral a.

Ant. spinal a.

Temporal br. of
post. cerebral a.

Post. anastomotic v.
(of Labbe)

Post. communicating a.
of cerebral arterial circle

Sup. cerebellar a.

Hypophyseal stalk

Post. inf. cerebellar a.

LATERAL ANGIOGRAM OF THE FETAL HEMICRANIUM

Here the cranium of the specimen shown in Plate 5 has been split along the midsagittal plane and then radiographed in the lateral position. Using only one half of the head avoids the bilateral duplications of the vessels that often prove confusing, especially in the interpretation of the finer branches.

The *common carotid artery* ascends the neck, and before bifurcating into the *external* and *internal carotids* it gives off the *superior thyroid artery,* which supplies the thyroid gland and other structures of the neck. The external carotid provides the major blood supply to the face and external cranial tissues. As it enters the facial region it abruptly elaborates three branches. The anterior member of these gives rise to the *lingual artery* and the *facial artery.* The first of these enters between the extrinsic muscles at the base of the tongue and runs along the inferior margin of the intrinisic muscles, and a *submental branch* runs under the chin. The facial artery courses around the external surface of the mandible and ascends to give *labial branches* to the mouth; eventually it reaches the region medial to the eyelids where it anastomoses with the *palpebral* and *supraorbital branches* of the *ophthalmic artery.*

The *internal maxillary artery* passes from the external carotid to the deeper regions of the face. It provides branches to the deep muscles of mastication, and gives off the *middle meningeal artery* to the internal skull. Its terminal branches enter the pterygopalatine fossa and supply the structures of the nasal cavity and its septum.

A large proximal branch of the internal maxillary ascends through the parotid region as the *superficial temporal artery* to supply the lateral regions of the scalp.

Another independent branch of the internal maxillary passes inferior to the ear toward the posterior cranium as the *occipital artery.* Here the ascending *pharyngeal artery* arises from its proximal part, but this vessel may arise from any closely related arterial source.

It is generally regarded that the *internal carotid artery* has no branches external to the cranial cavity. It enters the skull via the carotid canal and takes a tortuous course through the cavernous sinus, and its first branch of conspicuous caliber is the *ophthalmic artery* to the eye and orbital adnexa. It ascends to join the *cerebral arterial circle* and immediately sends off the *anterior* and *middle cerebral arteries.*

The *vertebral artery* ascends the spinal column and enters the cranial cavity through the foramen magnum. It converges with its bilateral counterpart to form the basilar artery that provides the *posteroinferior, anteroinferior* and *superior cerebellar arteries* in addition to numerous branches to the brain stem. Its terminal major branches are the *posterior cerebral arteries* and the *posterior communicating arteries* of the cerebral arterial circle.

From this angiogram one can determine the level of the corpus callosum by the position of the anterior cerebral arteries; the approximate direction and position of the lateral sulcus by the course of the middle cerebral artery; and the level of the tentorium and inferior surface of the temporal lobes by the location of the posterior cerebral artery.

Plate 161   Lateral Angiogram of Hemicranium   335

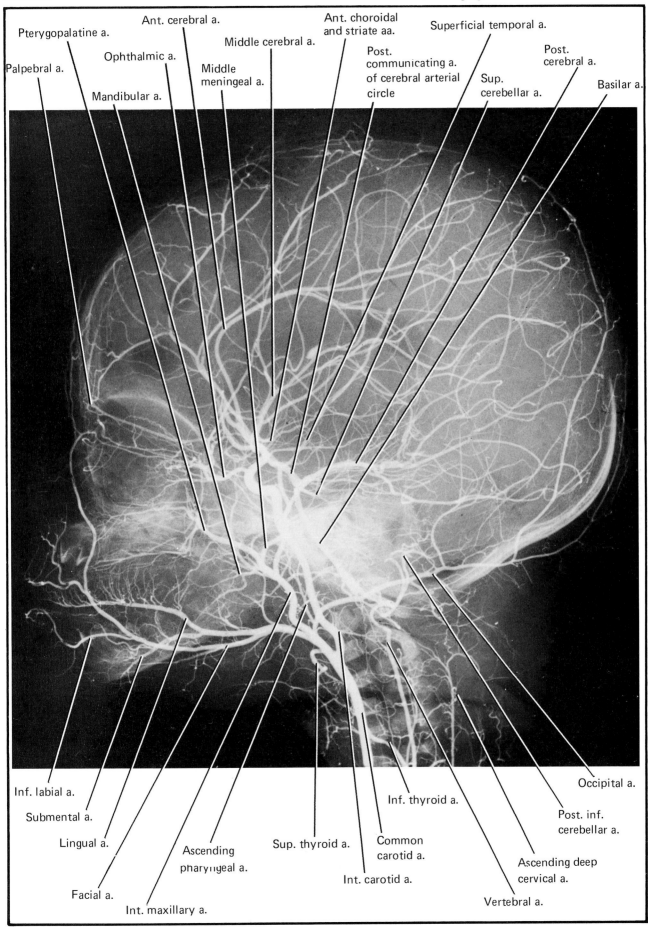

Pterygopalatine a.

Ant. cerebral a.

Palpebral a.

Ophthalmic a.

Middle cerebral a.

Ant. choroidal
and striate aa.

Superficial temporal a.

Post.
communicating a.
of cerebral arterial
circle

Post.
cerebral a.

Mandibular a.

Middle
meningeal a.

Sup.
cerebellar a.

Basilar a.

Inf. labial a.

Submental a.

Lingual a.

Ascending
pharyngeal a.

Sup. thyroid a.

Inf. thyroid a.

Common
carotid a.

Occipital a.

Post. inf.
cerebellar a.

Facial a.

Int. carotid a.

Ascending deep
cervical a.

Int. maxillary a.

Vertebral a.

ANTEROPOSTERIOR ANGIOGRAM OF THE FETAL HEAD

This radiogram was produced by rotating the neck 90 degrees to the right and exposing the head in an A-P position. It is particularly instructive of the intracranial distribution of the vertebral and internal carotid arteries and the facial relationships of the external carotid ramifications. When compared with the preceding lateral hemicranial view of the same specimen, it enhances the three dimensional interpretation of the vessels.

The *internal carotid* ascends to the base of the skull, where an abrupt medial turn indicates its entrance and passage through the carotid canal. Lateral to the body of the sphenoid, it runs a sigmoidal course through the cavernous sinus and emerges superolateral to the hypophyseal fossa to branch into the *middle* and *anterior cerebral arteries*. The middle cerebrals pass superolaterally deep within the lateral sulcus of the brain, and the anterior cerebral, after forming the anterior parts of the *cerebral arterial circle*, follows the sagittal fissure between the cerebral hemispheres.

The *vertebral arteries* ascend the vertebral column and turn medially to penetrate the dura at the atlanto-occipital interval. After giving off the *posteroinferior cerebellar arteries*, they converge to form the centrally positioned *basilar artery*. This vessel ascends the anterior surface of the brain stem and gives off numerous lateral pontine branches and the *posterosuperior cerebellar artery* (unlabeled). At the superior edge of the pons the *superior cerebellar arteries* branch laterally just before the basilar bifurcates into *posterior cerebral arteries*. From the proximal sections of the posterior cerebrals the *posterior communicating arteries* run anteriorly to form the lateral parts of the arterial circle.

The *external carotid artery* trifurcates into its linguofacial, internal maxillary and occipital branches, but only the first two are readily discernible here. The lingual arteries converge to run parallel courses within the tongue and the *facial artery* passes laterally external to the mandible and then turns medially toward the superior central regions of the face. Running deep in the facial tissues, the *internal maxillary artery* crosses the pterygoid fossa and approaches the lateral walls of the nasal cavity.

For technical interest, the quality of radiographic detail of this plate should be compared with that of the preceding angiogram. The lateral view is the result of direct x-ray exposure on industrial-quality film, whereas the A-P film was exposed in a fluorescent cassette. The finer, sharper lines of the lateral view were obtained with the use of much more prolonged and intense radiation.

Plate 162   Anteroposterior Angiogram of Head   337

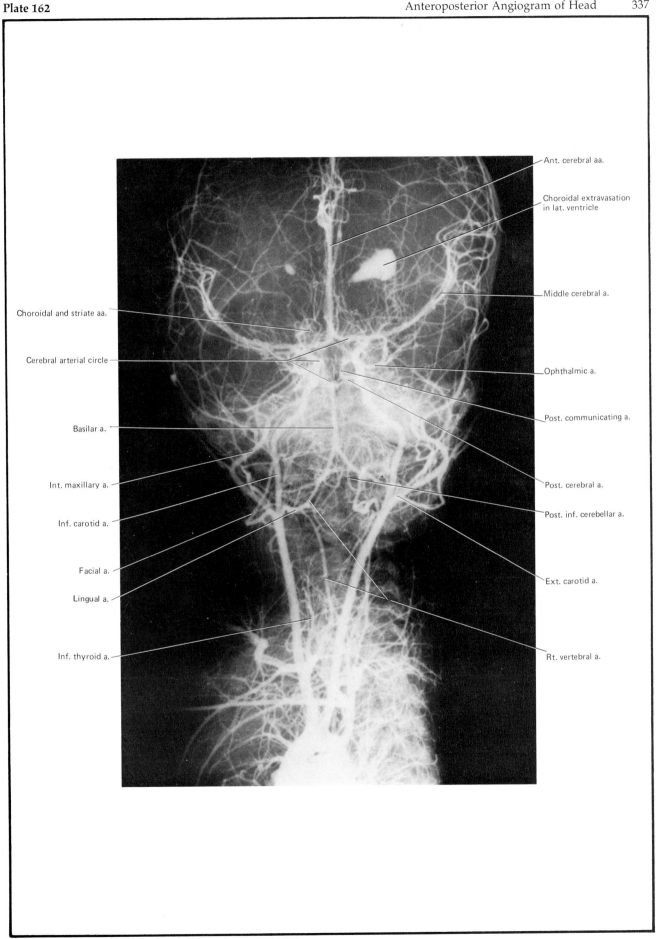

Ant. cerebral aa.

Choroidal extravasation
in lat. ventricle

Middle cerebral a.

Choroidal and striate aa.

Cerebral arterial circle

Ophthalmic a.

Post. communicating a.

Basilar a.

Int. maxillary a.

Post. cerebral a.

Inf. carotid a.

Post. inf. cerebellar a.

Facial a.

Ext. carotid a.

Lingual a.

Inf. thyroid a.

Rt. vertebral a.

VENOUS ANGIOGRAM OF THE DURAL SINUSES

In this illustration, the epidural sinuses were injected with a fine suspension of barium sulfate through a catheter introduced into the superior sagittal sinus at the posterior fontanelle. Since the catheter was directed posteriorly, the anterior part of the sagittal sinus was incompletely filled because of a back pressure of congested blood. Despite this, a very good filling of the sinuses at the base of the skull was obtained. Although the major sinuses are described as discrete channels, this venogram emphasizes that the dura is crosslaced with many minor diffuse channels, particularly in the floors of the middle and posterior cranial fossae, which help obscure the conventionally expected picture. Nevertheless, many informative aspects may be indicated.

The *superior sagittal sinus* receives the cerebral venous drainage from the superior parts of the hemispheres and conveys the blood to the confluence at the occiput. Here it passes into the *transverse sinuses* that carry to the *sigmoid sinus* and the jugular vein. The blood from deeper parts of the brain may converge toward the *great cerebral vein* located above the third ventricle. Cerebral veins from the inferior and lower lateral parts of the hemisphere drain through numerous connections to the *cavernous* and *petrous sinuses*. Peculiarly, this view shows an end-on approach to the carotid artery as it leads into the cavernous sinus producing a radiolucent hole.

The cavernous sinus receives numerous emissary veins through the foramina of the middle cranial fossa; these veins bring venous blood from the orbit via the *ophthalmic vein* and from the deep face through an intricate plexus in the pterygoid fossa. Because the ophthalmic and deep facial veins, like the sinuses, have no valves, blood may flow in any direction according to ambient pressures. Thus, infective processes of the face and orbit have unfortunate access to the epidural regions and particularly to the cavernous sinus.

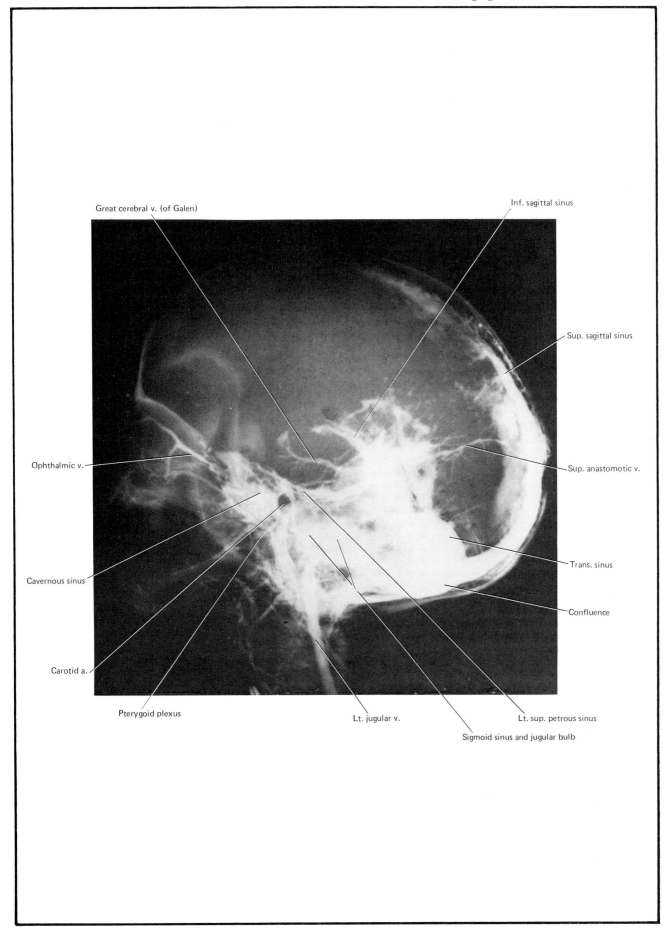

Great cerebral v. (of Galen)

Inf. sagittal sinus

Sup. sagittal sinus

Ophthalmic v.

Sup. anastomotic v.

Cavernous sinus

Trans. sinus

Confluence

Carotid a.

Pterygoid plexus

Lt. jugular v.

Lt. sup. petrous sinus

Sigmoid sinus and jugular bulb

SUPERFICIAL DISSECTION OF THE FACE AND SCALP: LATERAL ASPECT

This specimen was prepared from a 28-week-old fetus that had received an arterial injection of Neoprene latex via the umbilical artery. The dissection involved the careful removal of the entire dermal layer after incisions were made that left the skin intact around the eye, ear and nasolabial region. Unfortunately, artistic renderings of the facial muscles in most illustrated texts show idealized detail of the individual muscles that is seldom, if ever, approximated in the most careful dissections. The major technical difficulty lies in the facts that most of the muscles of expression insert into the skin around the orifices and that removal of the skin usually leaves a ragged exposure of the fibers beneath. Therefore, no pretense is made here of exposing the finer fasciculi to the camera, but rather this figure presents what a dissector would see on his own reasonably well dissected specimen.

A few simple facts must be kept in mind when superficially dissecting the face. (1) All of the muscles that move the skin of the face, scalp or ear are derived from the embryonic myotome of the second visceral (hyoid) arch, and the platysma is the primary derivative of this myotome. (2) All of these muscles receive motor innervation from the facial cranial nerve, which was phyletically and embryologically associated with the hyoid visceral arch and all of its derivatives. (3) The sensory distribution to most of the face (except proprioceptive distribution) comes from the branches of the trigeminal cranial nerve, but the finer ramifications of both of these cranial nerves intertwine and become indistinguishable. (4) The muscles of mastication that provide motion to the jaw are innervated by motor branches of the trigeminal nerve.

Starting in the neck region, the *platysma muscle* ensheathes its anterior surface and extends above the mandible to the cheek. Through its thin layer of fibers, the *great auricular* and *transverse cervical nerves*, sensory branches of the cervical plexus, may be seen extending to the skin of the *parotid region* and the anterior neck.

Small straps of muscle fasciculi converge upon the angles of the mouth to elevate or depress the angle and counteract the sphincter action of the *orbicularis oris*, a muscle that encircles the mouth deep to the lips. Of these straps, the *zygomaticus major* and *levator labii superioris muscles* are the most easily seen in the cheek region, where they arise on the zygomatic bone and maxilla, respectively, and insert on the angle and upper border of the lip. The *depressor anguli oris* is an antagonist of the above muscles and the sphincter that may be seen partially covered by the platysma near the point of the chin. The platysma extends to the skin over the parotid region, and unfortunately in this case covers the masseter, a muscle of mastication that inserts on the ramus and angle of the jaw. Another large muscle of mastication, the *temporalis*, is visible arising from the temporal region of the skull to insert on the coronoid process of the mandible, which it closes powerfully.

Part of the *orbicularis oculi* has been exposed near the lateral margin of the orbit. This muscle encircles the orbital opening and contracts the skin around the eyelids. A second set of fibers form the palpebral fasciculi that course transversely under the eyelids.

A mobile aponeurosis, the *galea aponeurotica* covers the calvaria and is actually the intermediate fibrous connection between a double bellied muscle of the scalp, the *occipitofrontalis* muscle. Its posterior belly pulls the galea backward and the frontal belly pulls it forward to wrinkle the scalp.

Between the galea and the skin of the scalp, branches of the external carotid artery and the superficial *temporal, occipital* and *posterior auricular arteries* supply the soft tissues to the height of the vertex. The *supraorbital artery* is a branch of the internal carotid via the ophthalmic artery. It supplies the skin of the forehead and anastomoses with the other vessels. Because no arteries penetrate the skull, all of the scalp tissues depend on these circumferential vessels. Their adequacy is often demonstrated by the profuse bleeding that may attend even minor injuries to the scalp. An equally adequate complex of veins ramify in the subcutaneous layer of the scalp, which, in the neonate, offers a very accessible system for venous cutdowns for infusions.

The *buccal fat pad* is a very prominent subcutaneous feature of the fetal face. It consists of well encapsulated adipose tissue that is readily shelled out to expose a deeper extension of the fat into the pterygoid fossa. Although it exists in a much smaller form in the adult, the disproportionate size in the fetus has been claimed to provide firmness to the check to assist in suckling.

Plate 164

Lateral Aspect of Face and Scalp

341

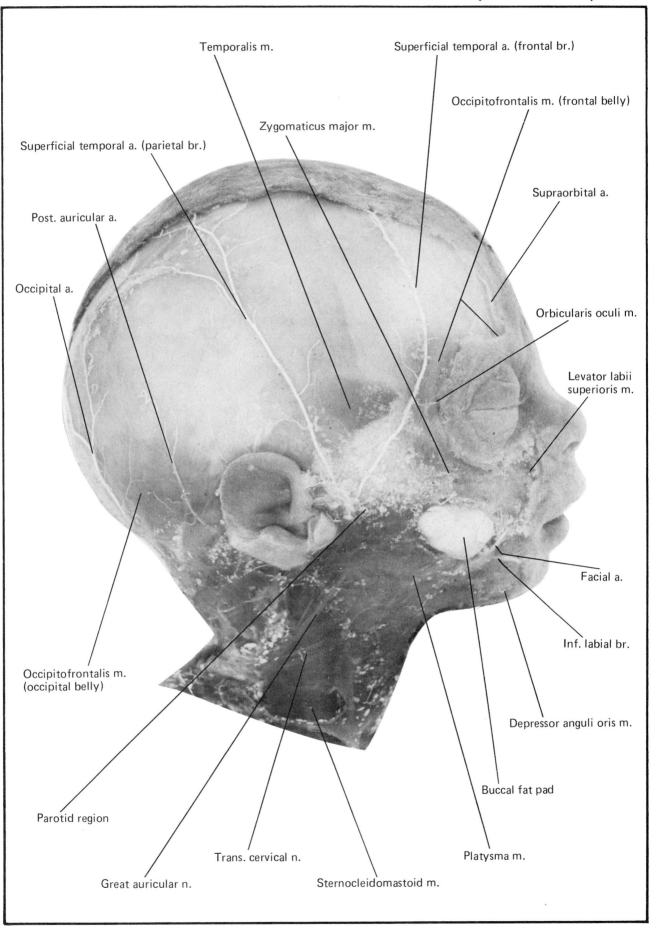

Temporalis m.

Superficial temporal a. (frontal br.)

Zygomaticus major m.

Occipitofrontalis m. (frontal belly)

Superficial temporal a. (parietal br.)

Supraorbital a.

Post. auricular a.

Orbicularis oculi m.

Occipital a.

Levator labii superioris m.

Facial a.

Inf. labial br.

Occipitofrontalis m. (occipital belly)

Depressor anguli oris m.

Parotid region

Buccal fat pad

Platysma m.

Great auricular n.

Trans. cervical n.

Sternocleidomastoid m.

DISSECTION OF THE DEEPER ARTERIES OF THE FACE

The zygomatic arch and the ramus and angle of the mandible have been removed to expose the major arteries of the face.

The injected external carotid artery enters the face medial to the hyoid attachments of the *digastric* and *stylohyoid muscles*. Here it makes a curve around the posterior border of the medial *pterygoid muscle* that had inserted on the medial surface of the mandibular ramus and angle. On the convexity of the curve arise the *posterior auricular* and *occipital arteries* that supply the posterior scalp. Anteriorly, at the commencement of the curve, the *facial artery* travels deep to the *submandibular gland* and around the external surface of the mandible. It passes anterosuperiorly along the cheek to the nasolabial region to disappear under the muscles.

The internal *maxillary artery* passes internal to the mandibular ramus between the insertions of *internal* and *external pterygoid muscles*, to which it supplies nutritive branches. The inferior *alveolar artery* and *nerve* pass over the anterior surface of the internal pterygoid to enter the mandibular foramen just distal to where it has been sectioned. The *middle meningeal artery*, which courses medially and deep to the external pterygoid, is not visible here, but the *deep temporal artery* that enters the infratemporal fossa to supply the deep surface of the *temporalis muscle* is shown as a stump that was cut when the muscle was retracted upward. The *masseter artery* was also cut with the removal of the ramus. It passed laterally through the mandibular notch to reach the deep side of the masseter muscle.

The internal maxillary continues to give numerous fine branches to the muscle and tissue of the pterygoid fossa as it approaches the pterygopalatine fossa. Before it enters the pterygopalatine fossa, it gives off the *superior alveolar artery* to the maxilla and the *infraorbital* artery to the infraorbital fissure. The major continuation, the *pterygopalatine branch*, enters the pterygopalatine fossa and is distributed to the nasal cavity and palate.

The *superficial temporal artery* ascends deep to the main part of the parotid gland to supply the scalp. A frontal branch can be seen passing to the lateral supraorbital region.

This plate should be compared with the angiograms of Plates 161 and 169.

Plate 165

Deeper Arteries of the Face   343

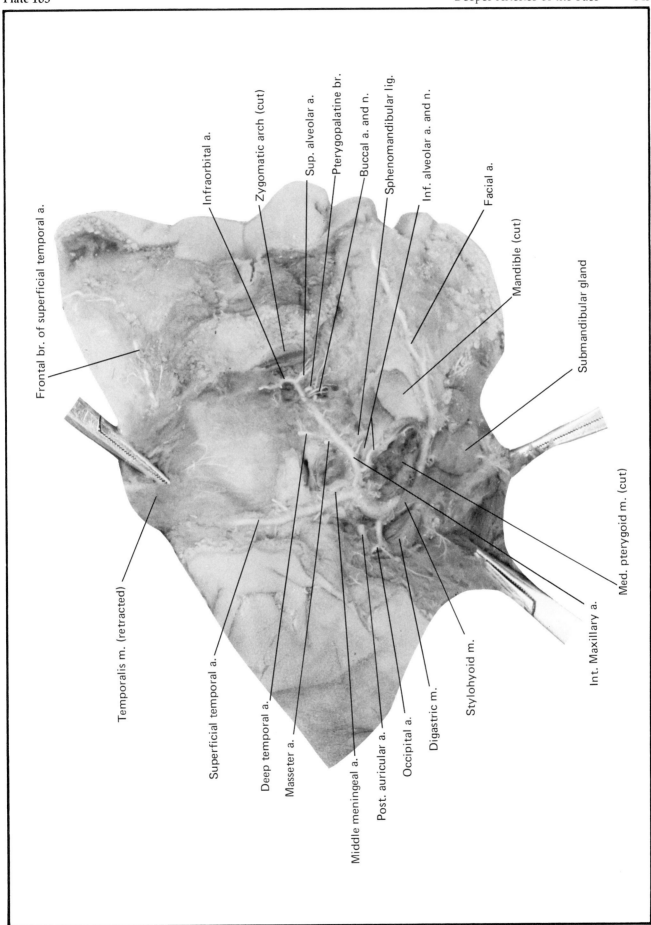

Frontal br. of superficial temporal a.

Infraorbital a.

Zygomatic arch (cut)

Sup. alveolar a.

Pterygopalatine br.

Buccal a. and n.

Sphenomandibular lig.

Inf. alveolar a. and n.

Facial a.

Mandible (cut)

Submandibular gland

Med. pterygoid m. (cut)

Int. Maxillary a.

Stylohyoid m.

Digastric m.

Occipital a.

Post. auricular a.

Middle meningeal a.

Masseter a.

Deep temporal a.

Superficial temporal a.

Temporalis m. (retracted)

SAGITTAL ASPECT OF THE FACE WITH THE NASAL SEPTUM

For this preparation an injected frozen fetus of approximately 33 weeks' gestation was sectioned along the midsagittal plane, splitting the nasal septum. The following two illustrations are progressive dissections of this specimen.

In the adult the nasal septum is a vertical plate of mucous membrane-covered bone and cartilage that midsagittally divides the nasal cavity. Its osseous elements are the perpendicular plate of the ethmoid superiorly and the vomer posteriorly. The anterior and inferior parts remain cartilaginous. In the perinatal human, however, only the inferior part of the vomer may be ossified, so that its greater part is still composed of cartilage. In the superior part of this fetal septum the cartilaginous *perpendicular plate of the ethmoid* is seen to be continuous with the *crista galli* that lies above the cribriform plate. The anterior and posterior ethmoidal arteries send a fine arterial plexus down each side of the plate to vascularize the greater part of the anterosuperior septum. The posteroinferior part of the septum receives arteries from the septal branches of the internal maxillary artery that passes through the pterygopalatine fossa. The terminal ramifications of both sets of vessels anastomose anteriorly with septal branches of the superior labial artery and the *greater palatine artery* where it ascends through the *incisive canal*.

Posterior to the septum, the incompletely ossified *body of the sphenoid* bears the chiasmatic groove and *hypophyseal fossa* on its superior surface, and the position of the sphenooccipital union is revealed by a broad band of cartilage posterior to the dorsum sellae.

The potential space that is the oral cavity is completely obliterated when the tongue is elevated against the palate. Between the gingival membrane and the lips, a slitlike space indicates the *vestibule* of the oral cavity.

Plate 166   Nasal Septum   345

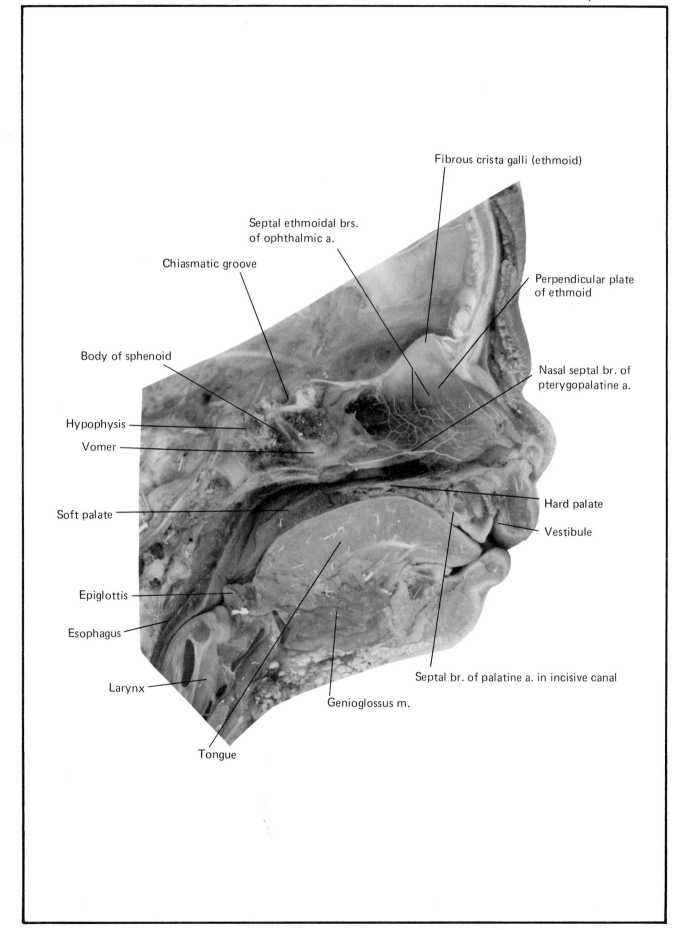

Fibrous crista galli (ethmoid)

Septal ethmoidal brs.
of ophthalmic a.

Chiasmatic groove

Perpendicular plate
of ethmoid

Body of sphenoid

Nasal septal br. of
pterygopalatine a.

Hypophysis

Vomer

Hard palate

Soft palate

Vestibule

Epiglottis

Esophagus

Septal br. of palatine a. in incisive canal

Larynx

Genioglossus m.

Tongue

MEDIAL ASPECT OF THE NASAL CAVITY: NASOPHARYNX AND OROPHARYNX

On the opposite side of the same specimen shown in the preceding plate, the septum has been cut away to expose the wall of the nasal cavity.

The *superior, middle* and *inferior conchae* are mucous membrane-covered scrolls of bone that project medially into each nasal passage. Inferior to each concha the respective *superior, middle* and *inferior meatus* are formed. (*Meatus* means passageway in Latin; the pleural and singular forms are spelled the same.) The resulting convoluted anatomy of the nasal cavity provides a greater surface area for preheating and moisturizing the aspired air, and in lower mammals it provides a larger area for olfactory sensitivity. In the human, however, the olfactory epithelium is confined to a small patch above the middle concha and a corresponding area on the opposing surface of the septum.

Superior to the soft palate, the *ostium* and its surrounding *torus* of the *auditory tube* are situated on the lateral wall of the nasopharynx anterior to the deep lateral *pharyngeal recess* that marks the most superior part of the pharynx. Here, the posterior pharyngeal wall has been gently pulled forward to reveal the potential space of the *retropharyngeal cleft* that exists between the prevertebral fascia and the fascia of the pharyngeal constrictors. This cleft follows the digestive tube from the pharyngeal region to the posterior mediastinum and permits motility of the pharynx and esophagus. Unfortunately, it also permits the inferior spreading of retropharyngeal abcesses.

Note the relationships of the craniovertebral articulations to the pharynx.

Plate 167   Nasopharynx and Oropharynx   347

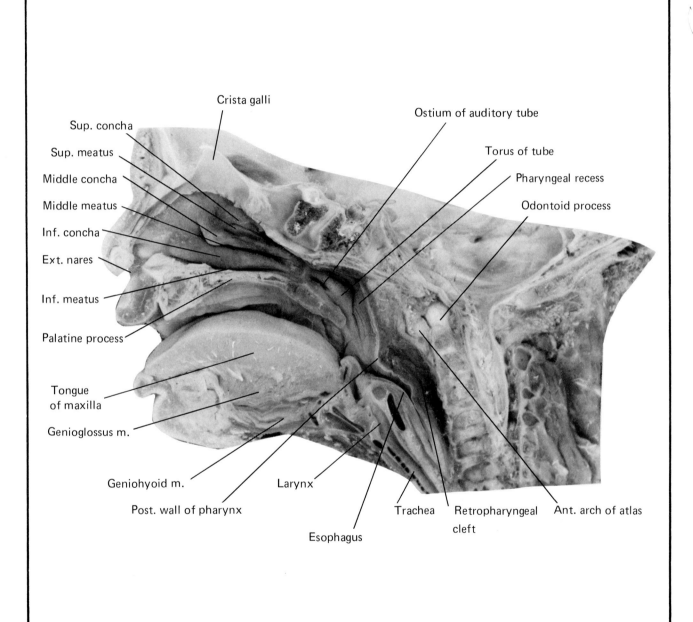

Crista galli

Ostium of auditory tube

Sup. concha

Torus of tube

Sup. meatus

Pharyngeal recess

Middle concha

Odontoid process

Middle meatus

Inf. concha

Ext. nares

Inf. meatus

Palatine process

Tongue
of maxilla

Genioglossus m.

Geniohyoid m.

Larynx

Post. wall of pharynx

Trachea   Retropharyngeal
cleft

Ant. arch of atlas

Esophagus

CONTINUED EXPOSURE OF THE NASAL CAVITY AND PHARYNGEAL REGION

The nasal conchae have been excised to expose underlying structures. Deep to the middle concha the *ethmoidal bulla* shows as an elongated, rounded eminence. As the ethmoid becomes pneumatized postnatally, several openings appear on the surface of the bulla; they communicate with the ethmoidal air cells.

Anteroinferior to the bulla a crescentic slit, the *semilunar hiatus*, contains the site of future communications with the frontal and maxillary sinuses (site of frontal communication is indicated by paper wedge). In the neonate, only the maxillary sinus shows any degree of pneumatization, which is expressed as a shallow evagination of the epithelium in the midregion of the semilunar hiatus.

The inferior meatus contains the distal opening of the *nasolachrymal duct* that carries the secretions of the lachrymal gland to the nasal cavity.

The tongue has been retracted inferiorly to expose the posterior oral cavity and the oropharynx. The narrowed entranceway between the oral cavity and the pharynx is called the *fauces*, whose lateral border is formed by two folds. Anteriorly, the *palatoglossal fold* connects the *soft palate* to the dorsum of the tongue, and its epithelium covers the fasciculi of the *palatoglossal muscle*. The free posterior edge of the soft palate is connected to the pharyngeal wall by a second *palatopharyngeal fold* that encases the *palatopharyngeus muscle*. Between these two folds lies the tonsilar fossa containing the *palatine tonsil*. Another *salpingopharyngeal fold* indicates the position of the *salpingopharyngeus muscle* that runs between the torus tubarium and the lateral pharyngeal wall. During swallowing, its contraction tends to open the ostium of the auditory tube to equalize internal and external pressures on the tympanum.

In the inferior part of the pharynx, the epiglottis guards the entrance to the *larynx* and helps to deflect swallowed material toward the more posterior *esophagus*.

Plate 168   Nasal Cavity and Pharyngeal Region   349

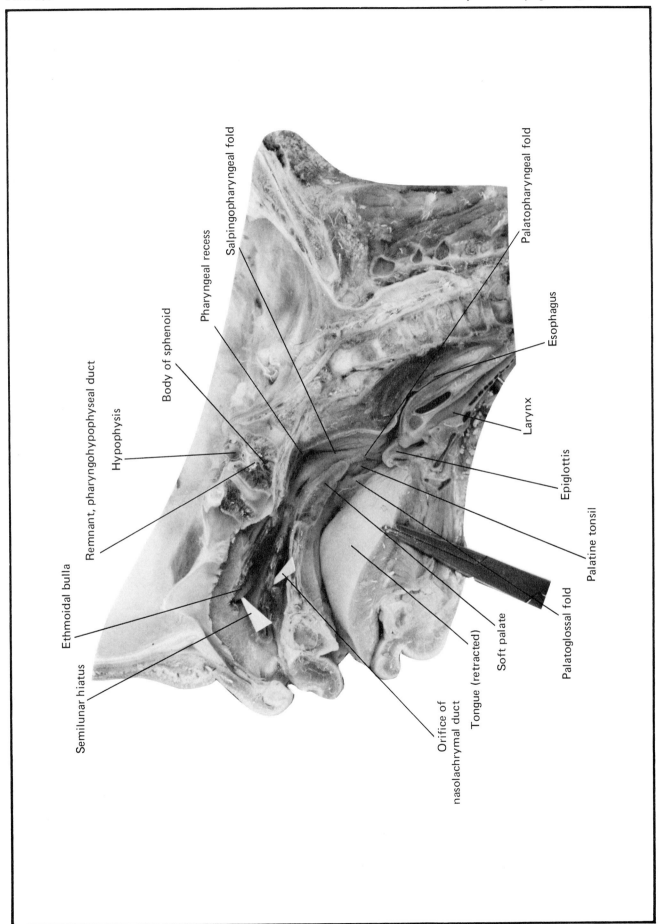

Salpingopharyngeal fold

Palatopharyngeal fold

Pharyngeal recess

Body of sphenoid

Esophagus

Hypophysis

Remnant, pharyngohypophyseal duct

Larynx

Ethmoidal bulla

Epiglottis

Palatine tonsil

Semilunar hiatus

Orifice of
nasolachrymal duct

Tongue (retracted)

Soft palate

Palatoglossal fold

ANGIOGRAM OF THE FETAL FACE

This is the opposite side of the head shown in the hemicranial angiogram of Plate 161. Here the cerebral hemisphere has been removed so that its vessels will not be confused with the branches of the external carotid that supply the face, scalp and calvaria.

As the *external carotid* ascends the neck, its first conspicuous branch in this specimen is the *superior thyroid artery*. Although this vessel more frequently arises from the *common carotid artery* just below the bifurcation, its origin may vary even between the two sides of the same body. Posterior to this vessel, the *occipital artery* courses posteriorly to supply the scalp in the occipital region. Its descending branch anastomoses with the ascending deep cervical branches of the *transverse cervical artery*. The ascending *pharyngeal artery* arises close to the occipital branch and travels upward along the pharyngeal wall to reach the level of the lateral pharyngeal recess.

The *lingual* and *facial arteries* usually arise independently from the external carotid artery, but here they leave the parent vessel as a common trunk. As the facial artery passes deep to the submandibular gland, which it supplies with fine branches, it gives a superior branch, the *tonsillar artery*, to the palatine tonsil and its fossa. It then proceeds obliquely across the external surface of the mandible and, near the angle of the mouth, sends the *inferior labial artery* to the lower lip and chin. The main vessel ascends the face toward the bridge of the nose. Lateral to the nostril the *superior labial artery* courses medially in the upper lip, giving a pair of significant branches to the anterior part of the nasal septum. Inferior to the orbit the facial artery receives fine anastomotic branches from the *infraorbital artery*, and deep to the internal canthus of the eye it terminates in anastomotic connections with branches of the ophthalmic artery.

The distribution of the lingual artery is well revealed here. It passes forward external to the hypoglossus muscle and enters the root of the tongue near the posterior edge of the mylohyoid muscle, at which point it gives off the *submental artery* to the anterior floor of the mouth. Within the substance of the tongue the lingual artery shows an array of fine vertical branches that ascend to its surface.

In the parotid region, the external carotid artery sends the *internal maxillary artery* anterosuperiorly deep to the ramus of the mandible. This vessel presents a very complex system of branches in its comparatively short course. Its first major derivative, the *middle meningeal artery*, passes into the infratemporal fossa to reach the foramen spinosum. Upon entering the cranium, it provides the primary arterial supply to the bones of the calvaria and the dura. A finer accessory meningeal artery (unlabeled) duplicates its proximal course to enter the foramen ovale.

At approximately the same level, an inferior branch, the *inferior alveolar artery*, descends to enter the mandibular foramen to supply the mandible and its dentition. A proximal branch of this vessel, the *buccal artery*, supplies the internal structures of the cheek. As the internal maxillary artery threads its way among the muscles of mastication, it provides each with nutritional branches that are assigned the name of the muscle.

In the midregion of the internal maxillary, a medium-sized branch, the *deep temporal artery*, passes upward on the internal surface of the temporalis muscle.

The internal maxillary artery ends in a spray of vessels as it enters the pterygopalatine fossa. The first of these, the *superior alveolar artery*, descends on the posterolateral aspect of the maxilla and enters the bone to provides branches to the superior molars. At the same level the parent vessel gives off the *infraorbital artery* that enters the infraorbital fissure and eventually terminates in the muscles and skin of the infraorbital part of the face. Within the fossa the major artery subdivides into palatine and septal branches. The *greater palatine* artery supplies the tissue covering the hard palate, and the *nasal branch* ramifies within the mucosa of the nasal conchae and the meatus.

The *superficial temporal artery* is formed by the upward continuation of the external carotid artery. This vessel becomes superficial above the parotid gland (where its pulse may be felt) and sends large frontal and parietal branches to the coverings of the skull that course between the galea and the scalp.

The *internal carotid artery* bears no conspicuous branches external to this cranium. Upon reaching the base of skull, it enters the carotid canal of the petrous bone and travels anteromedially until it reaches the lateral surface of the body of the sphenoid. It then takes a sigmoidal course within the cavernous sinus. At the final curvature, before it enters the dura, the internal carotid gives off the *ophthalmic artery*. This vessel enters the orbit through the superior orbital fissure to supply the retina and external structures of the bulb as well as meningeal nervous and epithelial structures related to the ethmoid bone. The ophthalmic artery also supplies the orbital adnexae and, via the *supraorbital artery*, provides internal carotid anastomoses to the face and scalp.

When viewing this angiogram, it should be remembered that postnatal growth would lengthen the face inferiorly and would proportionately "space out" the branches of the external carotid artery.

Plate 169   Angiogram of the Face   351

Supraorbital a.

Palpebral brs.

Deep temporal a.

Infraorbital a.

Int. maxillary a.

Sup. alveolar a.

Nasal and greater
palatine aa.

Sup. labial a.
and septal br.

Buccal a.

Inf. labial a.

Inf. alveolar a.

Tonsillar a.

Submental a.

Facial a.

Lingual a.

Ophthalmic a.

Sup. thyroid a.

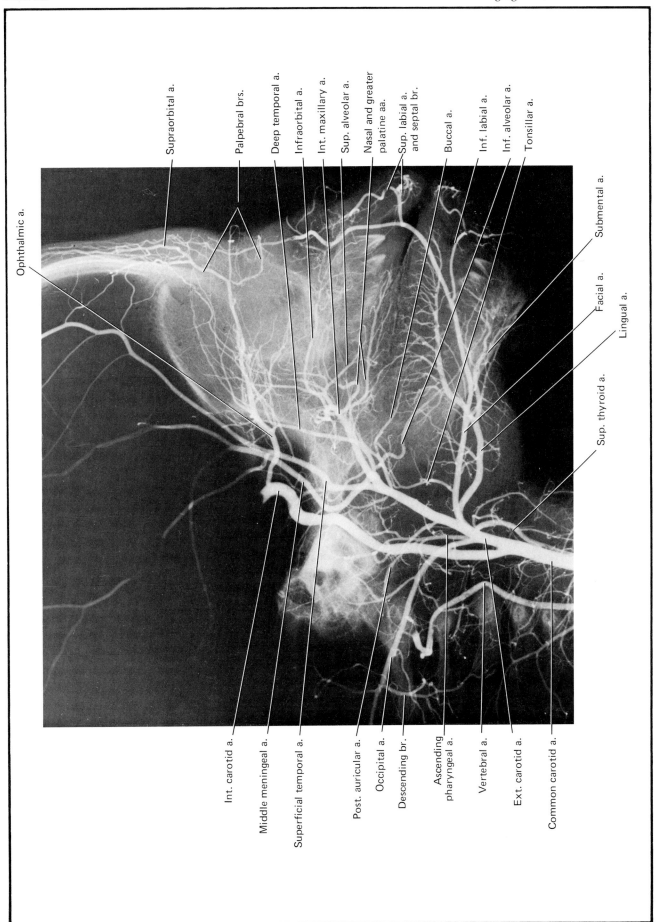

Int. carotid a.

Middle meningeal a.

Superficial temporal a.

Post. auricular a.

Occipital a.

Descending br.

Ascending
pharyngeal a.

Vertebral a.

Ext. carotid a.

Common carotid a.

FRONTAL SECTION OF THE FETAL FACE: MIDBULBAR PLANE

An injected fetus of approximately 29 weeks' gestation was sectioned to show the deeper structures of the face. In most sectioned material in this atlas, the planes of exposure were cut with an intentional slight obliquity to the true planes as anatomically defined. Thus it provides the viewer with a greater three dimensional appreciation of structural relationships by comparing the differences presented by two halves of the section.

In this section the right side of the head (left side of picture) is cut slightly posterior to the opposite side, as is revealed by the fact that the anterior edge of the temporalis muscle can be seen only on the right.

The orbital region shows the posterior half of the ocular bulb with its three major layers containing the fibrous, vascular and nervous components. Because the sensory structures of the eye are an outgrowth of the brain, the external layers of the bulb are homologous to the meninges. Although each may be histologically subdivided into finer laminae, the outer, thick fibrous layer, the *sclera*, corresponds to the dura, and the middle, highly vascularized *choroid* is the equivalent of the piarachnoid. The choroid, in combination with the more anterior ciliary body and iris, forms the *uveal tract*. The *retina* is formed from a double walled, cup-shaped vesicle of the embryonic brain, and so it presents two layers. The black, pigmented layer lies against the choroid, and the light-sensitive layer of nervous components is loosely attached to the internal surface. Here the sensory layer is wrinkled by the chemical fixation and indicates the ease with which it may spontaneously or traumatically become detached.

In the anterior supralateral part of each orbit lies the lachrymal gland. Its relations are better shown in subsequent dissections of this region.

The section of the nasal cavity at this level well illustrates the relations of the mucous membrane-covered conchae to meatus. On the right side of the cavity the *middle meatus* has been cut through the *semilunar hiatus* and presents the anterior part of the *ethmoidal bulla,* and in the center the continuity of the *crista galli* and the *perpendicualr plate of the ethmoid* can be appreciated.

The *tongue* occupies most of the oral cavity, and when the mouth is closed it lies against the *hard palate.* This latter structure separates the oral and nasal cavities and consists of two medially cantilevered processes of each maxilla. Between the thick mucous membrane and the bone, the major channels of the two *greater palatine arteries* run toward the anterior part of the structure.

In the sublingual region of the oral cavity, the anterior edges of the *genioglossus muscles* may be seen entering the base of the tongue at the center. Superolateral to these, the *lingual arteries* course to the lingual apex.

Gingival membranes cover the blunt alveolar processes that separate the *vestibule* of the mouth from the oral cavity proper. Lateral to the buccal mucous membrane, the *buccinator muscle* tenses the cheek during mastication or forcefully expelling air. Part of the *buccal fat pad* intervenes between this muscle and the more superficial *zygomaticus major* and *minor.*

In the upper part of the section, the frontal lobes of the brain extend forward over the orbital plates of the frontal bone to occupy the anterior cranial fossa.

Plate 170   Midbulbar Plane of the Face   353

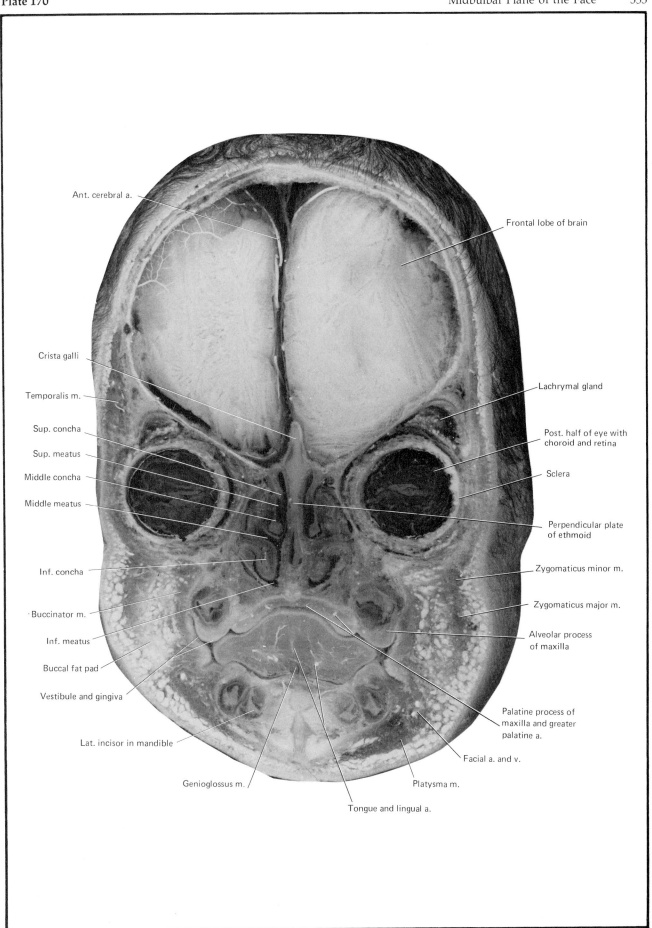

Ant. cerebral a.

Frontal lobe of brain

Crista galli

Lachrymal gland

Temporalis m.

Sup. concha

Post. half of eye with
choroid and retina

Sup. meatus

Middle concha

Sclera

Middle meatus

Perpendicular plate
of ethmoid

Inf. concha

Zygomaticus minor m.

Buccinator m.

Zygomaticus major m.

Inf. meatus

Alveolar process
of maxilla

Buccal fat pad

Vestibule and gingiva

Palatine process of
maxilla and greater
palatine a.

Lat. incisor in mandible

Facial a. and v.

Genioglossus m.

Platysma m.

Tongue and lingual a.

FRONTAL SECTION THROUGH THE FETAL FACE: RETROBULBAR PLANE

In this deeper section of the same specimen shown in the preceding plate, the retrobulbar parts of the orbit and more posterior parts of the oral and nasal cavities are revealed. Again, the cut is intentionally slightly oblique to a true frontal plane, showing the deeper relations on the right side of the head.

Retrobulbar fat and the ocular muscles fill the posterior part of the orbits, and the *optic nerve* is conspicuous particularly in the left orbit (right side of illustration. Within the nerve the central artery to the retina may be seen, and the fine *posterior ciliary arteries* that penetrate the posterior part of the bulb are shown sectioned around the nerve periphery. The ophthalmic artery lies above the nerve as it passes toward the superomedial part of the orbit. Description of the individual ocular muscles will be left to a subsequent section on the eye and orbit.

The section of the nasal cavity lies near the junction of the hard and soft palate where the vomer of the septum reaches the palatine bone. The individual conchae and meatus are not distinct where the nasal cavities enter their respective internal nares that lead to the pharynx.

Below the orbit on the right side of the head, the fat of the *pterygoid fossa* lies medial to the insertion of the temporalis muscle on the coronoid process of the *ramus* of the mandible. Between the temporalis and the fat body, the *internal maxillary artery* passes anteriorly.

The anterior part of the *masseter muscle* descends to insert on the external surface of the ramus and the mandibular angle. The posterior part of the buccal fat pad lies superficial to the masseter, but it communicates with the fat of the pterygoid fossa anterior to the mandibular ramus.

In the oral cavity the extrinsic muscles of the tongue may be identified in its base. The *hyoglossus muscle* runs superior to the *submandibular gland* as it extends from the hyoid bone to the lateral sublingual surface. Between it and the *genioglossus muscle,* the *lingual artery* sends branches into the lingual mass of intrinsic muscle.

The *geniohyoid muscles* extend from the chin to the hyoid bone and are covered externally by the transverse sheet of the *mylohyoid muscle.* Lateral to the geniohyoids, the *submental artery* of the main lingual branch supplies the sublingual musculature.

Inferior to the mylohyoid muscle, the *anterior belly* of the *digastric muscle* extends anteriorly from the hyoid region to the internal surface of the anterior part of the mandible.

Plate 171   Retrobulbar Plane of the Face   355

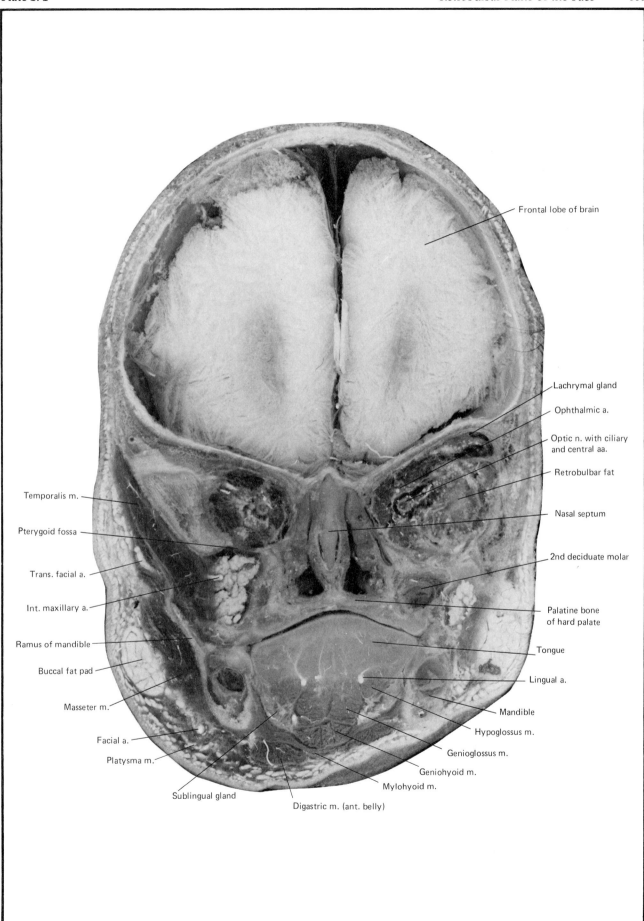

Frontal lobe of brain

Lachrymal gland

Ophthalmic a.

Optic n. with ciliary
and central aa.

Retrobulbar fat

Nasal septum

2nd deciduate molar

Palatine bone
of hard palate

Tongue

Lingual a.

Mandible

Hypoglossus m.

Genioglossus m.

Geniohyoid m.

Mylohyoid m.

Digastric m. (ant. belly)

Sublingual gland

Platysma m.

Facial a.

Masseter m.

Buccal fat pad

Ramus of mandible

Int. maxillary a.

Trans. facial a.

Pterygoid fossa

Temporalis m.

FRONTAL SECTION THROUGH THE DEEP FACE: MUSCLES OF MASTICATION

This particular posterior view of a deep frontal section was selected and enlarged to show the relations of the muscles of mastication to the skull and mandible. The posterior rather than anterior view better shows the positions of the cranial fossae relative to the infratemporal and pterygoid fossae at the base of the skull. This cut is also slightly biased in relation to the frontal plane, so that the plane of section on the left side of the hand (right side of illustration) lies posterior to the right.

At the top, the *lesser wings of the sphenoid* form the demarcation between the anterior and middle cranial fossae. From the *sphenoid body* the *greater wing of the sphenoid* sweeps across the floor and up the lateral wall of the middle fossa, forming the depression to contain the anterior pole of the temporal lobe of the brain. In the medial wall of the fossa, the subdural structures include the *ophthalmic artery* and the most anterior part of the *cavernous sinus.* Inferior to this area the anterior part of the *trigeminal ganglion* lies within a double fold of the dura (cave of Meckel).

The external surface of the greater wing is related to the three fossae. The first, the *temporal fossa*, is a lateral depression of the skull that lies above the *zygomatic arch* and contains the *temporalis muscle.* Below the zygomatic arch and inferior to the floor of the middle cranial fossa is the *infratemporal fossa.* Medial and slightly anterior to this, the depression between the pterygoid lamina that gives origin to the deeper muscles of mastication is the *pterygoid fossa.*

The section here passes through the *temporomandibular joint* and ramus of the mandible down to the mandibular angle. It thus cuts through all of the muscles of mastication that directly activate the temporomandibular articulation. Note that the powerful *masseter* and *medial pterygoid* muscles have widely separated origins from the zygomatic arch and pterygoid fossa, respectively, but they converge to insert on opposite sides of the ramus and angle. Thus this muscular configuration is known as the *mandibular sling.* The masseter, medial pterygoid and temporalis muscles all act synergistically to forcefully close the jaw, but the *external pterygoid* has a different role. It arises from the pterygoid lamina and infratemporal fossa and extends posterolaterally to insert on the neck of the *mandibular condyle* and the *articular disc* that intervenes between the condyle and the mandibular fossa. Therefore, its contraction pulls the condyle and disc forward in a gliding action and helps to open the jaw. It is obvious that since the temporomandibular joint is not a hinge-type articulation, the axis of rotation for the joint movement lies inferior to the condyle in the midregion of the *ramus.* The action of the external pterygoid also tends to dislocate the joint when the jaw is opened widely.

All of the muscles that activate the temporomandibular articulation, plus the mylohyoid and some small muscles associated with the pharyngeal and tympanic regions, are innervated by the motor division of the trigeminal nerve.

The *internal maxillary artery* with a section of its inferior alveolar branch may be identified on the internal surface of the ramus running between the two pterygoid muscles. Inferior to the mandible a section of the *facial artery* passes superficial to the *submandibular gland.*

The oral and nasal cavities have been exposed at the level of the soft palate, and on the right side of the illustration the tendon of the *tensor veli palatini,* a muscle that originates in the *pterygoid fossa,* can be seen making a 120-degree turn around the *hamulus* to insert into and tense the soft palate. This muscle is innervated by the trigeminal nerve.

Plate 172

Muscles of Mastication   357

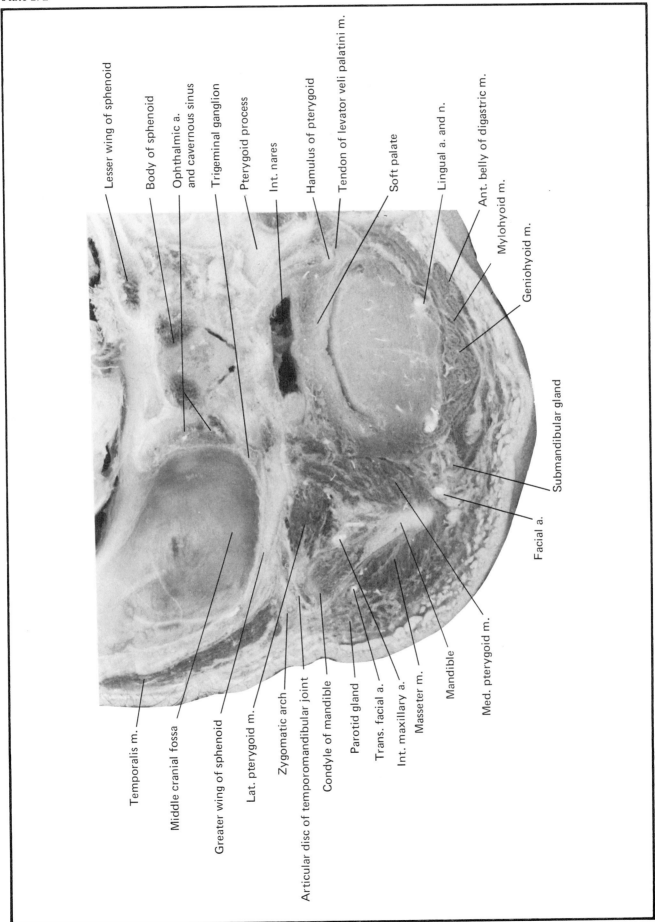

Lesser wing of sphenoid

Body of sphenoid

Ophthalmic a. and cavernous sinus

Trigeminal ganglion

Pterygoid process

Int. nares

Hamulus of pterygoid

Tendon of levator veli palatini m.

Soft palate

Lingual a. and n.

Ant. belly of digastric m.

Mylohyoid m.

Geniohyoid m.

Submandibular gland

Facial a.

Med. pterygoid m.

Mandible

Masseter m.

Int. maxillary a.

Trans. facial a.

Parotid gland

Condyle of mandible

Articular disc of temporomandibular joint

Zygomatic arch

Lat. pterygoid m.

Greater wing of sphenoid

Middle cranial fossa

Temporalis m.

HORIZONTAL SECTION THROUGH THE FETAL HEAD: MANDIBULAR REGION AND POSTERIOR CRANIAL FOSSA

The horizontal, like the frontal sections, have been deliberately cut slightly oblique to the true anatomic plane, and the exposure on the right side of the head (left in picture) lies inferior to the left. This section was selected to reinforce the three dimensional concepts of the muscles of mastication and the floor of the oral cavity.

The *masseter muscle* is situated external to the mandibular ramus, and the *medial pterygoid* lies on its internal surface. Between the medial pterygoid and the pharyngeal wall, the pterygoid fat body is evident. The section has cut through the body of the mandible and has exposed its medullary cavity, which lies deep to the developing tooth buds. Within the mandibular arch, the sublingual floor of the oral cavity shows the paired *genioglossus muscles* as they originate on the internal surface of the mandibular symphysis and extend into the base of the tongue. Lateral to these, the diffuse lobules of the *sublingual salivary glands* are strung along the surface of the mylohyoid muscle.

The dorsum of the tongue descends into the pharynx and the *palatopharyngeal* folds lie against its dorsolateral surface.

As this section passes horizontally through the petrous bone, it lays open (on the right side) the lower part of the tympanic cavity and parts of the cochlear and vestibular apparatus. Inasmuch as these structures are discussed in subsequent plates, they are mentioned here only as topically referential structures.

The section passes through the upper limits of the posterior cranial fossa and shows the intriguing fact that the arterial injection medium passes directly into epidural sinuses through numerous arteriovenous anastomoses, particularly around the upper cervical and posterior cranial regions.

The transverse sinuses, as they extend around the occiput, show clotted blood mixed with the injection medium. Laterally, they run into the *sigmoid sinuses*, where they approach the posterior surface of the petrous bone. On the left of the illustration, the *inferior petrous sinus* may be traced from the clivus to the sigmoid sinus.

The contents of the posterior cranial fossa are shown as the pons and cerebellar hemispheres at this level.

Plate 173   Mandibular Region and Posterior Cranial Fossa   359

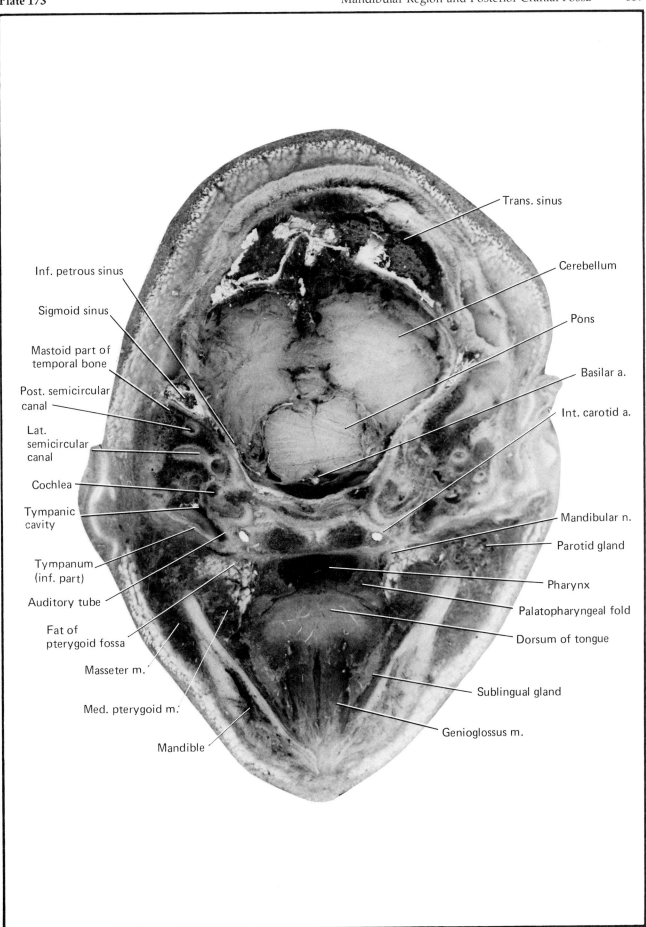

Inf. petrous sinus

Sigmoid sinus

Mastoid part of
temporal bone

Post. semicircular
canal

Lat.
semicircular
canal

Cochlea

Tympanic
cavity

Tympanum
(inf. part)

Auditory tube

Fat of
pterygoid fossa

Masseter m.

Med. pterygoid m.

Mandible

Trans. sinus

Cerebellum

Pòns

Basilar a.

Int. carotid a.

Mandibular n.

Parotid gland

Pharynx

Palatopharyngeal fold

Dorsum of tongue

Sublingual gland

Genioglossus m.

DORSUM OF THE TONGUE AND RELATED PHARYNGEAL STRUCTURES

The lingual surface and the pharyngeal structures have been displayed by splitting and retracting the palate and retracting the pharyngeal walls.

From the *lingual apex* to the V-shaped *sulcus terminalis*, the dorsum of the *lingual body* is covered with fine *filiform papillae* and more sparsely scattered larger *fungiform papillae*. Arranged in two rows parallel to the sulcus terminalis are the large *vallate papillae*. Two sets of *foliate papillae* are restricted to the posterior lateral margins of the tongue. The *foramen cecum* is a blind pit at the apex of the convergence of the *sulcus terminalis*. This marks the embryonic origin of the thyroglossal duct, whose inferior part gave origin to the thyroid gland.

Posterior to the foramen cecum the mucosa of the tongue bears irregular patches of lymphoid tissue that form the *lingual tonsils.*

Half of the soft palate with its split uvula is retracted to each side of the specimen and exposes the *palatoglossal* and *palatopharyngeal* folds that lie, respectively, anterior and posterior to the palatine tonsil. These form the *fauces,* a passage through which the oral cavity communicates with the pharynx. For this reason the folds are often referred to as the anterior and posterior pillars of the fauces.

The *palatine tonsils* are an aggregate of lymphoid follicles that virtually fill the interval between the anterior and posterior pillars in the young child, but in the fetus they are mostly embedded under a fold, the *plica semilunaris,* whose free edge hangs over the tonsil and produces a cleftlike space called the *tonsillar sinus.* The vascularity of the tonsil bed is shown by the superficial ramifications of the tonsillar arteries that are derivatives of the facial artery.

Posterior to the tongue the epiglottis projects upward to guard the entrance to the larynx. During deglutition, the *glottis* is closed and the epiglottis rises and leans posteriorly over the glottis to guide ingested matter through the *piriform recesses* that on each side lead to the *esophagus.*

Plate 174   Tongue and Pharyngeal Structures   361

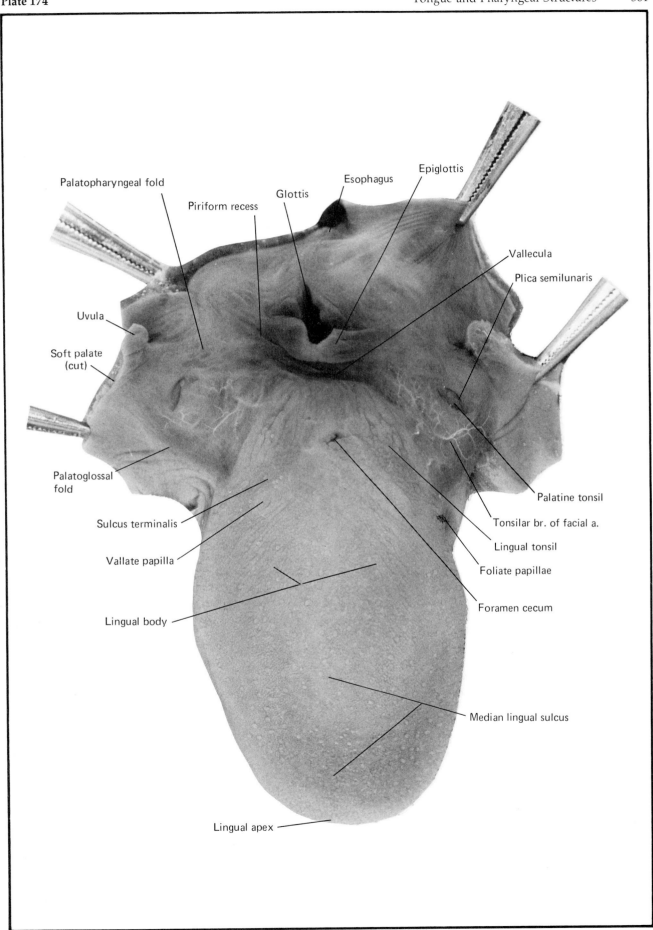

Palatopharyngeal fold

Piriform recess

Glottis

Esophagus

Epiglottis

Vallecula

Plica semilunaris

Uvula

Soft palate
(cut)

Palatoglossal
fold

Sulcus terminalis

Vallate papilla

Lingual body

Palatine tonsil

Tonsilar br. of facial a.

Lingual tonsil

Foliate papillae

Foramen cecum

Median lingual sulcus

Lingual apex

SAGITTAL SECTION OF THE TONGUE: PHARYNX AND LARYNGOTRACHEAL REGION

This specimen was dissected from an injected, frozen and sagittally sectioned fetus.

The base of the tongue reveals the arrangement of the fibers of the *genioglossus muscle*, which originates on the posterior surface of the anterior region of the mandible and extends fibers in a fanlike array to the entire base of the tongue. Contraction of this muscle depresses and protracts the tongue. Like all muscles of the tongue it is innervated by the hypoglossal nerve (CNXII). Inferior to the genioglossus, the *geniohyoid muscle* runs between the mandible and the body of the hyoid bone. It draws the hyoid forward or fixates it against the antagonistic infrahyoid muscles. A branch of the first cervical nerve provides its innervation through the hypoglossal nerve.

The soft palate follows the slope of the dorsum of the tongue and ends in the median *uvula,* which shows its branches of the *lesser* (posterior) *palatine artery.*

Ingested matter is propelled to the pharynx by the pressure of the tongue against the hard palate. It is deflected from the laryngeal opening toward the esophagus by the epiglottis. Simultaneous closure of the glottis and contraction of the pharyngeal constrictors forces the matter into the upper end of the esophagus, where local reflexes propel it toward the stomach.

The structure of the larynx is easily appreciated in sagittal section. The large, shield-shaped thyroid carti-lage is connected to the hyoid by the thyrohyoid membrane and is elevated or depressed with this bone.

In the posterior wall of the larynx the thick and broad *lamina* of the *cricoid cartilage* is evident. This cartilage is shaped like a signet ring with the band lying anterior beneath the thyroid cartilage and the bezel facing posteriorly. The superior edge of the lamina bears two articular facets that are surmounted by a pair of *arytenoid* cartilages. The fact that part of an arytenoid shows in this section indicates that the plane of incision lies a little to one side of the midline, for a true midsagittal cut would have simply separated the two arytenoids.

Each vocal fold is attached to the medial base of an arytenoid cartilage, and the rotation and lateral or medial movements of these cartilages tense and approximate or separate the folds. These actions close the glottis for swallowing or adjust the position and tension of the folds against the stream of expired air for phonation. On the medial surface of the laryngeal wall a superior *vestibular fold* lies above an upward directed chamber, the *laryngeal ventricle.* Immediately below the ventricle the true vocal fold stretches between the arytenoid and the internal surface of the thyroid cartilage.

The inferior chamber of the larynx leads directly into the *trachea,* which is supported against negative pressure by a series of C-shaped cartilaginous rings. The open part of each tracheal cartilage faces posteriorly against the anterior surface of the esophagus. Thus the cartilage is not evident in the sagittal section of the posterior tracheal wall. The interval between the ends of each cartilage is bridged by smooth muscle fasciculi forming the trachealis muscle that exerts some control over the lumen of the trachea by approximating the ends of each ring.

Plate 175   Pharynx and Laryngotracheal Region   363

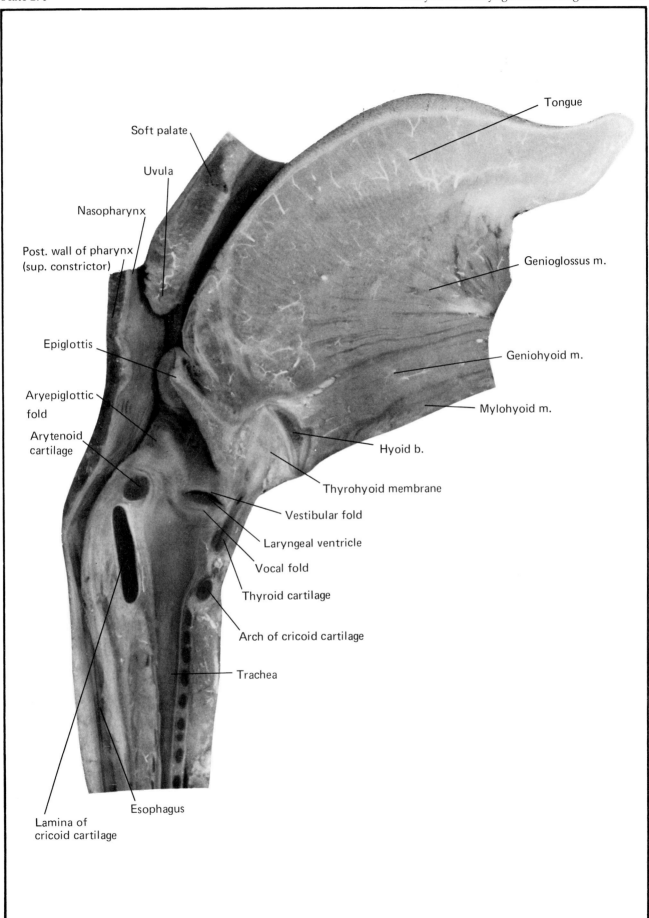

Tongue

Soft palate

Uvula

Nasopharynx

Post. wall of pharynx
(sup. constrictor)

Genioglossus m.

Epiglottis

Geniohyoid m.

Aryepiglottic
fold

Mylohyoid m.

Arytenoid
cartilage

Hyoid b.

Thyrohyoid membrane

Vestibular fold

Laryngeal ventricle

Vocal fold

Thyroid cartilage

Arch of cricoid cartilage

Trachea

Esophagus

Lamina of
cricoid cartilage

POSTERIOR EXPOSURE OF THE PHARYNGEAL REGION

Coronal cleavage of the posterior cranial fossa through the jugular foramen (thus exposing the jugular bulb) separates the cervical vertebral column from the pharynx along the retropharyngeal cleft.

Here the posterior pharyngeal wall and upper *esophagus* have been slit to provide a posterior view of the *nasopharynx* and *oropharynx*. It should be noted that the most superior part of the posterior pharyngeal wall was left attached to the skull to show the manner of its suspension from the base of the *occipital bone*. Just lateral to this attachment the pharynx is widest and extends almost to the jugular bulbs to produce the pharyngeal recesses that here lie above the two upper retractors.

The posterior edge of the *soft palate* separates the nasopharynx from the oropharynx and bears the median unpaired *uvula*. The arch of the palate is continued down each side of the pharyngeal wall as the *palatopharyngeal fold* that contains fasciculi of the *palatopharyngeal muscle* and forms the posterior pillar of the fauces. Through this arch the *dorsum of the tongue* can be seen lying anterior to the epiglottis, and the two lateral gutters formed by the *piriform recesses* indicate the path by which swallowed matter is shunted around the glottal opening.

From each side of the epiglottis the mucus membrane of the *aryepiglottic fold* extends to the apex of each *arytenoid cartilage*. An interarytenoid notch separates the superior parts of the two cartilages.

Longitudinal mucosal folds mark the commencement of the *esophagus,* and injected *esophageal branches* of the inferior *thyroid artery* provide its superior blood supply.

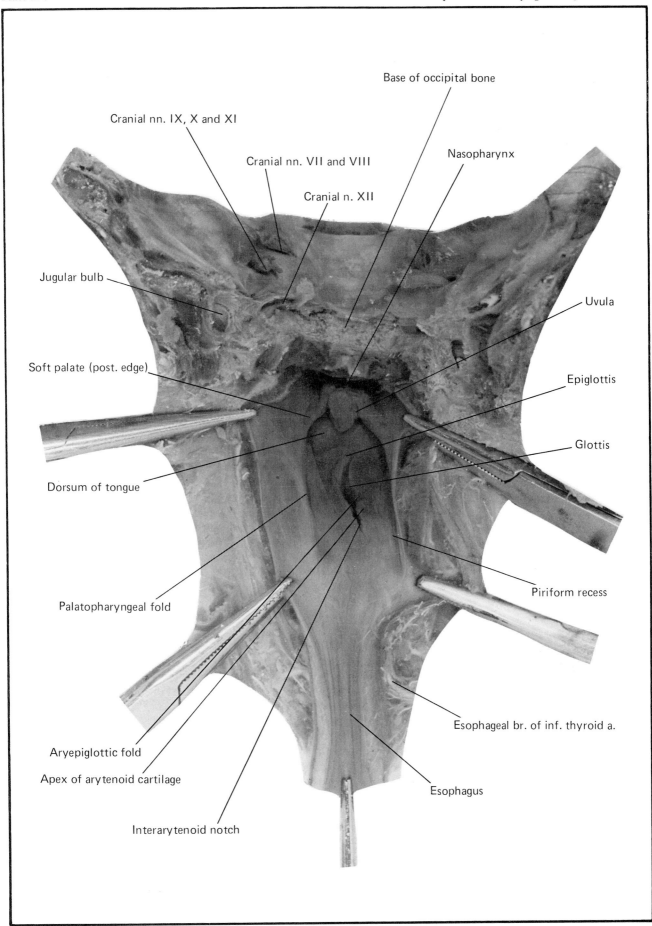

Base of occipital bone

Cranial nn. IX, X and XI

Cranial nn. VII and VIII

Nasopharynx

Cranial n. XII

Jugular bulb

Uvula

Soft palate (post. edge)

Epiglottis

Glottis

Dorsum of tongue

Piriform recess

Palatopharyngeal fold

Aryepiglottic fold

Esophageal br. of inf. thyroid a.

Apex of arytenoid cartilage

Esophagus

Interarytenoid notch

POSTERIOR REGION OF THE NECK: SUPERFICIAL DISSECTION

This exposure was made by incising the skin just below the ear and retracting it down over the shoulder and clavicle. It separated from the underlying tissues along the natural cleavage plane that occurs between the subcutaneous fascia and the deeper connective tissues. Because the fetal fascia is quite transparent and further dissection after taking the photograph only disrupted the finer subcutaneous nerves, this simple procedure was found sufficient to reveal the anatomy of most of the nerves found in the posterior cervical triangle. This triangle is bounded by the *trapezius muscle* posteriorly and the *sternocleidomastoid muscle* anteriorly, with the base formed by the clavicle. Here, the intact platysma covers the lower anterior part of the triangle.

The *cervical plexus,* which consists of a complex interweaving of the anterior primary divisions of the first four cervical nerves, provides motor and cutaneous branches to the neck and supraclavicular regions. Its ramifications emerge from between the anterior and middle scalene muscles, and those to the posterior triangle pass around the posterior border of the sternocleidomastoid where they become visible in this view.

In the superior part of the field the *great auricular, posterior auricular* and *lesser occipital nerves* send cutaneous branches to supply the scalp overlying the temporal fossa and the anterolateral occipital region. Near the same point where the great auricular nerve first becomes visible, the *anterior cutaneous nerve* may be seen passing superficial to the external jugular vein to give sensory branches to the anterior cervical skin. One centimeter inferior to this point, a large trunk gives rise to the *anterior, middle* and *posterior supraclavicular* nerves that supply a cutaneous area that covers the shoulder and clavicle like an epaulet.

The *accessory cranial nerve* (CNXI), in conjunction with branches from the cervical plexus, supplies motor fibers to the sternocleidomastoid muscle from its deep surface. The nerve then passes across the posterior triangle, where it receives more cervical contributions and can be seen entering the deep surface of the trapezius to provide its motor innervation.

Plate 177   Posterior Region of Neck   367

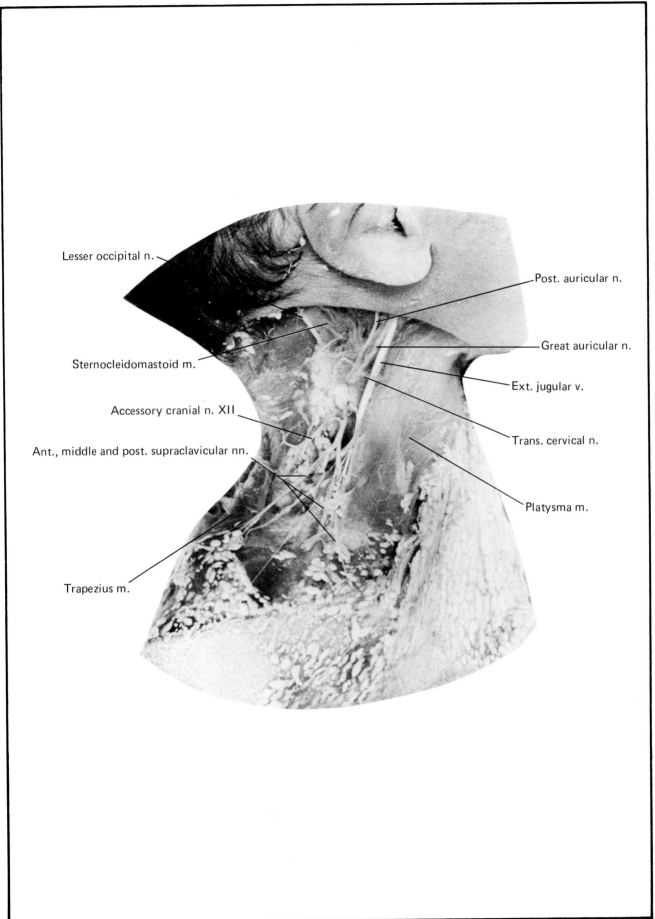

Lesser occipital n.

Post. auricular n.

Great auricular n.

Sternocleidomastoid m.

Ext. jugular v.

Accessory cranial n. XII

Ant., middle and post. supraclavicular nn.

Trans. cervical n.

Platysma m.

Trapezius m.

THE ANTERIOR CERVICAL TRIANGLE

The skin and investing fascia have been dissected from the anterior cervical region of this full term fetus. To further expose deeper structures, the central part of the *sternocleidomastoid muscle* has been removed, leaving the segments of its origin and insertion for reference. The *internal jugular vein* that ran a course lateral to the carotid artery has also been excised to better expose the arterial branches.

The sternocleidomastoid forms both the anterior border of the posterior triangle, and the posterior border of the anterior one. However, the positions of the triangles are reversed, with the base of the anterior being defined by the inferior border of the mandible and the anterior border being defined by the anterior midline of the neck. The anterior triangle is further subdivided into four smaller triangles, three of which use the digastric muscle in common borders. Superiorly, the *submandibular triangle* is formed between the angle of both bellies of the digastric with the mandible as the base. The *submental* triangle lies between the anterior digastric belly and the midline and has the hyoid as a base. The posterior digastric belly and the omohyoid muscle frame the *carotid triangle* with the sternocleidomastoid as a base, and the sternocleidomastoid and omohyoid muscles define the *muscular triangle* with the midline as its base.

In the superior part of the field the two bellies of the *digastric muscle* have a common insertion by an intermediate tendon to the hyoid bone. The posterior belly arises in a groove medial to the mastoid process of the temporal bone, whereas the anterior belly originates from the inner surface of the anterior part of the mandible. Their action elevates the hyoid. The two bellies are not derived from the same branchiomeric myotome because the anterior is innervated by the motor division of the trigeminal while the posterior receives a branch of the facial nerve.

Between the anterior digastric bellies, and also in the anterior floor of the submandibular triangle, the *mylohyoid muscle* forms a sling across the floor of the oral cavity. This muscle is innervated by a motor branch of the trigeminal and serves to elevate the tongue and hyoid apparatus. Deeper within the triangle and posterior to the mylohyoid, the *hyoglossus muscle* arises from the hyoid to insert into the lateral base of the tongue to depress it. A thin slip of muscle fibers arose from the styloid process to insert on the hyoid, encircling the central tendon of the digastric. The *stylohyoid muscle* has been retracted to expose the vessels around the *submandibular gland* more fully. The gland is a discrete, firm structure that, unlike the parotid, can be easily shelled out.

The *external carotid artery* enters the submandibular triangle medial to the digastric and stylohyoid tendons. Its *lingual artery* courses with the *hypoglossal cranial nerve* (CNXII) and enters the base of the tongue between the mylohyoid and hypoglossus muscles in the apex of the triangle. The *facial artery* passes anterior to the submandibular gland and gives off the *submental artery* to the floor of the mouth. It continues superiorly external to the mandible. Posterior to the gland the external carotid artery may be seen here descending into the parotid region.

Within the carotid triangle the *common carotid artery* bifurcates into the *external* and *internal carotids*. The latter, although more lateral in origin, curves medial and posterior to the former to enter the skull without giving off cervical branches. The slight swelling at the point of bifurcation indicates the *carotid sinus*, a baroceptor that reflexly influences the blood pressure. Near the apex of the carotid triangle the common carotid gives rise to the *superior thyroid artery* (which may variably arise from the external carotid.) Above this the *superior laryngeal* artery courses downward from the external carotid to supply the larynx. In most cases this vessel arises in common with the superior thyroid.

Where the sternocleidomastoid had been removed, the cervical plexus was exposed and has been retracted over the *medial* and *posterior scalene muscles*.

The *omohyoid muscle* ascends obilquely across the neck from its scapular origin to its insertion on the hyoid bone. It is somewhat digastric, with a thinner intermediate region that is attached to the clavicle by a fascial sling. It is innervated by branches from the first three cervical nerves and serves to depress the hyoid bone.

In the muscular triangle a set of straplike muscles of hypobranchial orgin lie anterior to the trachea, thyroid gland and larynx. The most superficial of these, the *sternohyoid muscle,* has been cut away on the left side of the specimen, leaving but a stump to show its origin from the inner surface of the sternal manubrium. It inserts into the body of the hyoid bone, which it depresses. Deep to this muscle, the *sternothyroid muscle* inserts into a line on the anterolateral surface of the thyroid cartilage. From this insertion the shorter *thyrohyoid muscle* originates and appears as a continuation of the former muscle as it ascends to insert on the hyoid. The sternothyroid depresses the larynx, and by continued action through the thyrohyoid it depresses the hyoid bone. The strap muscles receive innervation from the first two or three cervical nerves via a loop of the cervical plexus called the ansa cervicalis.

In the midline the strap muscles are separated and expose the underlying *isthmus* of the *thyroid gland*, which shows prominently injected branches of the *inferior thyroid artery.*

The fetal neck, like the fetal face, is much more compressed in relation to adult proportions, a fact that requires firm elevation of the chin and extension of the neck to give better access to the trachea for tracheotomies, a rather frequent emergency procedure in early infancy.

Plate 178　　　　　　　　　　　　　　　　　　　　　　Anterior Cervical Triangle　　369

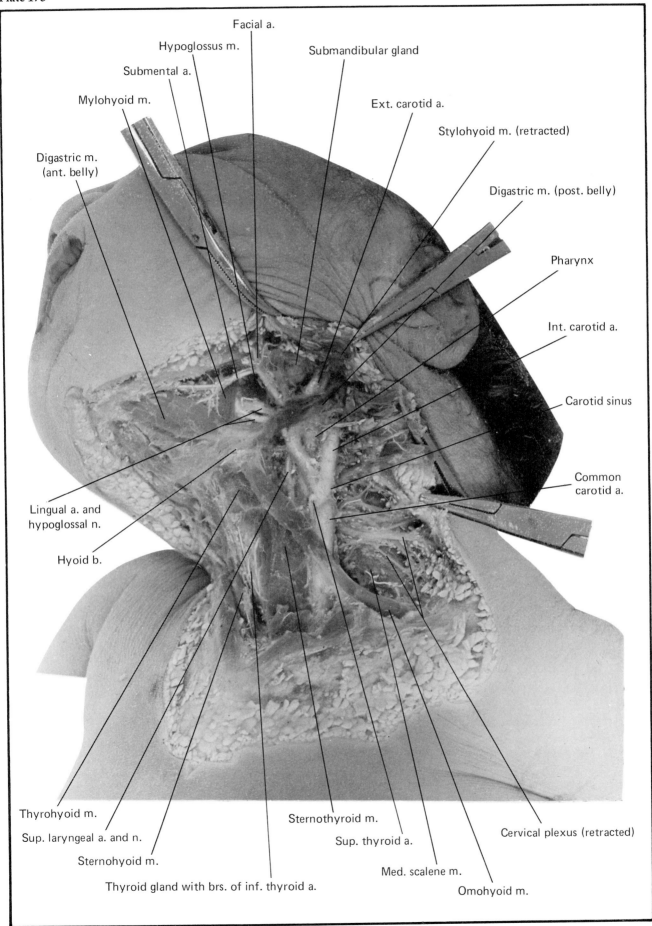

Facial a.

Hypoglossus m.

Submental a.

Submandibular gland

Mylohyoid m.

Ext. carotid a.

Stylohyoid m. (retracted)

Digastric m.
(ant. belly)

Digastric m. (post. belly)

Pharynx

Int. carotid a.

Carotid sinus

Common
carotid a.

Lingual a. and
hypoglossal n.

Hyoid b.

Thyrohyoid m.

Sup. laryngeal a. and n.

Sternohyoid m.

Sternothyroid m.

Sup. thyroid a.

Cervical plexus (retracted)

Med. scalene m.

Omohyoid m.

Thyroid gland with brs. of inf. thyroid a.

RETROPHARYNGEAL EXPOSURE OF THE DEEP CERVICAL STRUCTURES

The preparation of this specimen is similar to that shown in Plate 176. However, here the frontal (coronal) section through the posterior cranial fossae lies slightly posterior to the jugular foramen so as not to destroy the jugular vein and associated cranial nerves. The anterior deep structures were separated from the prevertebral fascia along the natural retropharyngeal cleft, and the cervical vertebral column, along with its dorsal muscle mass, has been severed at the level of the first thoracic segment and removed. Retraction of the lateral cervical skin and muscles then spread the contents of the vascular (carotid) sheath that bound the nerves, arteries and veins in common.

In the upper part of the field, the posterior pharyngeal wall is shown attached to the basiocciput that bears a central *pharyngeal tubercle*, to which the posterior raphe of the superior pharyngeal constrictor is attached. The lateral expansions of the *pharyngeal recesses* are particularly evident here. The muscular fibers of the pharyngeal constrictors unfortunately are not individually discernible, but under water immersion, the posterior pharyngeal wall became translucent, so that the superior part related to the naso- and oropharynx appears darker in the photograph.

Branches of the *ascending pharyngeal artery* (from the facial artery) can be seen with associated veins of a coarser nature forming a vascular plexus on the pharynx. The arteries anastomose with the *esophageal branches* of the *inferior thyroid artery*.

On the surface of the constrictors fine nerves follow the distribution of the vessels to create the *pharyngeal nervous plexus,* composed of contributions from the vagus, glossopharyngeal and, to a small extent, the accessory nerves.

In the column of vascular and nervous structures flanking the pharynx, the most posterior structure is the *cervical sympathetic trunk.* This normally lies in direct contact with the prevertebral fascia and bears three irregularly shaped ganglia. The *superior cervical sympathetic ganglion* is the large fusiform swelling at the upper part of the trunk, and the *middle cervical sympathetic ganglion* lies at the level of the esophageal arteries. The *inferior cervical sympathetic ganglion* may be identified near the origins of these arteries. The cervical trunk transmits the sympathetic fibers from the upper thoracic segments into the neck and head. Just above the superior ganglion, a plexus of fine fibers enters the skull entwined on the surface of the carotid artery. It ramifies with the vessels primarily to provide vasomotor control and to dilate the pupil of the eye.

The *carotid arteries* lie anterior to the sympathetic trunk. The common carotid is visible diverging (because of retraction) from the esophagus as it travels up the neck. At the level of the pharynx the external carotid branches forward, and the internal carotid curves medially as it approaches the skull. Between the bifurcation of these vessels the *stylopharyngeus muscle* descends from the styloid process and inserts into the pharynx between the superior and middle constrictors. This is best seen and labeled on the right side. The *glossopharyngeal nerve* (CNIX) leaves the jugular fossa and innervates the stylopharyngeus as it passes around its posterior border to enter the pharyngeal plexus.

Since this is a doubly injected specimen (produced inadvertently by the rupture of the aortic or pulmonary valves that let the latex enter the larger veins), the internal jugular veins are the large lateral vessels filled with the injected medium. Across the posterosuperior aspect of each vein, the *accessory nerve* (CNXI) travels from the jugular fossa to the internal surface of the retracted sternocleidomastoid muscles. The *vagus nerve* (CNX) leaves the fossa and courses inferiorly between the internal carotid and jugular vessels, and in its most superior segment it gives off a pharyngeal branch that here, on the right side, may be seen accompanying the glossopharyngeal nerve into the pharyngeal wall. The two vagi follow the common carotid arteries to enter the mediastinum anterior to the fourth aortic arch derivatives on both sides.

Plate 179

Deep Cervical Structures   371

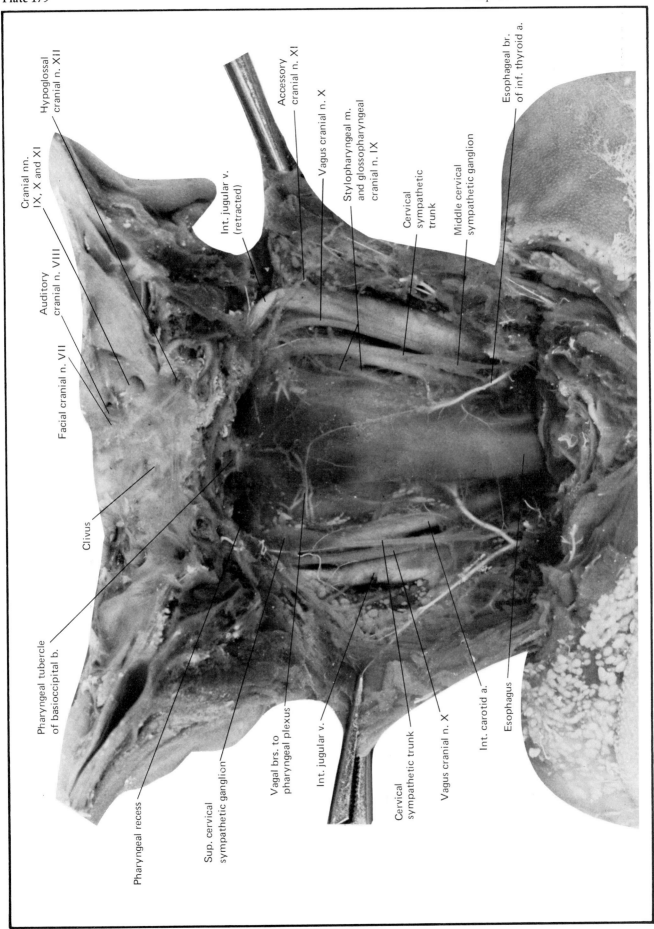

Hypoglossal cranial n. XII

Cranial nn. IX, X and XI

Accessory cranial n. XI

Vagus cranial n. X

Int. jugular v. (retracted)

Stylopharyngeal m. and glossopharyngeal cranial n. IX

Cervical sympathetic trunk

Middle cervical sympathetic ganglion

Esophageal br. of inf. thyroid a.

Auditory cranial n. VIII

Facial cranial n. VII

Clivus

Pharyngeal tubercle of basioccipital b.

Pharyngeal recess

Sup. cervical sympathetic ganglion

Vagal brs. to pharyngeal plexus

Int. jugular v.

Cervical sympathetic trunk

Vagus cranial n. X

Int. carotid a.

Esophagus

ANGIOGRAM OF THE CERVICAL REGION

The cervical region is longitudinally traversed by three sets of arteries. The *carotid arteries* are the most conspicuous pair and ascend the anterior cervical region to supply visceral and muscular structures in the neck. At its bifurcation, the *external carotid* ramifies to the deep and superficial facial areas while the *internal carotid* enters the skull to supply the diencephalon and most of its derivatives. Its cerebral branches are distributed to the greater part of the cerebral hemispheres, and the ophthalmic branch supplies the ocular bulb and its orbital adnexa, eventually anastomosing with facial branches around the eye.

In the base of the neck, the *thyrocervical trunk* sends the *inferior thyroid artery* to supply the gland and surrounding muscles and the superior section of the esophagus. The *superior thyroid artery* recurves downward into the anterior cervical viscera from above.

The vertebral arteries form the second cervical arterial system. These vessels arise from the subclavians and pass abruptly posterosuperiorly to enter the transverse foramen of the sixth cervical vertebra to ascend the column through the successive foramina. They supply the vertebral elements and the cervical part of the spinal cord and dura by a series of segmental branches. At the level of the atlantooccipital membrane, the arteries penetrate the dura and converge to form the single basal artery of the upper brain stem. Although it is smaller than the carotid system, the vertebral system nourishes the more primitive but more vital areas of the brain.

The third system of longitudinal cervical arteries is formed by the anastomoses of the main channels of the *ascending deep cervical arteries* of the *costocervical trunk* with the *descending cervical branch* of the *occipital artery*, a branch of the external carotid. These vessels supply the dorsal musculature of the neck and send segmental laminar branches to the neural arches of the cervical vertebrae.

Plate 180   Angiogram of Cervical Region   373

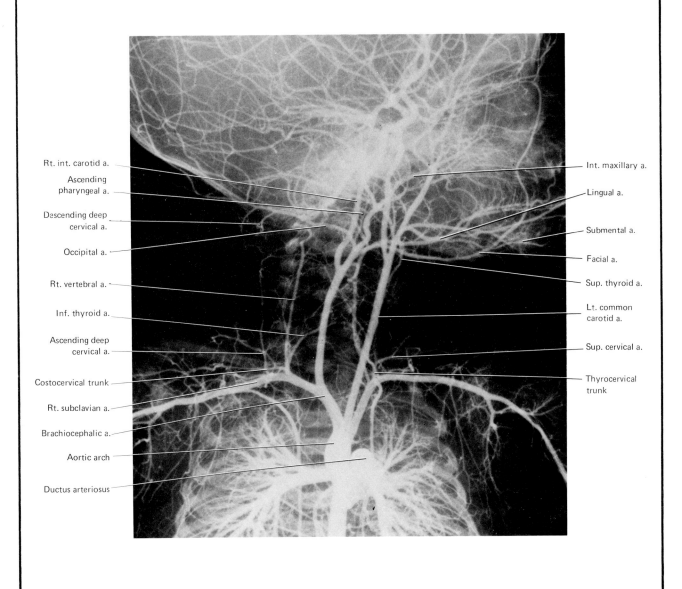

Rt. int. carotid a.

Ascending
pharyngeal a.

Descending deep
cervical a.

Occipital a.

Rt. vertebral a.

Inf. thyroid a.

Ascending deep
cervical a.

Costocervical trunk

Rt. subclavian a.

Brachiocephalic a.

Aortic arch

Ductus arteriosus

Int. maxillary a.

Lingual a.

Submental a.

Facial a.

Sup. thyroid a.

Lt. common
carotid a.

Sup. cervical a.

Thyrocervical
trunk

HORIZONTAL SECTION THROUGH THE CRANIOCERVICAL ARTICULATION

In the plane of section shown here, the submental triangle reveals the pair of *geniohyoid muscles* passing under the tongue. On either side the anterior bellies of the *digastric muscle* lie inferior to sections of the lateral parts of the *mylohyoid* at the point where the mylohyoid covers the *lingual artery* and *nerve* at the base of the tongue.

In the *pharynx* the *epiglottis* is situated medial to the two piriform recesses. The loose, connective tissue between the posterior pharyngeal wall and the prevertebral muscles indicates the plane of the retropharyngeal cleft. Lateral to this potential space, the large vessels of the neck are ensheathed in common with several nerves. Anterior to the carotid sheath, which contains the jugular vein and carotid artery, the structures that pass through the skull in the region of the infratemporal fossa are gathered around the *mandibular branch of the trigeminal nerve*.

The lateral masses and anterior arch of the atlas enclose the *odontoid process* and its *transverse ligaments*. Posterior to this, the dura contains the upper cervical *spinal cord*.

A fragment of the posterior occipital bone indicates that most of the surrounding nuchal muscles insert on the posterior base of the skull.

Plate 181   Horizontal Section through Craniocervical Articulation   375

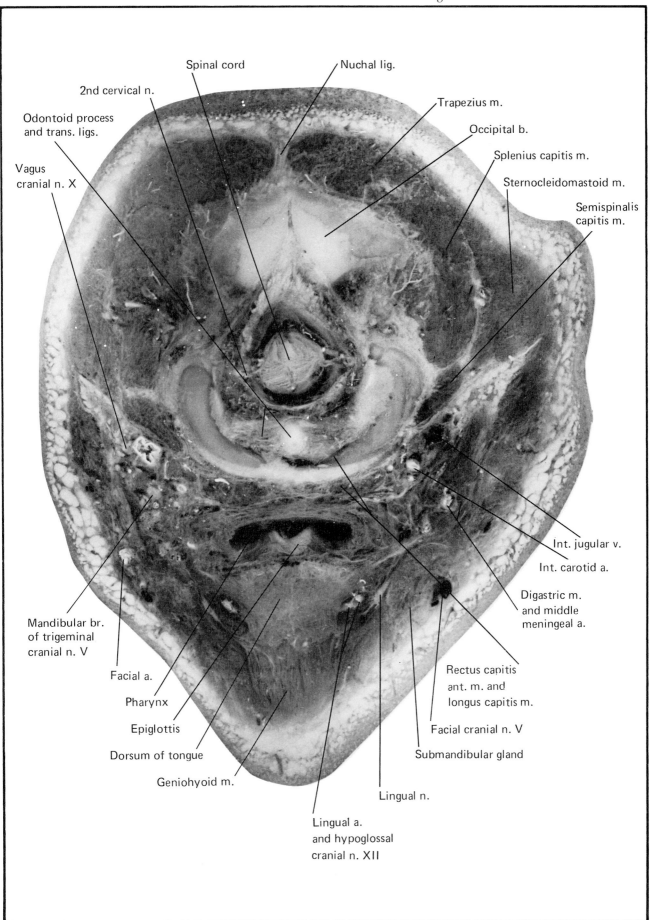

Spinal cord

Nuchal lig.

2nd cervical n.

Trapezius m.

Odontoid process
and trans. ligs.

Occipital b.

Splenius capitis m.

Vagus
cranial n. X

Sternocleidomastoid m.

Semispinalis
capitis m.

Int. jugular v.

Int. carotid a.

Mandibular br.
of trigeminal
cranial n. V

Digastric m.
and middle
meningeal a.

Facial a.

Rectus capitis
ant. m. and
longus capitis m.

Pharynx

Epiglottis

Facial cranial n. V

Dorsum of tongue

Submandibular gland

Geniohyoid m.

Lingual n.

Lingual a.
and hypoglossal
cranial n. XII

HORIZONTAL SECTION THROUGH THE NECK AT THE LEVEL OF THE THIRD CERVICAL VERTEBRA: INFERIOR ASPECT

In the anterior part of this section the larynx has been exposed below the *rima epiglottis* (glottal opening), and the relations of the two major cartilages of the larynx are revealed. Since this is an inferior view of the section, the *vocal folds* attach posteriorly above (superior) to the thick *lamina of the cricoid* and anteriorly to the inner surface of the thinner thyroid cartilage. Posterior to the cricoid the *posterior cricoarytenoid muscles* rotate and adduct the arytenoid cartilages to change the size of the glottal opening and tension of the cords. Between these muscles and the prevertebral *longus capitis muscles*, the commencement of the *esophagus* is shown as a transverse slit.

Anterior to the larynx the thin, straplike *thyrohyoid* and *sternohyoid* muscles lie between the thyroid cartilage and the skin.

The carotid sheath is situated lateral to the larynx and forms a common container for the *carotid artery* and the *jugular vessels* that are flanked by the *sternocleidomastoid muscle*.

The cartilaginous part of the third cervical vertebra has been cut below the ossification center, but the characteristic configuration of a cervical vertebra is indicated by the large lateral pillars between the articular facets and the *vertebral arteries* in the *transverse foramina*.

The deep dorsal cervical muscles are continuations of the series that form the *erector spinae* muscles of the back. These include the *splenius, semispinalis capitis* and *multifidus*, all of which are innervated by dorsal primary divisions of the spinal nerves. The superficial *trapezius* and *sternocleidomastoid muscles* both are innervated by a combination of nerves from the cervical plexus and the accessory nerve (CNXI). The *levator scapulae* receives motor fibers from the cervical plexus only.

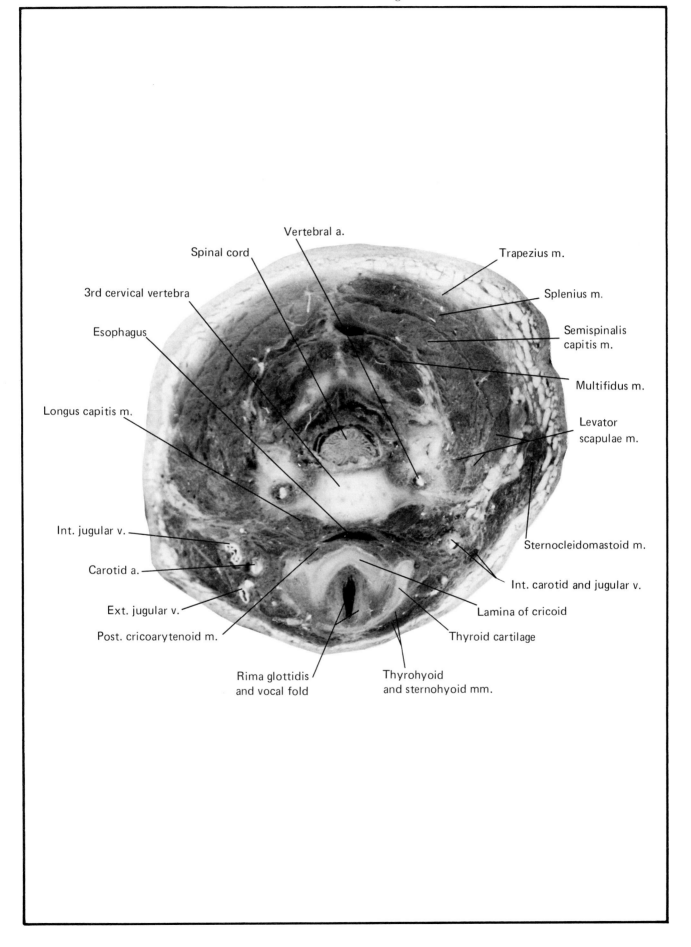

Vertebral a.

Spinal cord

3rd cervical vertebra

Esophagus

Trapezius m.

Splenius m.

Semispinalis
capitis m.

Multifidus m.

Longus capitis m.

Levator
scapulae m.

Int. jugular v.

Carotid a.

Sternocleidomastoid m.

Ext. jugular v.

Int. carotid and jugular v.

Post. cricoarytenoid m.

Lamina of cricoid

Thyroid cartilage

Rima glottidis
and vocal fold

Thyrohyoid
and sternohyoid mm.

HORIZONTAL SECTION THROUGH THE NECK AT THE LEVEL OF THE FIFTH CERVICAL VERTEBRA

This section passes through the trachea at the level where the isthmus of the *thyroid gland* connects its two lateral lobes. The extensive vascularity that is characteristic of all endocrine tissue is here indicated by the numerous injected branches of both the *inferior* and *superior arteries* that ramify through the substance of the gland. Between the thyroid and the esophagus, the *inferior laryngeal nerves,* recurrent branches of the vagus, ascend to supply the trachea, esophagus and most of the intrinsic muscles of the larynx.

Anterior to the thyroid the sternohyoid and omohyoid muscles may be distinguished, particularly on the left side.

The carotid sheath on the right contains the medial *carotid artery* and the more lateral thin-walled *jugular vein,* which shows some of the latex medium because of double injection. Posterior to the carotid the large vagus nerve (CNX) descends to the thorax.

In the prevertebral region lie the *longus colli muscles* of the cervical vertebrae, and the more lateral *anterior* and *middle scalene muscles* arise from the transverse processes of the vertebrae and attach to the uppermost ribs. Between these muscles, the nerves of the lower cervical and brachial plexus leave the cervical intervertebral foramina. The dorsal cervical muscles are the same as indicated in the preceding illustration.

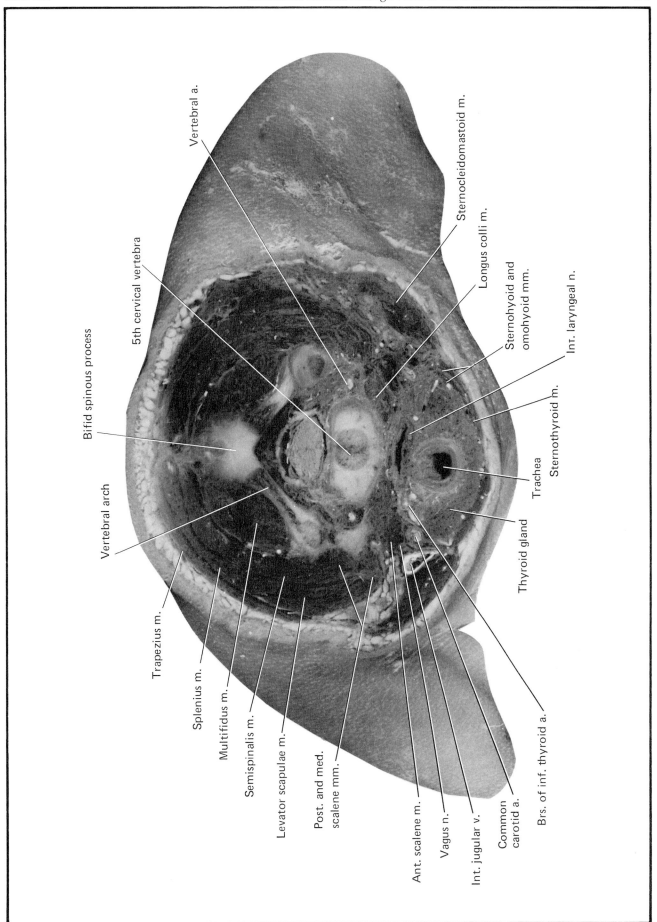

Vertebral a.

Sternocleidomastoid m.

Longus colli m.

5th cervical vertebra

Sternohyoid and omohyoid mm.

Int. laryngeal n.

Bifid spinous process

Sternothyroid m.

Trachea

Vertebral arch

Thyroid gland

Trapezius m.

Splenius m.

Multifidus m.

Semispinalis m.

Levator scapulae m.

Post. and med. scalene mm.

Ant. scalene m.

Vagus n.

Int. jugular v.

Common carotid a.

Brs. of inf. thyroid a.

HORIZONTAL SECTION THROUGH THE NECK AT THE LEVEL OF THE FIRST THORACIC VERTEBRA: INFERIOR VIEW

Because the ribs slant downward anteriorly, the plane at which the base of the neck joins the thoracic inlet is obliquely inclined to the horizontal. Thus, in the adult the anterior margin of the thoracic inlet that is marked by the notch of the manubrium lies at the level of the second thoracic vertebra. This permits structures in the upper extremes of the pleural cavities and mediastinum to occupy space in the base of the neck. Despite the fact that the ribs are less oblique in the perinatal body and the manubrial notch lies at the lower level of the first thoracic vertebra, thoracic viscera are still discernible in the lower neck region. On the left side of the specimen (which coincides with the left side of the picture because this is an inferior view of the section), the *apex of the left pleural cavity* extends above the level of the first rib. A similar situation is not apparent on the right only because the cut is transversely oblique and shows more superior aspects of the structures on that side.

The presence of the lung apex in the base of the neck is of considerable anatomic and pathologic significance. Apical lung sounds are readily auscultated above the clavicle, and the pathology of the lung that is common to this region may also affect the nerves and vessels that lie in close approximation to the apical pleura.

On both sides the *eighth cervical nerve* may be traced from the spinal canal to where it passes over the lung apex to contribute to the inferior trunk of the brachial plexus.

Anteriorly, the upper poles of the bilobed *thymus gland* intrude into the base of the neck. The relative size of these structures diminishes within the first postnatal decade and they become confined to the anterior mediastinum.

The right *glenohumeral joint* is well displayed with its synovial cavity. Although this area is topologically treated with the upper extremity, the muscles and joints of the pectoral girdle revealed here should be compared with the views shown in the previous section of this book.

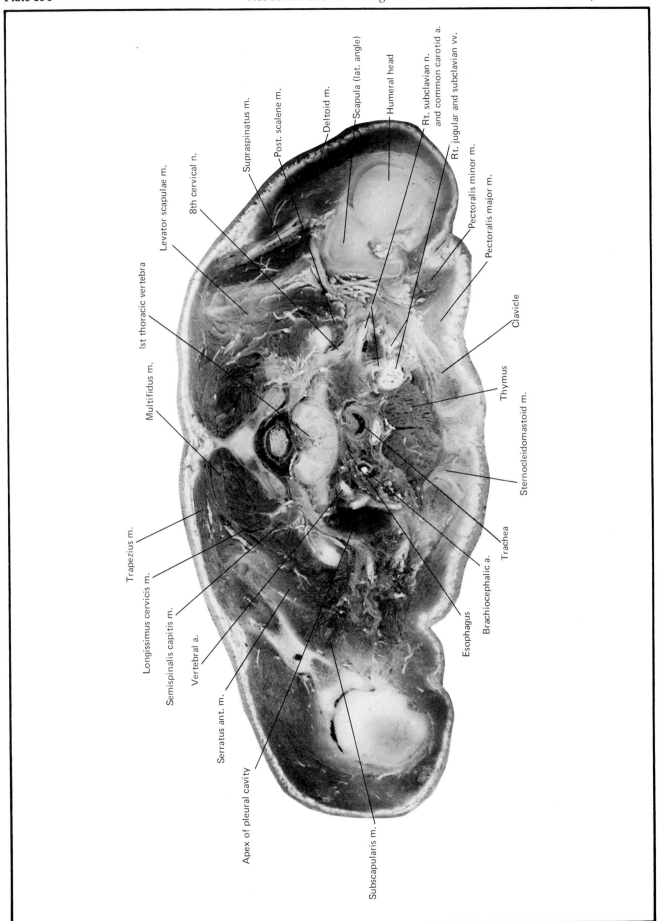

Supraspinatus m.

Post. scalene m.

Deltoid m.

Scapula (lat. angle)

Humeral head

Rt. subclavian n. and common carotid a.

Rt. jugular and subclavian vv.

8th cervical n.

Levator scapulae m.

Pectoralis minor m.

Pectoralis major m.

1st thoracic vertebra

Clavicle

Multifidus m.

Thymus

Sternocleidomastoid m.

Trapezius m.

Trachea

Longissimus cervicis m.

Brachiocephalic a.

Semispinalis capitis m.

Esophagus

Vertebral a.

Serratus ant. m.

Apex of pleural cavity

Subscapularis m.

THE PALPEBRAL FISSURE

The slit between the superior and inferior palpebrae constitutes the palpebral fissure. In the stillborn perinate and earlier fetal cadavers the eye is firmly closed, and instrumental retraction of the lids is required to open the fissure and expose the bulb.

The medial commissure of the fissure, the *internal canthus,* is more acute than the *external canthus* and serves as the apex for a triangular space called the *lachrymal lacuna.* The base of this triangle is produced by the *superior* and *inferior lachrymal papillae* that form opposing prominences on their respective palpebrae. Each of the papillae bears a small orifice, the *lachrymal puncta,* that drains the accumulation of tears from the lacuna and transfers the fluid through a pair of ducts to the lachrymal sac that lies in the fossa of the lachrymal bone. From there the secretions of the lachrymal gland pass through the nasolachrymal duct to drain into the inferior nasal meatus.

Deep to the lacuna the *medial caruncle* forms a fleshy protuberance that is delineated from the sclera by a pink crescent of tissue, the *semilunar fold.*

The superior and inferior palpebrae are forcefully opposed by fibers of the *orbicularis oculi muscle,* and each is given additional firmness by an internal fibrous plate of connective tissue. These *tarsal plates* are of unequal size; the *superior tarsus* is larger and receives the insertion of the *levator palpebrae superioris muscle.*

The *conjunctiva,* an epithelium lining the internal surface of the eyelids, is reflected over the exposed anterior surface of the bulb, covering both sclera and cornea. Thus all structures visible through the palpebral fissure are covered by this continuous membrane.

Plate 185   Palpebral Fissure   383

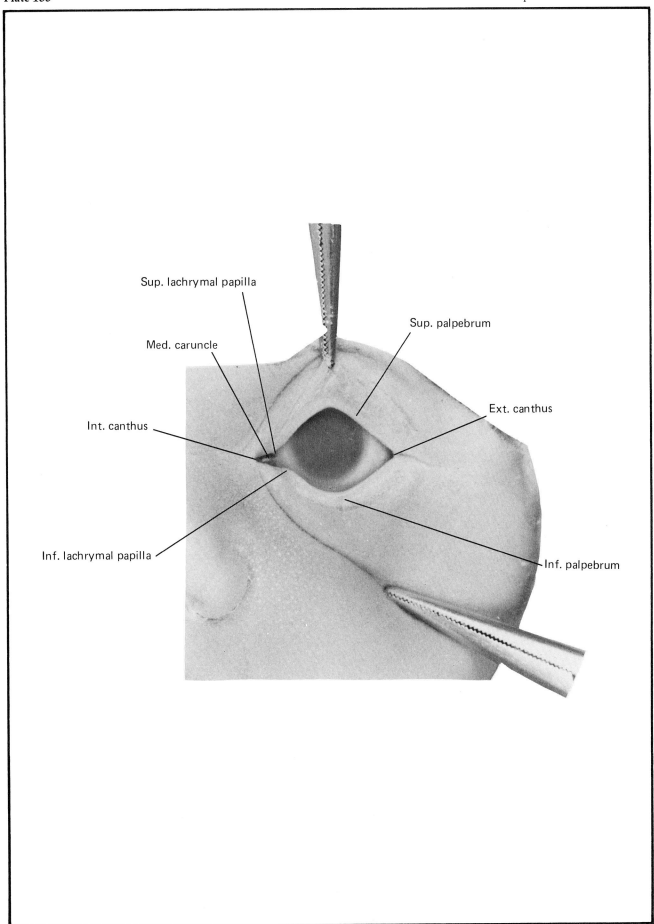

Sup. lachrymal papilla

Med. caruncle

Sup. palpebrum

Int. canthus

Ext. canthus

Inf. lachrymal papilla

Inf. palpebrum

THE OCULAR BULB AND ITS MUSCLES

The eye of the late fetal or neonatal cadaver is seldom obtained when the *cornea* is as clear as in the vital state. This normally transparent structure that forms the first of the several refractive media of the ocular optical system rapidly becomes cloudy after death, but in most fetal cadavers close inspection usually will still reveal the *iris* and the outline of the *pupil.*

Aqueous humor fills the space between the cornea and the lens and acts as the second refractive medium. The iris intervenes between these two structures and divides the aqueous space into the preirideal *anterior chamber* and the postirideal *posterior chamber.* The lens and the bulbar space behind it that is filled with the gelatinous *vitreous humor* form the third and fourth refractive media.

The ocular bulb fits into the orbital adnexa like the ball and socket arrangement of an enarthrodial joint. The differential actions of the extrinsic muscles then provide a circumduction or universal motion to the ocular bulb.

The four rectus muscles are equidistantly inserted on the anterior half of the bulb and arise from a fibrous cuff, the *anulus tendineus,* which is attached around the optic canal and medial part of the orbital fissure, whereas the levator palpebrae and superior oblique muscles arise just above this structure. Through the aperture in the anulus all retrobulbar nerves except the trochlear enter the orbit. Because this common origin of the muscles lies medial to the longitudinal (optical) axis of the bulb, the *superior* and *inferior recti,* in addition to their respective elevation and depression of the bulb, also provide a synergistic adduction and antagonistic rotation. The *medial* and *lateral recti* reciprocally adduct and abduct the bulb.

Both oblique muscles insert on the lateral part of the posterior half of the bulb. The *superior oblique* passes forward above the medial rectus to reach a fibrous loop of tissue, the *trochlea* (pulley), that is attached to the superomedial rim of the orbit. Its tendon hooks around the trochlea and passes obliquely posterolaterally over the bulb to insert on its lateral posterior half. Thus, despite its origin in the posterior orbit, this muscle functions as though its origin were the trochlea and depresses, abducts and medially rotates the eye. The *inferior oblique* is unique in that it arises from the inferomedial part of the orbit just inferior to the lachrymal fossa. It passes posterolaterally under the bulb and superficial to the inferior rectus to insert on the lateral posterior bulb surface to elevate, abduct and laterally rotate the eye. The two oblique muscles also tend to protract (protrude) the bulb whereas the four recti retract it. The superior, inferior and medial recti and the levator palpebrae are innervated by the *oculomotor nerve* (CNIII), and the lateral rectus exclusively receives innervation from the *abducens nerve* (CNVI). The *trochlear nerve* (CNIV), as its name implies, is solely responsible for the motor action of the superior oblique.

Plate 186   Ocular Bulb and Muscles   385

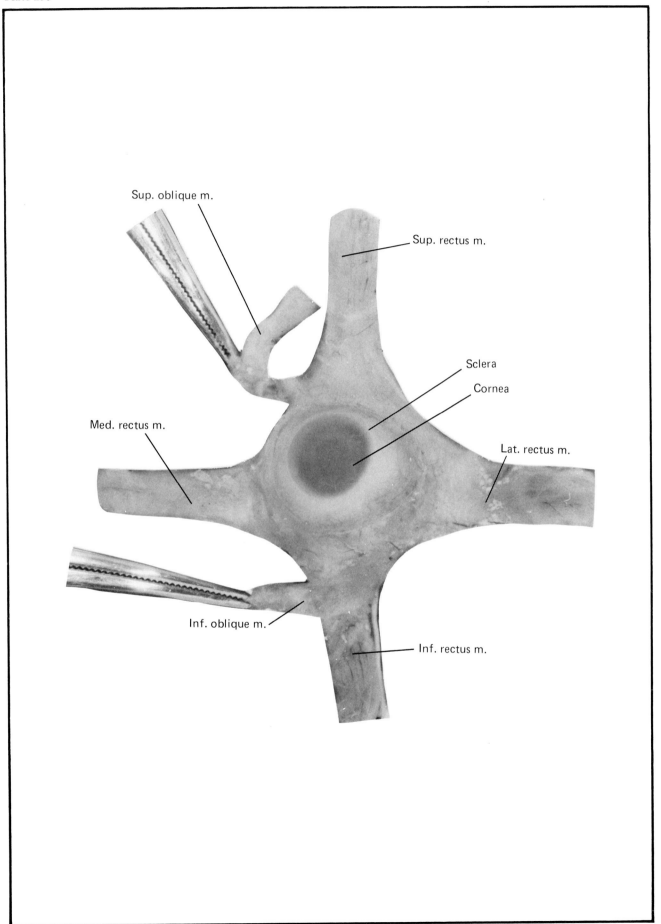

Sup. oblique m.

Sup. rectus m.

Sclera

Cornea

Med. rectus m.

Lat. rectus m.

Inf. oblique m.

Inf. rectus m.

SUPERFICIAL DISSECTION OF THE SUPERIOR ASPECT OF THE ORBIT

Exposure of the orbital contents is best effected by removing the orbital plate of the frontal bone. The orbital *periosteum* or *periorbita* is the first soft tissue encountered. It is firmly attached around the optic canal, the orbital fissures and the anterior orbital rim. A fold of the periorbita attaches to the ciliary region of the anterior bulb and forms the *orbital septum,* a fibrous membrane that helps to anchor the bulb within the orbit. The periorbita is rather thick and easily separated from the bone in the midorbital regions and is here reflected to the nasal side. In the undisturbed underlying structures the amorphous *lachrymal gland* occupies the superolateral region. This organ secretes the tears that lubricate and wash the conjunctiva. Medially, the *levator palpebrae* overlies the *superior rectus muscle,* and the large *supraorbital nerve,* a branch of the ophthalmic division of the trigeminal, shows a gentle curving course across the roof of the orbit. The *supraorbital artery* emerges from fatty depositions to parallel the course of the nerve and emerge in the skin of the brow. The anterior part of the *supratrochlear nerve* is visible coursing to the superior oblique muscle.

In the region lateral to the body of the sphenoid, the sectioned optic nerve (CNII) enters the optic canal, and the *oculomotor nerve* penetrates the dura more posteriorly. The *abducens nerve* (CNIV) pierces the dura below the dorsum sellae medial to the large root of the *trigeminal nerve* (CNV).

Plate 187   Superficial Dissection of Superior Aspect of Orbit   387

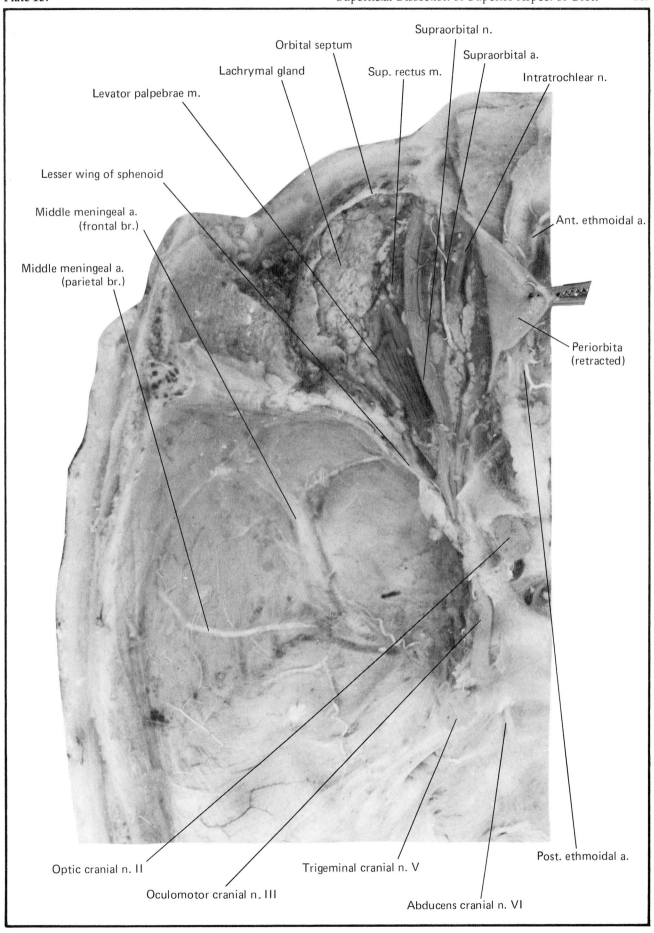

Orbital septum

Supraorbital n.

Lachrymal gland

Supraorbital a.

Levator palpebrae m.

Sup. rectus m.

Intratrochlear n.

Lesser wing of sphenoid

Ant. ethmoidal a.

Middle meningeal a.
(frontal br.)

Middle meningeal a.
(parietal br.)

Periorbita
(retracted)

Optic cranial n. II

Trigeminal cranial n. V

Post. ethmoidal a.

Oculomotor cranial n. III

Abducens cranial n. VI

DEEPER DISSECTION OF THE SUPERIOR ASPECT OF THE ORBIT

In the continued dissection of the preceding specimen, the lachrymal gland has been removed to expose the *lachrymal artery* and *nerve*. The anterior part of the *levator palpebrae muscle* has been sectioned, revealing the large orbital venous plexus that drains via the ophthalmic vein to the cavernous sinus. On the superior anterior surface of the bulb the insertion of the superior rectus contains numerous fine arteries and veins.

Medially, the removal of the fat bodies shows the relations of the *superior oblique* and *medial rectus muscles* more clearly.

On the medial wall of the middle cranial fossa, the dura of the cavernous sinus has been opened to show the *ophthalmic division* arising from the *trigeminal nerve* (CNV), and the fine *trochlear nerve* (CNIV) may be discerned passing deep to the *oculomotor nerve* (CNIII).

Plate 188   Deeper Dissection of Superior Aspect of Orbit   389

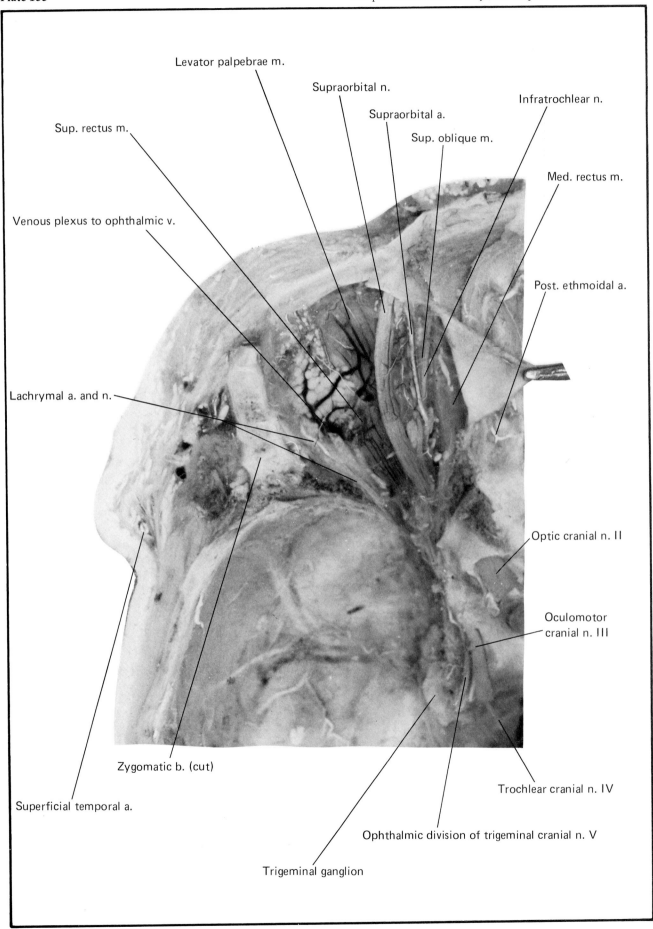

Levator palpebrae m.

Supraorbital n.

Supraorbital a.

Infratrochlear n.

Sup. rectus m.

Sup. oblique m.

Med. rectus m.

Venous plexus to ophthalmic v.

Post. ethmoidal a.

Lachrymal a. and n.

Optic cranial n. II

Oculomotor cranial n. III

Zygomatic b. (cut)

Trochlear cranial n. IV

Superficial temporal a.

Ophthalmic division of trigeminal cranial n. V

Trigeminal ganglion

DEEP DISSECTION OF THE SUPERIOR ASPECT OF THE ORBIT

Reflection of the *levator palpebrae* and *superior rectus* muscles and the dissection and removal of the orbital fat have exposed the posterior half of the bulb, the optic nerve and related vessels.

The positions of the *lateral* and *medial recti* are well displayed, and the convergence of the muscles to their origin in the fibrous tissue around the optic nerve can be appreciated.

The orbital portion of the bulb is covered with an uninterrupted capsule of connective tissue that here exhibits a fine plexus of vessels. This *bulbar fascia* is also reflected around the insertions of the muscles to extend over them like a sheath and also blends with the dura covering the optic nerve. The capsule is loose and separated from the underlying sclera by a periscleral space that is, in effect, a bursa that enhances the analogy that the eye and the orbital adnexa form a ball and socket joint.

Where the optic nerve enters the bulb it is surrounded by several fine *posterior ciliary arteries*. These pierce the sclera and supply the uveal tract and external one third of the retina. The *central artery* enters the bulb embedded in the optic nerve and supplies the inner two thirds of the retina with nonanastomosing end arteries. Two *long posterior* ciliary arteries enter the medial and lateral aspects of the posterior bulb surface (only the lateral member is visible here) and pass around the bulb between the sclera and choroid to anastomose with *anterior ciliary arteries* from muscular branches.

Deep and lateral to the posterior ciliary arteries a small mass of cells makes up the *ciliary ganglion,* visible here as a stellate body about 1 millimeter in diameter. This ganglion provides the postsynaptic parasympathetic fibers to the iris and ciliary muscles.

The medial branches of the ophthalmic artery include the *supraorbital artery* and a more medial vessel that gives off the *anterior* and *posterior ethmoidal branches* and continues forward to anastomose with facial branches as the *supratrochlear* artery (see Plates 193 and 194).

Plate 189   Deep Dissection of Superior Aspect of Orbit   391

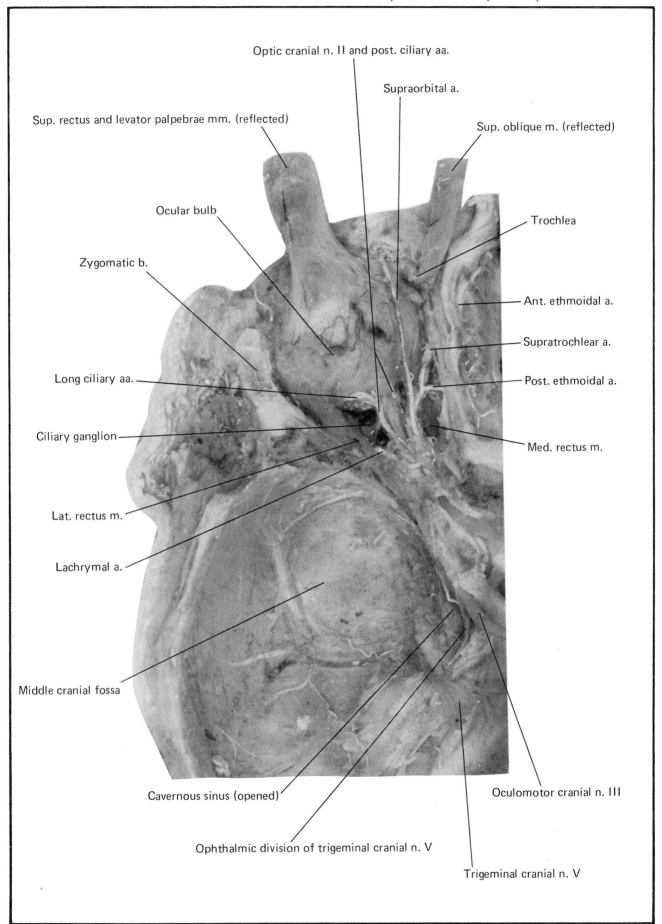

Optic cranial n. II and post. ciliary aa.

Supraorbital a.

Sup. rectus and levator palpebrae mm. (reflected)

Sup. oblique m. (reflected)

Ocular bulb

Trochlea

Zygomatic b.

Ant. ethmoidal a.

Supratrochlear a.

Long ciliary aa.

Post. ethmoidal a.

Ciliary ganglion

Med. rectus m.

Lat. rectus m.

Lachrymal a.

Middle cranial fossa

Cavernous sinus (opened)

Oculomotor cranial n. III

Ophthalmic division of trigeminal cranial n. V

Trigeminal cranial n. V

FRONTAL SECTION THROUGH THE ORBIT AND POSTERIOR HALF OF THE OCULAR BULB

This section shows the spatial arrangement of the ocular muscles as they approach the coronal equator of the bulb. The *levator palpebrae* and *superior rectus* course together in the 12-o'clock position at the top of the bulb. Proceeding clockwise, a slight episclerotic thickening at the 2-o'clock position is the only indication of the tendinous section of the superior oblique muscle at this level. The lateral rectus appears as a strap of muscle at the 3-o'clock position where it lies medial to the posterior pole of the *lachrymal gland* and *lachrymal artery*. At the 5-o'clock position the *inferior oblique* muscle passes diagonally across the floor of the orbit toward its insertion medial to the lateral rectus. The *inferior rectus* approaches the bulb in the 6-o'clock position and the medial rectus lies at the 9-o'clock. Superior to the medial rectus, the *superior oblique* runs toward the trochlea accompanied by the *supratrochlear artery*.

Inferomedial to the orbit a slight invagination of epithelium from the middle meatus indicates the extent of the maxillary sinus in the late fetus. Postnatally this will expand to fill a large space between the orbital floor and the alveolar processes of the maxilla.

Plate 190   Frontal Section through Orbit and Ocular Bulb   393

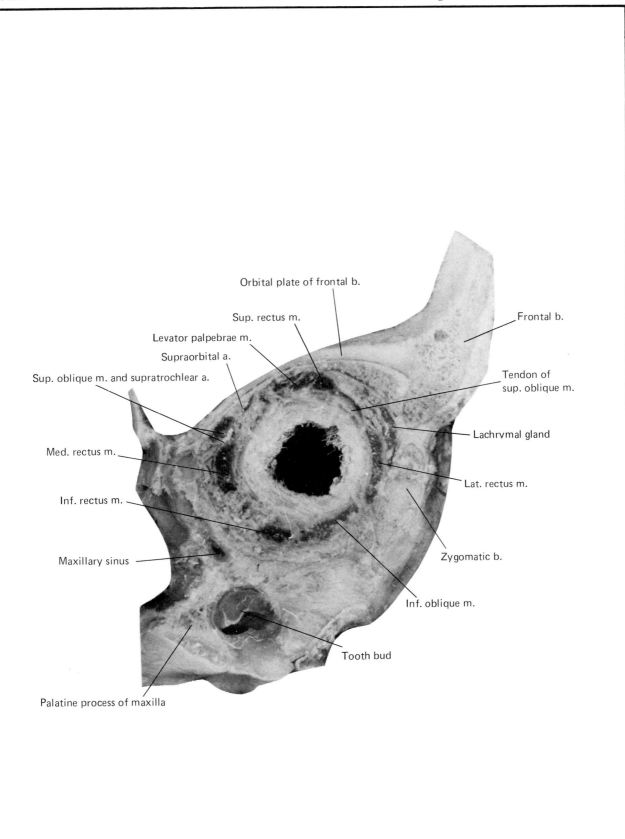

Orbital plate of frontal b.

Sup. rectus m.

Levator palpebrae m.

Supraorbital a.

Frontal b.

Sup. oblique m. and supratrochlear a.

Tendon of
sup. oblique m.

Med. rectus m.

Lachrymal gland

Inf. rectus m.

Lat. rectus m.

Maxillary sinus

Zygomatic b.

Inf. oblique m.

Tooth bud

Palatine process of maxilla

FRONTAL SECTION THROUGH THE POSTERIOR ORBIT AND THE OPTIC NERVE

Being farther posterior than the preceding section, this view indicates the convergence of the ocular muscles toward a common fibrous origin on the posteromedial wall of the orbit. The *superior oblique* muscle and the *four recti* muscles display their thicker, contractile bellies and indicate the rich vascularity of the muscular tissue. The prominent mass of dense *retrobulbar fat* is not simply a site of fat storage; it functions to provide a firm bed for the bulbar socket that resists the combined pull of all of the muscles shown here and serves as a universal fulcrum for their differential actions.

The section of the optic nerve here lies distal to the point where the central artery leaves the ophthalmic artery and pierces the dural sheath of the optic nerve. It then assumes a position in the center of the fiber tracts and enters the bulb through the optic disc to supply the retina. Around the dural sheath several *posterior ciliary arteries* may be discerned.

In the 5-o'clock position the inferior *orbital fissure* is shown bridged with connective tissue. The *infraorbital artery,* derived from the *internal maxillary,* courses forward toward the infraorbital foramen.

Plate 191   Frontal Section through Orbit and Optic Nerve   395

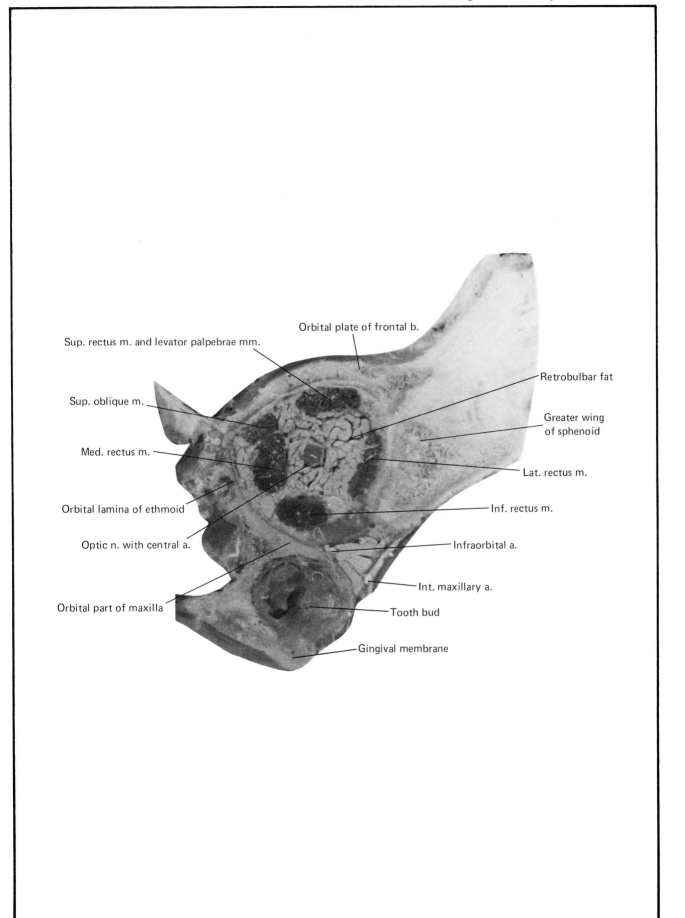

Orbital plate of frontal b.

Sup. rectus m. and levator palpebrae mm.

Retrobulbar fat

Sup. oblique m.

Greater wing
of sphenoid

Med. rectus m.

Lat. rectus m.

Orbital lamina of ethmoid

Inf. rectus m.

Optic n. with central a.

Infraorbital a.

Int. maxillary a.

Orbital part of maxilla

Tooth bud

Gingival membrane

HORIZONTAL SECTION THROUGH THE HEAD AT THE LEVEL OF THE OPTIC CHIASM

The primary value of this exposure lies in its display of the intimate relationship between the nasal and orbital cavities and the convergent course of the optic nerves toward the chiasm.

Although the thin *orbital lamina of the ethmoid* eventually will become pneumatized by a number of anatomically separate sinuses, the bone intervening between the nasal mucosa and the orbit will always be paper thin. Thus the frequent septic situations in the upper respiratory regions might gain access to the orbital cavity by eroding through the "lamina papyracea" of the ethmoid.

On both sides of the sphenoid the plane of section has passed through the *optic canals* and has exposed the entire course of the nerve on the left side.

The *optic nerve* is actually an afferent tract of fibers that originates in the ganglionic layers of the retina and leaves the bulb in a dural sheath. In the posterior orbit the nerve has a slightly sinuous course that provides slack to allow for the rotation of the bulb. It passes through the *anulus tendineus,* from which the rectus muscles arise to enter the optic canal. In the chiasmatic groove of the sphenoid the fibers from the nasal half of each retina interweave and cross to the opposite tract forming the *optic chiasm.* The tracts then continue lateral to the *cerebral peduncles* to synapse in the metathalamic lateral geniculate bodies from where projections to the visual cortex arise.

In the relations of the chiasm shown here, it is seen that pathologic enlargement of the hypophysis which lies below the *tuber cinereum,* or aneurysms of the carotid or its regional branches could affect the chiasm. Tumors of the hypophysis would interfere primarily with the crossed fibers and alter neural transmissions from the nasal retina that perceives the temporal visual field.

Plate 192   Horizontal Section through Head at Level of Optic Chiasm   397

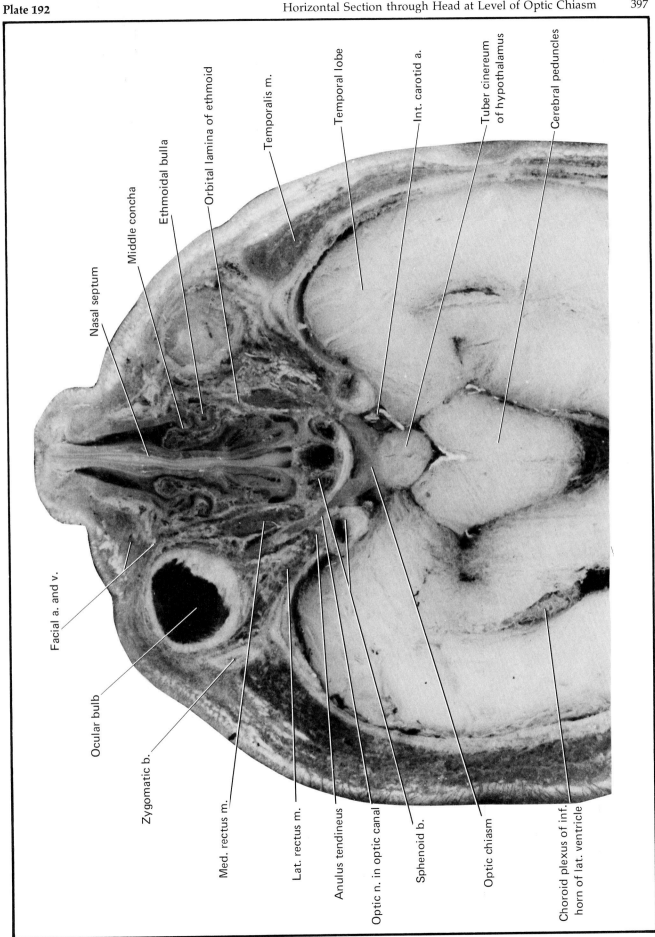

Nasal septum

Middle concha

Ethmoidal bulla

Orbital lamina of ethmoid

Temporalis m.

Temporal lobe

Int. carotid a.

Tuber cinereum of hypothalamus

Cerebral peduncles

Facial a. and v.

Ocular bulb

Zygomatic b.

Med. rectus m.

Lat. rectus m.

Anulus tendineus

Optic n. in optic canal

Sphenoid b.

Optic chiasm

Choroid plexus of inf. horn of lat. ventricle

ANGIOGRAM OF THE ORBITAL REGION: SUPRAORBITAL VIEW

In this vertical projection of one half of the fetal head with the mandible and neck removed, both internal and external carotid arteries were cut above the level of bifurcation. The contrast medium reveals the *internal carotid artery* where it enters the carotid canal and runs medially to enter the cavernous sinus. As it ascends posterior to the optic canal, the carotid gives off the *ophthalmic artery.* This vessel enters the orbit inferior to the optic nerve but within its dural sheath. Where it leaves the dura it provides a spray of fine *posterior ciliary arteries* to the bulb and the important *central artery* to the nerve. This latter vessel repenetrates the dura to assume its position in the center of the optic nerve fibers.

A conspicuous branch leaves the ophthalmic artery and runs along the medial wall of the orbit in association with the belly of the superior oblique muscle. It gives large *anterior* and *posterior ethmoidal arteries* to the nasal cavity and olfactory fossa and continues anteriorly as the *supratrochlear artery* to anastomose with the *facial artery* above the internal canthus. The *supraorbital artery* travels superior to the bulb and supplies the adjacent muscles and the parallel supraorbital nerve. It then passes to the forehead where, with facial anastomoses, it supplies the anterior scalp. The *lachrymal artery* courses along the superior surface of the lateral rectus muscle, supplying it and the lachrymal gland. This artery receives anastomotic branches from the *middle meningeal* and *deep temporal arteries.*

All of the vessels that supply vascularity to the ocular muscles contribute fine *anterior ciliary arteries* to the bulb. These, like their posterior counterparts, vascularize the sclera choroid and the more peripheral part of the retina.

Plate 193   Angiogram of Orbital Region: Supraorbital View   399

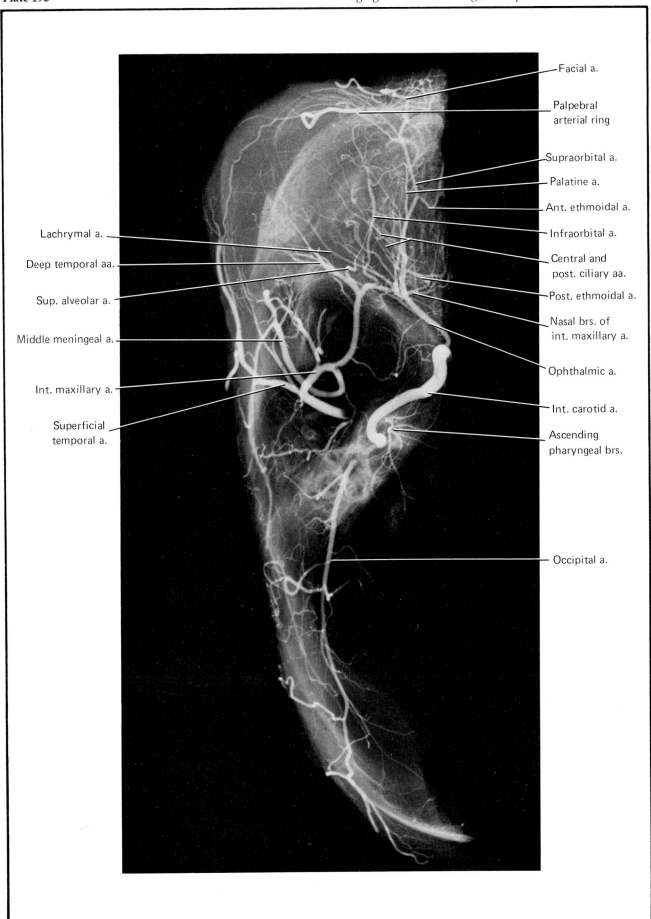

Facial a.

Palpebral
arterial ring

Supraorbital a.

Palatine a.

Ant. ethmoidal a.

Infraorbital a.

Central and
post. ciliary aa.

Post. ethmoidal a.

Nasal brs. of
int. maxillary a.

Ophthalmic a.

Int. carotid a.

Ascending
pharyngeal brs.

Occipital a.

Lachrymal a.

Deep temporal aa.

Sup. alveolar a.

Middle meningeal a.

Int. maxillary a.

Superficial
temporal a.

ANGIOGRAM OF THE ORBITAL REGION: LATERAL VIEW

This illustration was prepared from the opposite side of the same fetal specimen shown in the preceding angiogram. It is a lateral projection of the hemicranium with the brain removed.

The edgewise opacity of the orbital plates of the frontal bone superiorly and the maxilla inferiorly clearly give radiologic definition to the orbit in the lateral aspect, and comparison with the supraorbital view provides three dimensional comprehension.

The inferior relations of the *infraorbital, greater palatine* and *superior alveolar arteries,* which were easily confused with ophthalmic branches in the supraorbital view, are easily identified at their proper levels here, and the anastomotic relations between the larger branches of the *ophthalmic artery* and the *facial artery* in the anteromedial part of the orbit are well illustrated. Note that the apposition of the superior and inferior parts of the *palpebral arterial ring* indicates that the eyelids are firmly closed.

Posterior ciliary arteries may be detected entering the lower posterior half of the bulb, and a fine subscleral plexus is evident. In the anterior half of the bulb, fine derivatives of the *supraorbital artery* form *anterior ciliary arteries* that enter the bulb near the insertions of the recti muscles.

Plate 194   Angiogram of Orbital Region: Lateral View   401

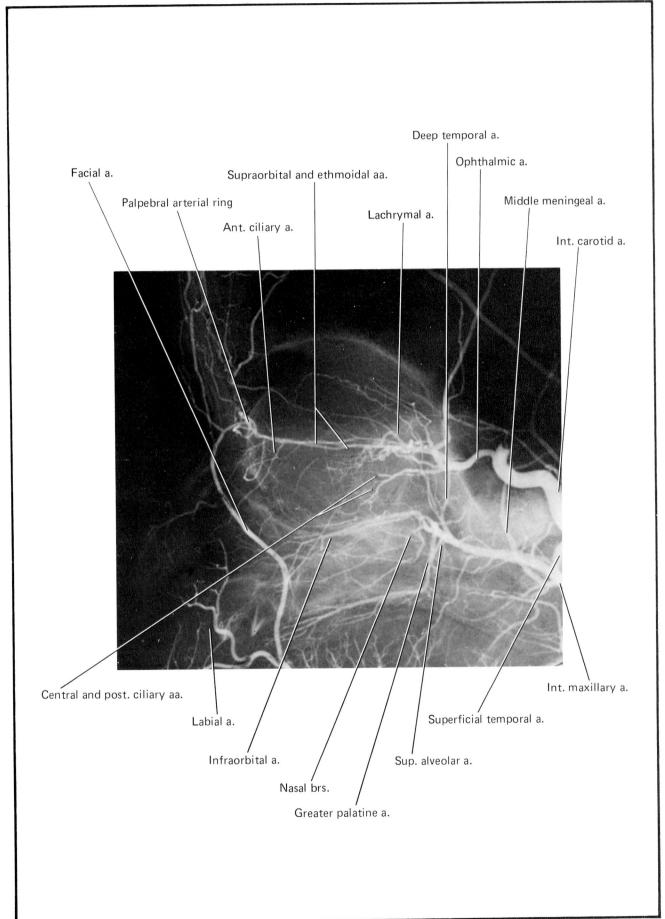

Deep temporal a.

Ophthalmic a.

Facial a.

Middle meningeal a.

Supraorbital and ethmoidal aa.

Palpebral arterial ring

Lachrymal a.

Int. carotid a.

Ant. ciliary a.

Central and post. ciliary aa.

Int. maxillary a.

Labial a.

Superficial temporal a.

Infraorbital a.

Sup. alveolar a.

Nasal brs.

Greater palatine a.

EXTERNAL ASPECT OF THE FETAL TYMPANIC CAVITY AND ITS OSSICLES

The left tympanic cavity of a prepared fetal skull of approximately 32 weeks' gestation was photographed from a lateral angle 35 degrees below the horizontal plane. The *tympanic ring* is an anular part of the temporal complex that has an independent evolutionary and osteogenic history. The ring is C-shaped, with the deficiency directed superiorly. Postnatally it grows into a long tube that forms the skeletal part of the proximal external auditory meatus.

In fresh specimens the *tympanic membrane* is stretched across the ring like the head of a drum and forms part of the inferolateral wall of the *tympanic cavity* or middle ear. Sound wave induced vibrations of the membrane are transmitted to the neurosensory apparatus in the internal ear by a complicated system of articulations among the three middle ear ossicles. The *malleus,* the initial bone in the conduction chain, is attached to the upper central region of the membrane by its *manubrium.* It has a pivotal articulation with the superolateral wall of the middle ear through its *lateral* and *anterior* processes. The rounded head of the malleus forms a diarthroidal joint with the body of the incus, which in turn transmits the motion to the stapes through its *long* and *lenticular* processes. The stirrup-shaped *stapes* receives the vibrations from the incus through its *head,* which passes them via the *anterior* and *posterior crura* to the stapedial *base.* The base almost completely obturates the *fenestra ovalis,* being fixed in this foramen by a membrane. The sound vibrations are thus transmitted to the liquid-filled vestibule of the osseous labyrinth, from where they reach the cochlea to excite the neurosensory *organ of Corti.* This structure transduces the sound waves into nerve impulses that are relayed to the cortex of the temporal lobe of the brain where sound is consciously appreciated.

Between the anterosuperior part of the ring and the *mandibular fossa,* the *petrotympanic fissure* is enlarged medially to form the *anterior iter chordae* that provides the *chorda tympani* with an exit from the tympanic cavity.

Plate 195   Tympanic Cavity and Ossicles   403

Squamous part of temporal b.

Body ⎤
Long process ⎬ Incus
Lenticular process ⎦

Petrotympanic fissure

Ant. iter chordae

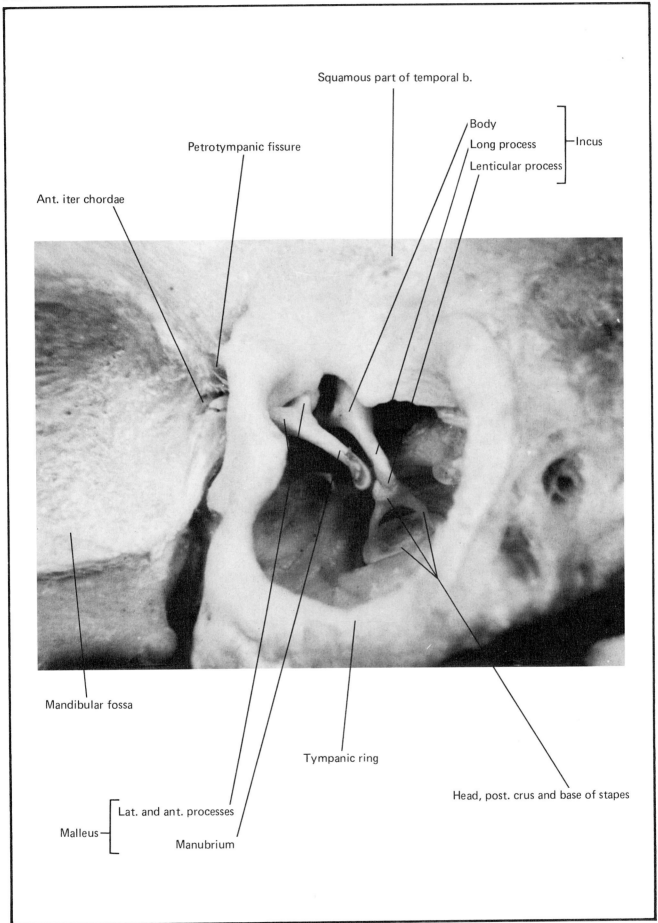

Mandibular fossa

Tympanic ring

Head, post. crus and base of stapes

Lat. and ant. processes

Malleus

Manubrium

THE OSSICLES OF THE MIDDLE EAR

The left otic ossicles of the term fetus shown here have been photographed in a separated arrangement of their functional sequence, but their true anatomic positions (see Plate 195) have been altered to display their individual characteristics in more detail.

The triple chain of ossicles is found only in the ear of mammals. The lower terrestrial vertebrates accomplished a similar function with a single ossicle, the columnella, which, being derived from the second visceral (hyoid) arch, is a homologue of the stapes but directly connects the tympanic membrane or its equivalent to the internal ear. The mammalian malleus and incus are derivatives of the first visceral (mandibular) arch, and their homologues are still parts of the jaw articulation in the nonmammalian vertebrates.

The *malleus,* so called because of its resemblance to a hammer, is attached to the tympanic membrane by the inferior end of the *manubrium.* It has a pivotal action around the articulations formed by its *anterior* and *lateral processes.* The former has a ligamentous fixation to the petrotympanic fissure, and in the earlier fetus still shows attachment to its parent cartilage (Meckel's) of the mandible through this opening. The lateral process is ligamentously attached to both the upper edge of the tympanic membrane and the notch of Rivinus.

The *head* of the *malleus* has a *superior ligament* that suspends it from the roof of the epitympanic recess, and it bears an *articular facet* for the diathrodial articulation with the incus.

The *incus* (Latin for anvil, so named because of its relation to the hammer) has a thick body and a stout, short process that pivots in the incudal fossa of the epitympanic recess. Its long *process* terminates in a medially directed hook, the *lenticular process,* that bears a minute facet for articulating with the head of the stapes. The *stapes* (Latin for stirrup, named because of its obvious resemblance) has an articular *head* that receives the tendon of the stapedius muscle on its posterior side, and an *anterior* and a *posterior crus.* These crura bear the base that has a peripheral membranous attachment to the edges of the fenestra ovalis.

The otic ossicles, like every other structure within the middle ear, are completely covered with the vascular mucosa. The malleoincudal and incudostapedial articulations are miniaturized diarthroses complete with cartilage-bearing surfaces, joint capsules and synovial membranes. The ossicles receive their vascular nutrition through fine vessels in the ligamentous attachments and membranous coverings.

It is rather remarkable that the otic ossicles and the osseous and membranous labyrinth systems have virtually reached their definitive size in the term fetus. This may be related to the fact that the extremely dense bone of the osseous labyrinth is not as likely to undergo further osteoblastic and osteoclastic remodeling once these systems become functional at birth.

Plate 196

Ossicles of Middle Ear   405

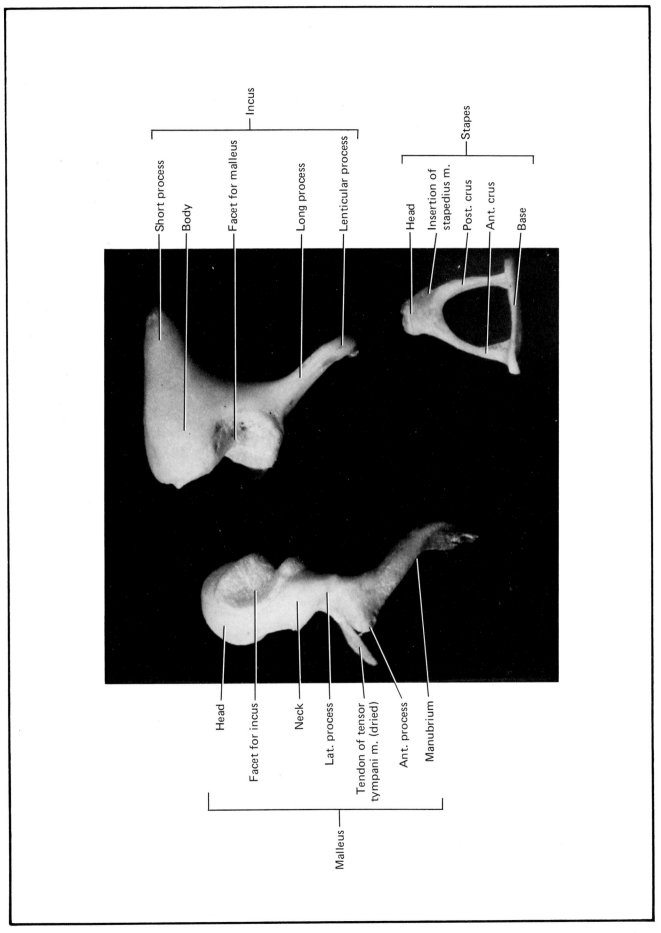

Incus

Short process

Body

Facet for malleus

Long process

Lenticular process

Stapes

Head

Insertion of stapedius m.

Post. crus

Ant. crus

Base

Head

Facet for incus

Neck

Lat. process

Tendon of tensor tympani m. (dried)

Ant. process

Manubrium

Malleus

THE MEDIAL WALL OF THE TYMPANIC CAVITY

Compare this view of the 32-week-old fetal right middle ear with Plate 195 to note that the inside edges of the tympanic ring in the inferior and inferoposterior quadrants have been ground away with a dental drill to give greater exposure to the medial wall of the tympanic cavity.

The *promontory* is a bullous eminence on the medial wall that conforms to the first turn of the cochlea. It lies between the superior *fenestra ovalis* (here occluded by the base of the stapes) and the inferior large *fenestra rotunda*. The surface of the promontory is scored by the grooves of the *tympanic plexus*, a fine ramification of sensory nerves derived from the *glossopharyngeal nerve* (CNIX), which courses between the mucosa and the bone.

Here the roof of the tympanic cavity, the *tegmen tympani*, has also been removed by a dental drill without disturbing the underlying anatomy.

As would be expected, all of the structures of the adult middle ear are expressed in the fetus, but like the tympanic bone, the extent of their ossification is not complete. This is particularly true of the coverings of the origins of two small muscles that are associated with the middle ear ossicles. The *cochlear process* is a thin, tubular shell of bone that houses in the adult the entire *tensor tympani muscle*, except its tendon. In the fetus, however, this tube is mostly cartilaginous, and a *groove of the cochlear process* indicates its position. The tensor tympani inserts into the manubrium of the malleus and alters the tension of the tympanic membrane. Because the malleus is derived from the first or mandibular visceral arch, it is logical that this muscle is derived from the mandibular myotome and is hence innervated by a fine motor branch of the mandibular (trigeminal) nerve.

The smallest discrete skeletal muscle of the body,

however, is the *stapedius,* which inserts near the head of the stapes and varies its tension on the membrane occluding the fenestra ovalis. This little muscle originates in the *pyramid,* a completely ossified cone in the adult, but a rather irregular bony container seen here in the fetus. Its superior aperture gives egress to the tendon of the stapedius.

The stapes, like the malleus, is of branchiomeric origin and is derived from the second or hyoid visceral arch. Thus the stapedius is innervated by a fine branch of the *facial nerve* (CNVII) as it passes adjacent to the pyramid.

The facial nerve passes across the superomedial wall of the middle ear in a tube of bone, the *facial canal*. In the adult this tube is completely ossified, but here the canal was partly cartilaginous anteriorly where it received the nerve (represented by some dried fibers) from the more medially situated part of the canal that lies within the petrous bone. The facial canal makes a 90-degree curve down the rear wall of the middle ear to exit from the stylomastoid foramen. As it passes posterior to the pyramid it gives off an acutely recurrent branch, the *chorda tympani*. This nerve reenters the tympanic cavity through the *posterior iter chordae* in the anterior base of the pyramid and crosses the superior part of the tympanic membrane medial to the manubrium of the malleus. It then exits through a special aperture, the *anterior iter chordae* (see Plate 195), in the petrotympanic fissure. The chorda tympani is distributed to taste receptors on the anterior two thirds of the tongue.

It should be remembered that all of the structures in the middle ear are covered with a vascularized mucous membrane that, by way of the auditory tube, is continuous with that of the upper respiratory spaces. With postnatal pneumatization of the mastoid processes, this membrane extends into its sinuses. Thus, a continuous route for infective processes connects the mastoid air cells and middle ear with the nasopharynx.

Plate 197   Medial Wall of Tympanic Cavity   407

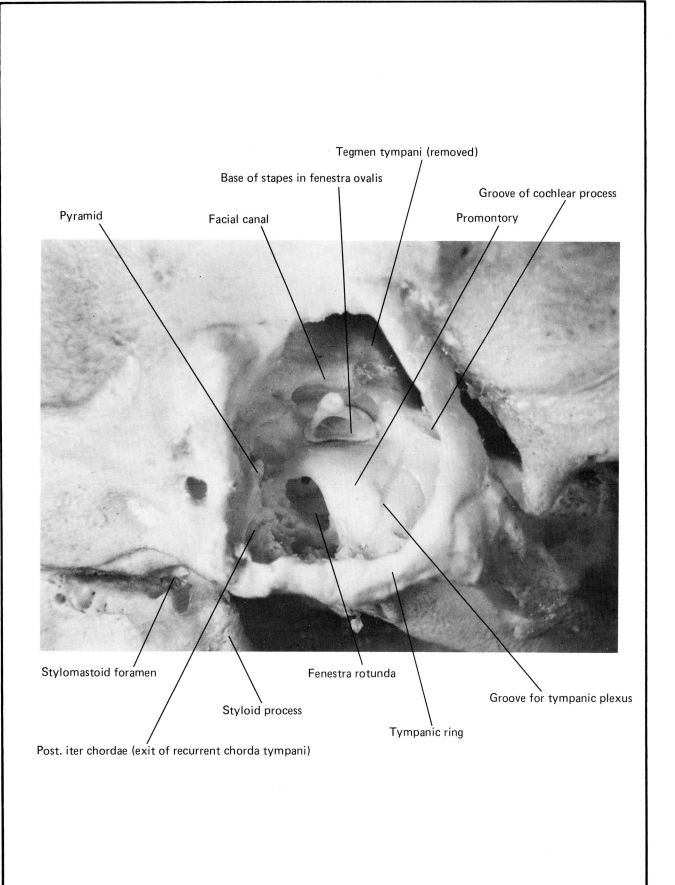

Tegmen tympani (removed)

Base of stapes in fenestra ovalis

Groove of cochlear process

Pyramid   Facial canal   Promontory

Stylomastoid foramen   Fenestra rotunda

Groove for tympanic plexus

Styloid process

Tympanic ring

Post. iter chordae (exit of recurrent chorda tympani)

SUPERIOR EXPOSURE OF THE INTERNAL EAR AND ITS RELATED ANATOMY

The internal ear or labyrinth is a complex system of membranous and bony ducts contained within the very dense osseous matrix of the petrous part of the temporal bone. It consists of two interconnected sensory systems of diverse function. The phyletically older *vestibular system* senses movement and postural changes through sensory endings in the ampullae of the *semicircular canals,* and the more recently evolved *cochlear system* transduces sound waves from the external environment. Despite this disparity of function, the two systems, because of a common developmental homology, show much similarity in their structure. Each consists of a basic double tubular design composed of the outer, epithelium-lined *osseous labyrinth* that contains, in an almost coaxial fashion, the inner *membranous labyrinth.* Both labyrinthine systems are filled with a serous fluid. That which is within the channels of the osseous labyrinth is called the *perilymph,* and the *endolymph* fills the membranous tubes.

The vestibular system is comprised of three closed loops of osseous-membranous tubules. Each loop, or semicircular canal, lies in a plane at right angles to the other two, and thus each defines the side of a three dimensional rectilinear object. All three loops share common chambers where they converge upon each other.

The *vestibule* is a common chamber for the osseous labyrinth and contains within separate recesses the *utricle* and *saccule* of the membranous labyrinth. The utricle is connected to the three semicircular canals, and one end of each canal is expanded into an *ampulla* that contains the neurosensory *crista ampullaris.* The utricle and saccule both contain in their *maculae* neurosensory projections that are activated by suspended concretions called *otoconia.* With this morphology in mind, the physical rationale behind the arrangement of the three canals and the chambers becomes obvious. Motion in any direction will cause an inertial response in the fluid of the canals that disturbs the sensory cristi, and changes in posture will vary the relation of the otoconia in respect to the projections in the maculae. Thus, a differential neurologic "reading" of the output of all of the sensory components of the membranous labyrinth gives the central nervous system a continuous appraisal of the body motion and position.

The cochlear system, an evolutionary derivative of the vestibular mechanism, consists of a tightly coiled expression of the osseous-membranous arrangement. The double tubular ducts are twisted into a two and three quarter turn about a common axis, with the endolymphatic duct and its peripheral membrane separating the perilymphatic space into two channels, the *scala vestibuli* and the *scala tympani.* Within the endolymphatic duct, the *organ of Corti* receives vibrations transmitted from the ossicles to the perilymph of the scala vestibuli and recurrently down the scala tympani. Different frequencies of sonic vibrations activate various regions of the organ of Corti and eventually provide cortical appreciation of the auditory range of the sonic spectrum.

In this figure the petrous bone has been ground away with a dental drill to expose the three semicircular canals. This procedure is not as technically difficult as it may seem because the softer parts of the petrous bone are easily abraded. As the tool approaches the solid, ivory-like consistency of the osseous labyrinth, one can easily outline its structure.

Here, the tool was driven into each semicircular canal to show its internal tubular duct. Medial to the vestibular apparatus, the *internal auditory meatus* has been opened to reveal the osseous bed of the *cochlear* and *vestibular ganglia* of the *auditory nerve* (CNVIII).

The roof of the *facial canal* has been opened to show its connection with the *hiatus of the facial canal* that transmits the *greater petrous nerve* to the middle cranial fossa.

Medially, the superior part of the petrous bone that overlies the cochlea has been abraded to expose its first turns. The central post of the cochlea, the *modiolus,* bears the screw-thread arrangement of the helical projection of the *osseous lamina,* which supports the central part of the organ of Corti.

Medial to the cochlea, the petrous bone has been eroded to display the normal trabeculations of cancellous bone where it is not supporting the labyrinthine system.

Anterolateral to the petrous bone the dental drill has opened the roof, or *tegmen tympani,* of the middle ear. The cavity has been extended medially to the *foramen spinosum* to show the underlying direction of the auditory tube.

Laterally, the roof of the *aditus,* which leads into the *tympanic antrum,* has been removed. A slight "honeycombing" of the lateral wall of the antrum presages the pneumatization that eventually will penetrate the developing mastoid sinuses.

Plate 198   Internal Ear and Related Anatomy   409

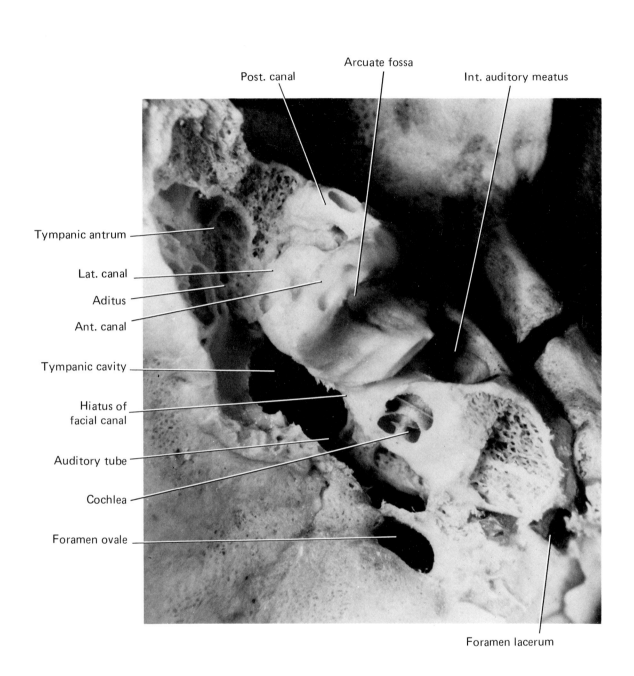

Post. canal

Arcuate fossa

Int. auditory meatus

Tympanic antrum

Lat. canal

Aditus

Ant. canal

Tympanic cavity

Hiatus of
facial canal

Auditory tube

Cochlea

Foramen ovale

Foramen lacerum

SUPERIOR ASPECT OF THE UNDISSECTED PETROUS BONE

The opposite side of the dissected specimen shown in the preceding plate was photographed for this comparative topographic reference.

The petrous bone in the fetus gives more superficial clues about its underlying internal morphology than it does in the adult. This indicates that the basic neurosensory structures are laid down first, and the remaining, less compact areas of the petrous formation undergo a growth through continued postnatal ossification that more deeply buries the osseous labyrinth. Thus the arcuate eminence is decidedly more pronounced in the fetus, and the *subarcuate fossa*, a cavity in the ring of the *anterior semicircular canal*, is completely filled with bone by the middle of the second decade. The *hiatus of the facial canal* is also disproportionately large, being nearly its definitive size.

The *tegmen tympani* that roofs the middle ear is very thin in the fetus and often reveals the position of the underlying cavity by a series of minute perforations.

Although the tympanic cavity, the ossicles and the osseous labyrinth are virtually adult size, the perinatal auditory tube is quite short but eventually lengthens with postnatal growth of the head. This situation may help to explain the much higher incidence of the transmission of pharyngeal infections to the middle ear in infants as opposed to adults.

Plate 199   Superior Aspect of Undissected Petrous Bone   411

Arcuate fossa

Int. auditory meatus

Arcuate eminence

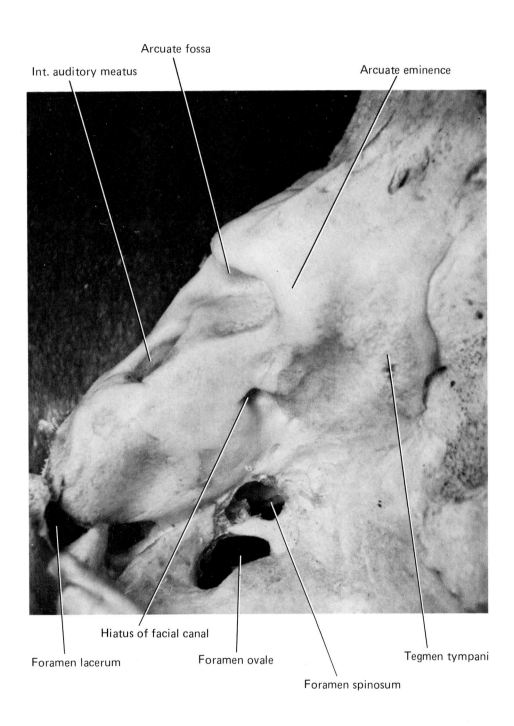

Hiatus of facial canal

Foramen lacerum

Foramen ovale

Foramen spinosum

Tegmen tympani

FRONTAL SECTION OF THE HEAD THROUGH THE LEVEL OF THE PETROUS BONE

In this posterior aspect of a frontal section of a fetal head from a specimen of approximately 30 weeks' gestation, the relationship of the other cranial structures to the petrous bone, and hence to the middle and internal ear, is amply illustrated. The section is slightly oblique to the frontal plane with the right side of the head (right side of picture) being cut slightly anterior to the left.

On the right, the internal ear has been cut through the first turn of the cochlea that is bulging toward the medial wall of the middle ear and thus produces its *promontory*. On the left, the more posterior section shows the *anterior canal* forming the *arcuate eminence*, and the lateral canal connecting to the *vestibule*, a chamber connected to the confluence of all the ducts. Below this the posteroinferior part of the tympanic cavity is manifest and part of the epitympanic recess may be discerned external to the lateral canal.

The posteroinferior parts of the temporal lobes of the brain lie just above the petrous bones where the scroll-like infolding of primitive cortical structures produces the *hippocampus*. Between the temporal lobe and the *basilar artery* on the left side, the *auditory nerve* (CNVIII), in combination with the *facial nerve* (CNVII), may be seen entering the internal auditory meatus.

Superiorly, the frontal section of the cerebral hemispheres shows the two *lateral ventricles* and the median slitlike *third ventricle* of the diencephalon. Between the pair of membranes that form the *septum pellucidum* is the "fifth ventricle," a space that becomes much attenuated in the adult. The *choroid plexuses*, highly vascularized structures found in each ventricle, produce the major quantity of the cerebrospinal fluid.

Plate 200   Frontal Section of Head through Level of Petrous Bone   413

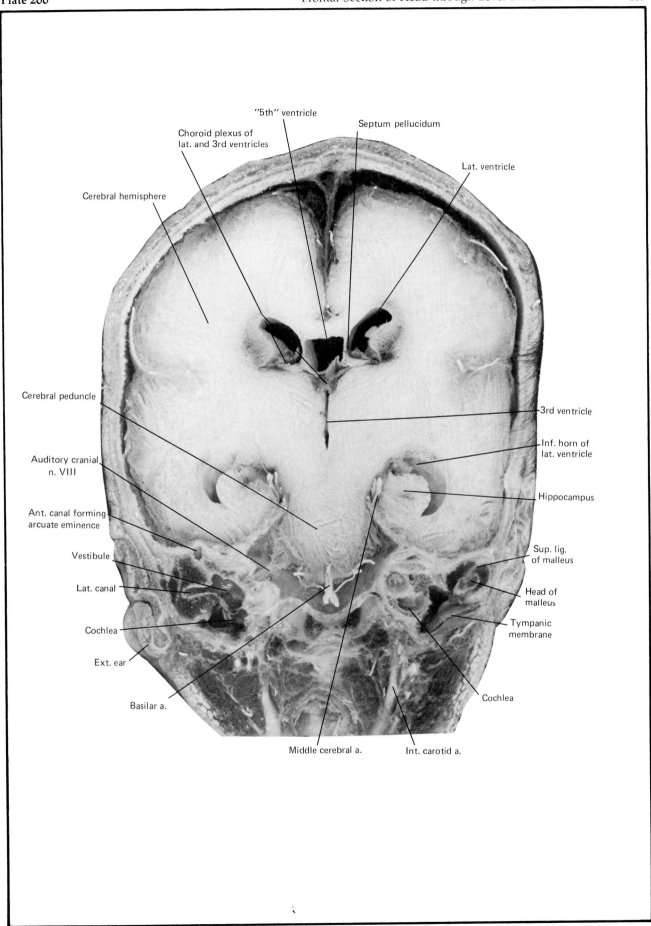

"5th" ventricle

Septum pellucidum

Choroid plexus of
lat. and 3rd ventricles

Lat. ventricle

Cerebral hemisphere

Cerebral peduncle

3rd ventricle

Inf. horn of
lat. ventricle

Auditory cranial
n. VIII

Hippocampus

Ant. canal forming
arcuate eminence

Vestibule

Sup. lig.
of malleus

Lat. canal

Head of
malleus

Cochlea

Tympanic
membrane

Ext. ear

Cochlea

Basilar a.

Middle cerebral a.

Int. carotid a.

ENLARGED DETAIL OF THE FRONTAL SECTION THROUGH THE PETROUS BONE

This plate shows an enlarged quadrant of the preceding illustration to provide detail of the internal and middle ear.

The osseous labyrinth of the *cochlea* is divided by the *spiral lamina* into the *scala vestibuli* and the *scala tympani,* and the bulge of the first turn produces the promontory on the medial wall of the tympanic cavity. Above the cochlea, the anterior part of the internal auditory meatus shows part of the facial nerve in tangential section, but the part of the facial canal crossing the medial wall of the middle ear again shows this nerve (accompanied by a fine artery) in cross section.

The epitympanic recess provides a sectional view of the *head of the malleus* and its *superior ligament.* Across the neck of the malleus, the sectioned *chorda tympani* can be identified.

Note that the *manubrium of the malleus* is attached to the *tympanic membrane* and both structures are covered with a continuous sheet of mucous membrane.

Plate 201

Internal and Middle Ear 415

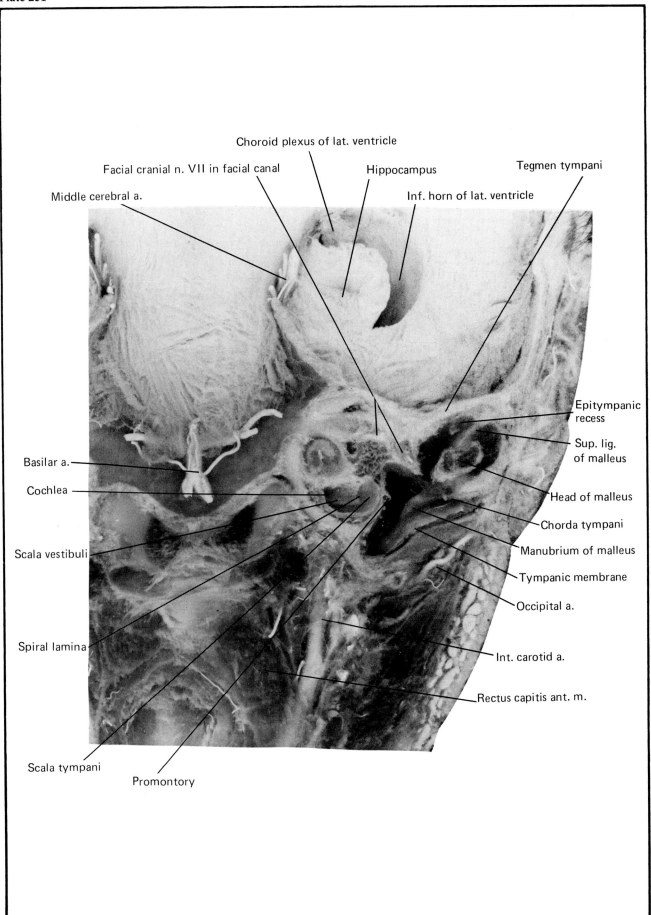

Choroid plexus of lat. ventricle

Facial cranial n. VII in facial canal

Hippocampus

Tegmen tympani

Middle cerebral a.

Inf. horn of lat. ventricle

Epitympanic recess

Sup. lig. of malleus

Basilar a.

Cochlea

Head of malleus

Chorda tympani

Manubrium of malleus

Scala vestibuli

Tympanic membrane

Occipital a.

Spiral lamina

Int. carotid a.

Rectus capitis ant. m.

Scala tympani

Promontory

ENLARGED SECTION THROUGH THE FIRST TURN OF THE COCHLEA

Here the plane of section has exposed most of the first cochlear turn of the osseous labyrinth and its connection to the *vestibule*. The membranous lining of the osseous labyrinth is shown to be vascularized by a centrifugal arrangement of vessels arising in the *modiolus*. Within the core of this bony center of the cochlear spiral, the fibers of the *cochlear nerve* and their *spiral ganglia* receive the afferents from the organ of Corti. Superior to the modiolus, the combined facial and acoustic nerves are shown in section. The vestibular part of the auditory nerve is terminally distributed to the three ampullae of the semicircular canals, and the facial component passes through the middle ear and out the stylomastoid foramen.

Plate 202   Enlarged Section through 1st Cochlear Turn   417

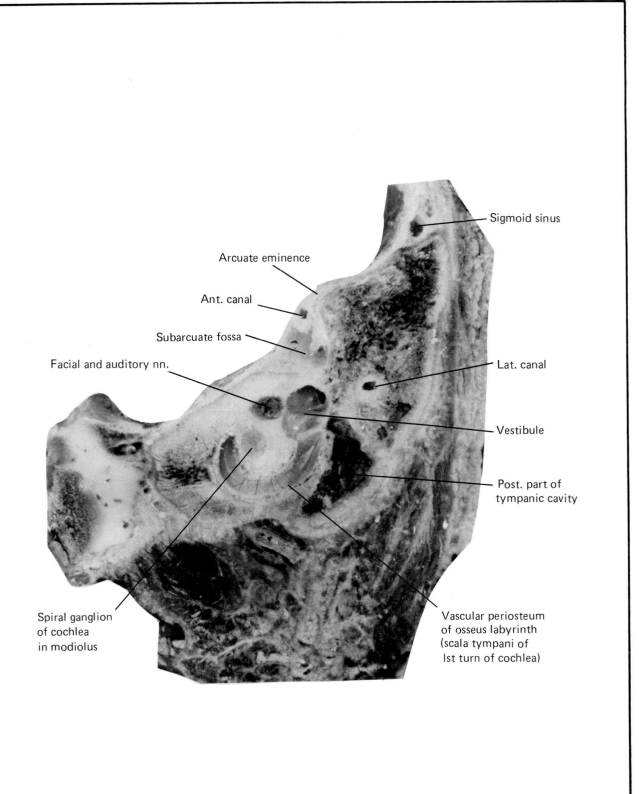

Sigmoid sinus

Arcuate eminence

Ant. canal

Subarcuate fossa

Facial and auditory nn.

Lat. canal

Vestibule

Post. part of
tympanic cavity

Spiral ganglion
of cochlea
in modiolus

Vascular periosteum
of osseus labyrinth
(scala tympani of
Ist turn of cochlea)

RADIOGRAM OF THE RIGHT HALF OF THE FETAL SKULL BASE: VERTICAL PROJECTION

In this specimen the calvaria and mandible have been removed and the vertical radiographic projection outlines the petrous bone in the same aspect as viewed in Plates 198 and 199. The x-rays readily reinforce the previous statements concerning the relative density of the osseous labyrinth. Although the rest of the skull is but faintly outlined by the radiation, and only the thin osseous plates presented in edge-on views show much radiopacity, the bone surrounding the vestibular and cochlear parts of the labyrinth demonstrates considerable resistance to x-ray penetration. However, the internal duct systems provide sufficient radiolucency to identify the various components and their positions within the bone.

Plate 203   Radiogram of Right Half of Skull Base   419

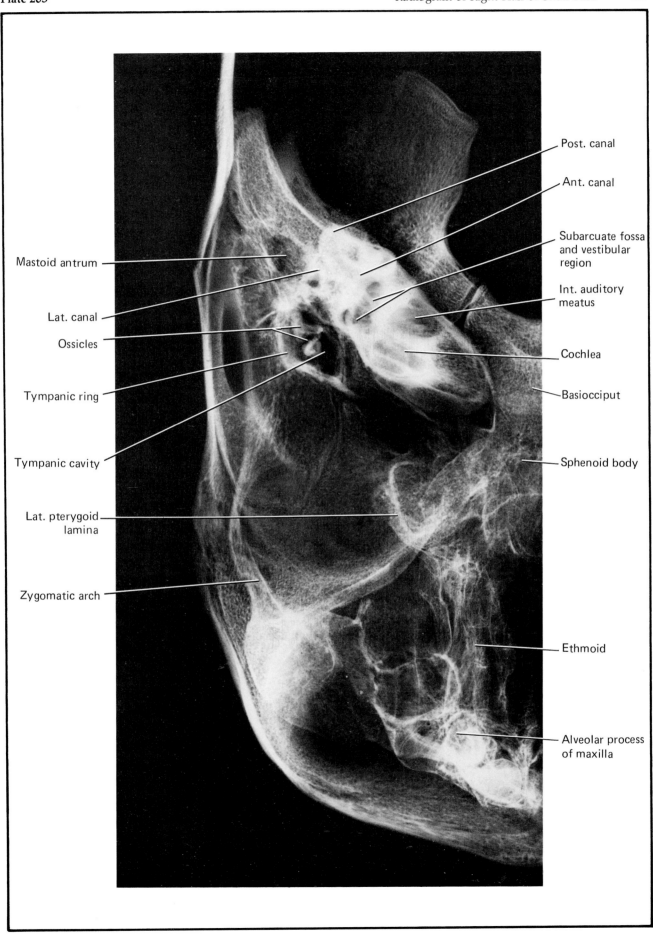

Post. canal

Ant. canal

Subarcuate fossa
and vestibular
region

Int. auditory
meatus

Cochlea

Basiocciput

Sphenoid body

Ethmoid

Alveolar process
of maxilla

Mastoid antrum

Lat. canal

Ossicles

Tympanic ring

Tympanic cavity

Lat. pterygoid
lamina

Zygomatic arch

ENLARGEMENT OF THE RADIOGRAM OF THE PETROUS REGION OF THE FETAL SKULL: VERTICAL PROJECTION

In this x-ray of a dried fetal skull with the mandible still attached, the internal osseous features of the middle and internal ear have been sufficiently enlarged to identify many of the individual components.

Within the middle ear, the *malleus,* its head and its faintly discernible manubrium may be identified, and its articular position in relation to the body of the *incus* can be determined by the *bony* and *short incudal* processes.

The internal ear reveals the more medial *internal auditory meatus* as a radiolucent area posterior to the *cochlea.* At least two of the two and three quarter turns of this organ can be identified, and the central *modiolus,* although hollowed to pass the cochlear nerve fibers, can still be identified in the first turn.

The spherical and elliptical recesses of the osseous labyrinth, together with the closely associated ampullae of the semicircular canals, can be noticed as a cluster of round, radiolucent areas medial to the otic ossicles. The posterior part of the *anterior canal* can be seen near the posterior border of the petrous bone, and the very faint outline of the *lateral canal* can be identified by its horizontal arc.

The thin roof of the tympanic cavity and the bone over the auditory tube have their radioluceny reinforced by the presence of the carotid canal inferior to these areas.

Plate 204   Radiogram of Petrous Region of Skull   421

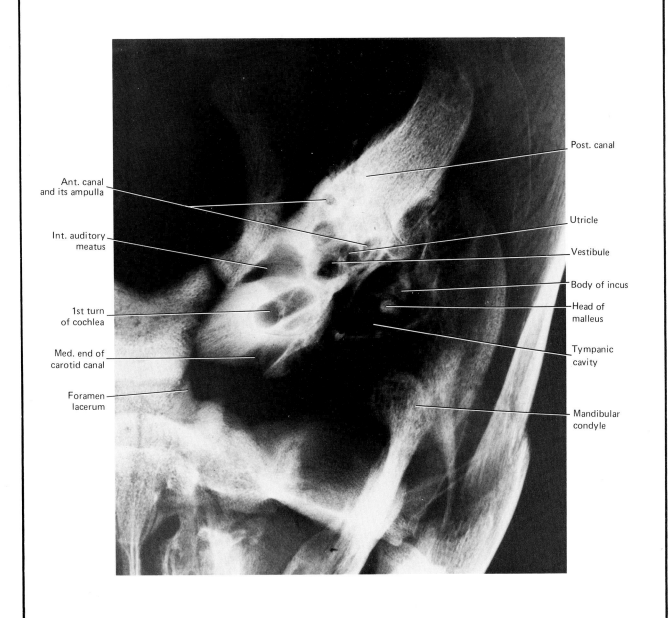

Ant. canal
and its ampulla

Int. auditory
meatus

1st turn
of cochlea

Med. end of
carotid canal

Foramen
lacerum

Post. canal

Utricle

Vestibule

Body of incus

Head of
malleus

Tympanic
cavity

Mandibular
condyle

RADIOGRAM OF THE FETAL SKULL HEMISECTION: LATERAL PROJECTION

In this view the individual semicircular canals are readily distinguished by virtue of the denser matrix of their osseous labyrinth. Because the *anterior* and *posterior* canals monitor motion in vertical planes, they stand above the bone mass surrounding the vestibular and cochlear areas and cast distinct shadows. The shadow of the *lateral canal,* however, is complicated by the cumulative densities of the other parts of the labyrinth. Nevertheless, it may be identified at the level of the confluence of the other canals.

The radiolucent area within the loop of the anterior canal indicates the *subarcuate fossa,* and anteroinferior to this the end-on view of the *internal meatus* shows another radiolucent area. The cochlea barely can be discerned lying anterior to the internal auditory meatus.

In comparison to the adult skull, the fetal osseous labyrinth is disproportionately large because it has already achieved its definitive dimensions.

Plate 205   Radiogram of Skull Hemisection   423

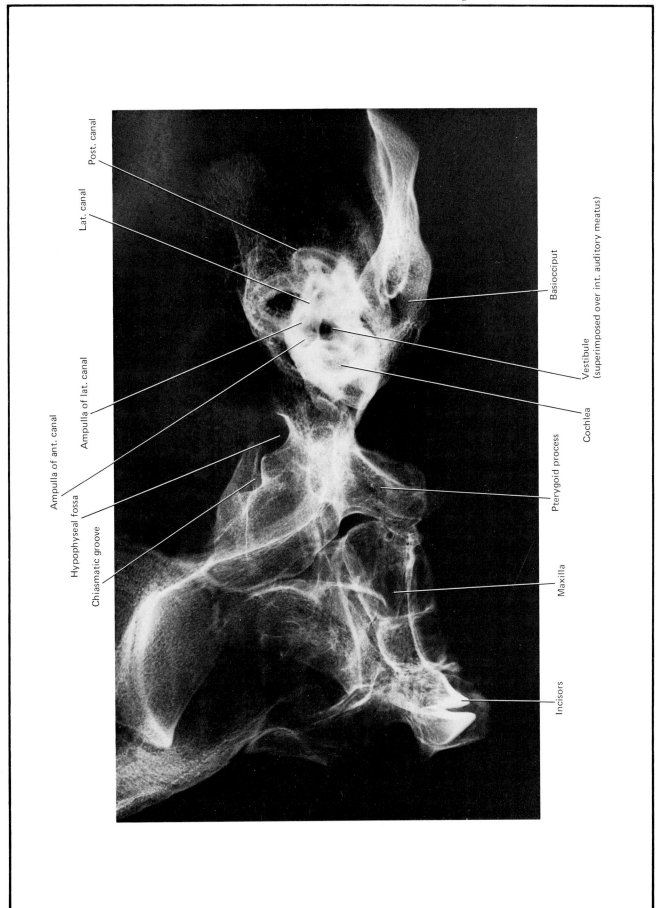

Post. canal

Lat. canal

Basiocciput

Vestibule
(superimposed over int. auditory meatus)

Ampulla of ant. canal

Ampulla of lat. canal

Cochlea

Hypophyseal fossa

Pterygoid process

Chiasmatic groove

Maxilla

Incisors

Index

Because this book is designed so that all illustrations are on the odd numbered pages with their descriptive text located on the opposing even numbered pages, the number of page entries required in the index is reduced considerably by referring to only one member of each page set. Therefore, this index directs the reader to only the even numbered, or text page, whether the information sought lies only in the text, only in the illustration, or in both.

Photographic Atlas of Fetal Anatomy

Designed by Sheila Humphreys

Text composed by Mid-Atlantic Composition,
Baltimore, Maryland,
in Palatino medium and semi-bold

Display type composed by Service Composition,
Baltimore, Maryland,
in Palatino semi-bold

Nomenclature typography by Lynne H. Apperson,
University Park Press,
Baltimore, Maryland

Printed by The Maple Press Co.,
York, Pennsylvania,
on Consolidated Productolith

Bound by The Maple Press Co.,
York, Pennsylvania,
in Columbia Bayside Linen

Special effect art by Graphic Image, Inc.,
Baltimore, Maryland

Book jackets printed by Bay Printing,
Baltimore, Maryland